CLINICAL HANDBOOK OF
MEDICAL-SURGICAL NURSING

WILMA J. PHIPPS, R.N., Ph.D., F.A.A.N.

Professor and Chairperson of Medical-Surgical Nursing
Frances Payne Bolton School of Nursing,
Case Western Reserve University;
Director of Medical-Surgical Nursing,
University Hospitals of Cleveland, Cleveland, Ohio

BARBARA C. LONG, R.N., M.S.N.

Associate Professor Emerita of Medical-Surgical Nursing,
Frances Payne Bolton School of Nursing,
Case Western Reserve University, Cleveland, Ohio

NANCY F. WOODS, R.N., Ph.D., F.A.A.N.

Professor and Chairperson,
Department of Parent and Child Nursing,
University of Washington, Seattle, Washington

Coordinating Editor

JUDITH K. SANDS, R.N., Ed.D.

Assistant Professor of Nursing
University of Virginia School of Nursing, Charlottesville, Virginia

CLINICAL HANDBOOK OF
MEDICAL-
SURGICAL
NURSING

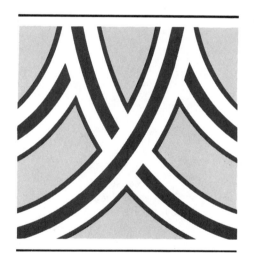

THE C.V. MOSBY COMPANY

ST. LOUIS · TORONTO · WASHINGTON, D.C.   1987

A TRADITION OF PUBLISHING EXCELLENCE

Editor: Don E. Ladig
Assistant Editor: Audrey Rhoades/Maureen Slaten
Editing and Production: Editing, Design & Production, Inc.
Design: Diane M. Beasley

Printed in the United States of America

The C.V. Mosby Company
11830 Westline Industrial Drive, St. Louis, Missouri 63146

Library of Congress Cataloging-in-Publication Data

Phipps, Wilma J., 1925-
    Clinical handbook of medical-surgical nursing.

    Includes bibliographies and index.
    1. Nursing—Handbooks, manuals, etc. 2. Surgical
nursing—Handbooks, manuals, etc. I. Long, Barbara C.,
1926-   . II. Woods, Nancy Fugate. III. Sands,
Judith. [DNLM: 1. Nursing—handbooks. 2. Surgical
Nursing—handbooks. WY 39 P573c]
RT51.P46 1986   610.73   86-23766
ISBN 0-8016-3850-X

GW/VHP/VHP   9 8 7 6 5 4   02/C/232

CONTRIBUTORS

VIRGINIA L. CASSMEYER, R.N., M.S.N.
Associate Professor, Medical-Surgical Nursing
School of Nursing
University of Kansas College of Health Sciences
Kansas City, Missouri

DOROTHY A. JONES, Ed.D., R.N., C., F.A.A.N.
Associate Professor
Boston College
Chestnut Hill, Massachusetts

DIANA MILLER, R.N., Dip. Teaching & Supervision
Co-ordinator, R.N. Refresher Programme
Centennial College of Applied Arts & Technology
Toronto, Ontario

DOROTHY L. SEXTON, Ed.D., R.N.
Associate Professor and Chairperson
Medical-Surgical Nursing Program
Yale School of Nursing
New Haven, Connecticut

PREFACE

The *Clinical Handbook of Medical-Surgical Nursing* is a concise yet thorough clinical reference book that presents the essential nursing care involved in most common medical-surgical conditions. It is designed to serve not as a textbook but rather as a valuable resource book for nursing students, new graduates, part-time and returning nurses, and active practitioners in various settings.

Medical-surgical nursing is an enormous, complex field whose knowledge base continues to expand at an unbelievable pace. Most practicing nurses out of necessity are specialists. It is difficult to keep up and stay comfortably current with the scope of knowledge needed for safe practice. New graduates face this problem as they attempt to prepare for licensure examination from textbooks many thousands of pages long. Float and part-time nurses are regularly sent to a wide variety of practice areas. Nurses returning to practice must polish rusty skills and replace out-of-date references. Practitioners commonly have the challenge of caring for diabetics admitted to the Psychiatry Department, patients with endocrine disorders in cardiac units, eye surgery patients transferred to Orthopedics, and so on.

The Clinical Handbook of Medical-Surgical Nursing fulfills the need for a concise and easy-to-use reference guide to medical-surgical nursing. A modified outline format is used to present the most comprehensive information in the smallest possible space. Only the common medical surgical conditions are fully described in the body of the book. Tables present the less common but related conditions in each area. Twenty sample nursing care plans have been included.

The book is organized by body systems to help the reader find material quickly and easily. Chapters on fluid and electrolyte imbalances and care of oncology patients are also included, since these are commonly occuring clinical situations.

Each chapter begins with a brief overview of the pathophysiology and typical medical management of the conditions described. The nursing care is presented using a nursing process format to assist the reader in developing care plans for day-to-day practice situations. The assessment data include essential factors, both subjective and objective, to be considered for each condition. Commonly encountered nursing diagnoses, typical etiologies, and related expected outcomes are listed. The associated nursing interventions are fully described with explanatory rationale where appropriate. The presentation for each condition concludes with a list of typical evaluation criteria.

The book makes liberal use of charts and tables to highlight content, present additional related material, and increase the reader's access to important information. Data throughout are readily available and easy to apply directly in practice. These features make the *Clinical Handbook of Medical-Surgical Nursing* a useful resource for both planning and delivering care.

I thank the editorial staff of The C.V. Mosby Company for their commitment to and assistance in completing the book, and my children for their patience in dealing with "another one of Mom's projects."

JUDITH SANDS

CONTENTS

CHAPTER 12

ENDOCRINE DISORDERS 156

CHAPTER 13

DISORDERS OF THE URINARY SYSTEM 176

CHAPTER 14

DISORDERS OF THE REPRODUCTIVE SYSTEM 189

CHAPTER 1

Fluid and Electrolyte Imbalance

The monitoring of fluid and electrolyte balance is a major nursing responsibility since this homeostatic balance may be threatened by virtually any medical or surgical disorder. It is also threatened by many common medical therapies. The nurse must be able to:

1. Recognize situations likely to cause imbalances
2. Identify patients at risk for developing imbalances
3. Initiate measures to prevent imbalances from occurring
4. Recognize the signs and symptoms of common imbalances
5. Carry out therapeutic measures prescribed by the physician
6. Monitor patient responses to the interventions

Fluid and electrolyte imbalances are commonly categorized for discussion as specific excesses or deficits although more than one may, and commonly does, exist in any clinical situation. Table 1-1 lists normal serum values for the body's major electrolytes and fluid osmolality.

PRIMARY FLUID IMBALANCES

Although sodium and water imbalances are frequently encountered together, it is important to differentiate between them. The treatments used for disturbances in balances vary substantially depending on the specific cause. Table 1-2 summarizes the normal daily fluid intake and output of an adult.

EXTRACELLULAR WATER DEFICIT (HYPEROSMOLAR IMBALANCE): DEHYDRATION

An extracellular water deficit occurs when the amount of water is decreased in proportion to the amount of solute in the water, causing the osmolality to exceed 300 mOsm/L.

Pathophysiology

Hyperosmolality causes water to move from the cells to the vascular compartment to help maintain the circulating blood volume. Osmotic diuresis occurs as the kidneys attempt to excrete the excess solute. Dehydration worsens caused by the loss of fluid used to flush out solutes in the urine.

TABLE 1-1 Normal serum electrolyte and fluid osmolality values

Electrolyte or Fluid	Serum Value
Sodium (Na^+)	135–145 mEq/L
Potassium (K^+)	3.5–5.0 mEq/L
Chloride (Cl^-)	100–106 mEq/L
Phosphate (PO_4^{2-})	2.8–4.5 mEq/L
Calcium (Ca^{2+})	4.5–5.8 mEq/L
Bicarbonate (HCO_3^-)	20–30 mEq/L
Body fluid osmolality	275–295 mOsm/L

TABLE 1-2 Approximate daily fluid intake and output for an adult eating 2,500 calories

Intake		Output	
Method	Amount (ml)	Method	Amount (ml)
Water in food	1,000	Skin	500
Water from oxidation	300	Lungs	350
Water as liquid	1,200	Feces	150
		Kidneys	1,500
TOTAL	2,500	TOTAL	2,500

Without intervention:

Intracellular fluid compartment becomes depleted, markedly impairing cell function. NOTE: Brain cells are particularly sensitive and mental status changes may be among the first signs.

Extracellular fluid losses impair circulation, further interrupting cellular metabolism and possibly leading to vascular collapse.

Water deficit is not usually a problem for an alert individual who has sufficient fluid available and is able to swallow. The box below lists risk factors that can lead to extracellular water deficit. Table 1-3 presents common signs and symptoms.

Medical Management

Medical management consists of replacing lost fluid plus supplying current daily need. The amount of fluid loss can be estimated from weight loss: 1 kg of body weight equals 1 L of fluid. The method of fluid delivery may be

RISK FACTORS LEADING TO EXTRACELLULAR WATER DEFICIT

Inability to recognize thirst:
  Confusion
  Altered consciousness
Inability to obtain fluids:
  Aphasia (person cannot request fluids)
  Paralysis, either general or restricted to swallowing
Inability to conserve fluids:
  Profuse sweating
  Vomiting or diarrhea, or gastrointestinal suctioning
  Profuse diuresis, as in diabetes insipidus
Hyperosmolar dietary intake:
  Tube feedings with concentrated protein, electrolytes, or glucose
Build-up of solutes secondary to a disease process:
  Renal failure
  Diabetic ketoacidosis
  Other endocrine and metabolic disorders

TABLE 1-3 Signs and symptoms of extracellular water deficit

Body System	Signs and Symptoms
Skin	Flushed, dry, poor turgor
Mouth	Dry, sticky mucous membranes
Eyes	Decrease in tears
	Soft, sunken eyeballs
Cardiovascular	Orthostatic hypotension
	Rapid pulse
Central nervous	Apprehension, restlessness, weakness
Blood (values)	Increased Na^+ and Hct (hematocrit), higher osmolality
Urine	Decreased output, higher osmolality, increased specific gravity (spg)
Other	Thirst, weight loss

oral, IV, or both. Initial fluid replacement is frequently glucose and water, supplemented by electrolyte solutions once patient's renal function is ensured. Replacement may take place over several days to avoid overtaxing the heart.

EXTRACELLULAR WATER EXCESS (HYPOSMOLAR IMBALANCE): WATER INTOXICATION

An extracellular water excess occurs when the amount of water is increased in proportion to the amount of solute in the water, causing the osmolality to fall below 275 mOsm/L.

Pathophysiology

Extracellular water excess rapidly becomes intracellular water excess as fluid moves into the cells to equalize the solute concentration, causing the cells to swell. NOTE: Brain cells are particularly sensitive to water increases, and the most common symptoms are changes in the patient's mental status.

Water excess rarely occurs under normal conditions since a falling osmolality usually suppresses the antidiuretic hormone (ADH), allowing the excess water to be excreted by the kidney. The box below lists risk factors

RISK FACTORS AND CONDITIONS LEADING TO EXTRACELLULAR WATER EXCESS

Excessive water intake:
  Instillation of a hyposmolar solution into a body cavity from which it is absorbed through mucous membrane, such as multiple tap water enemas, or continuous irrigation of bladder after prostatic surgery
  Psychiatric disorder characterized by excessive drinking of water or other hyposmolar fluids
  Excessive administration of hyposmolar fluids
Excessive water retention:
  Increase in antidiuretic hormone (ADH) in response to stress, drugs, anesthesia, inflammatory conditions, or tumors of brain or other organs
  Renal disease

TABLE 1-4 Signs and symptoms of extracellular water excess

Body System	Signs and Symptoms
Skin	Warm, moist, good turgor
	Slight peripheral edema
Cardiovascular	Bounding pulse, widened pulse pressure
Central nervous	Lethargy, confusion, convulsions
Gastrointestinal	Anorexia, nausea, vomiting
Blood (values)	Decreased Na^+ and Hct, lower osmolality
Urine	Increased output and lower osmolality, decreased specific gravity
Other	Sudden weight gain

and conditions that can lead to extracellular water excess. Table 1-4 presents common signs and symptoms.

Medical Management

Most patients respond well to simple water restriction. If severe symptoms are present the patient may be treated with small amounts of hypertonic saline given IV in addition to fluid restriction.

ISOTONIC VOLUME DEFICIT

An isotonic volume deficit occurs in conditions in which both extracellular water and electrolytes are lost from the body. Volume is decreased, but the osmolality remains in the normal range.

RISK FACTORS AND CONDITIONS LEADING TO ISOTONIC VOLUME DEFICIT

Hemorrhage
Profuse sweating
Excessive gastrointestinal losses from
    Vomiting or diarrhea
    Ileostomy drainage or gastrointestinal fistulas
    Nasogastric suctioning
Systemic infection

TABLE 1-5 Signs and symptoms of isotonic volume deficit

Body System	Signs and Symptoms
Skin	Cool, poor turgor
Mouth	Dry mucous membranes
Cardiovascular	Postural hypotension (early sign): Blood pressure of client when sitting or standing is more than 10 mm Hg lower than when client is lying down
	Low blood pressure, tachycardia, decreased vein filling
Respiratory	Increased respiratory rate
Urine	Low output, increased specific gravity
Other	Weight loss, weakness, fatigue

TABLE 1-6 Osmolality of common IV solutions

Type of Solution	Osmolality	Use
5% Dextrose in water (D5W)	Hyposmolar *goes in*	Replacement of water losses
Normal saline (0.9% NaCl)	Isotonic	Hyponatremia (sodium deficit)
Lactated Ringers' solution	Isotonic	Extracellular volume deficit
5% Dextrose in 0.45% saline (D5½NS)	Hyperosmolar *pulls out*	Maintenance of fluid levels

Pathophysiology

An isotonic volume loss does not disturb serum osmolality and the deficit is therefore restricted to the extracellular compartment. Severe losses can deplete the extracellular volume rapidly, leading to vascular collapse. The box on this page lists risk factors and conditions that can lead to isotonic volume deficit. Table 1-5 presents common signs and symptoms.

Medical Management

Treatment consists of identifying and correcting the underlying cause of fluid loss and then replacing the fluids and electrolytes that have been lost with appropriate isotonic fluids or blood products. See Table 1-6 for the osmolality of common IV solutions.

ISOTONIC VOLUME EXCESS

An isotonic volume excess occurs in conditions in which both extracellular water and electrolytes are retained by the body. Volume is increased but the osmolality remains in the normal range.

Pathophysiology

Isotonic volume excess involves the extracellular fluid compartment. Osmotic fluid movement does not occur across cell walls and the fluid accumulates in the vascular and interstitial spaces. Interstitial fluid overload (edema) results from hydrostatic and osmotic pressures that move fluid from the blood stream to the interstitial spaces. The box on p. 4 lists common causes of edema by their physiologic mechanism. Table 1-7 presents common signs and symptoms of isotonic volume excess.

Medical Management

The treatment of isotonic volume excess depends on the underlying condition. The management of congestive heart failure, cirrhosis, renal failure, and other conditions that result in isotonic volume excess is dealt with in depth in other portions of the book.

TABLE 1-7 Signs and symptoms of isotonic volume excess

Body System	Signs and Symptoms
Skin and superficial tissues	Edema, especially dependent edema; skin may be tight, smooth, and shiny, or cool, and pale
Cardiovascular	Neck vein engorgement (vein distention even in upright position)
Respiratory	Rales; dyspnea, frothy cough, and cyanosis indicate pulmonary edema, a medical emergency
Other	Weight gain is best early sign of volume excess, since several liters of fluid may be retained without visible evidence of edema

CAUSES OF EDEMA ACCORDING TO UNDERLYING PHYSIOLOGIC MECHANISM

FLUID PRESSURE
Increased capillary fluid pressure
Increased venous pressure
  Vein obstruction
    Varicose veins
    Thrombophlebitis
    Pressure on veins from casts, tight bandages, or garters
  Increased total volume with decreased cardiac output
    Congestive heart failure
  Fluid overloading: too rapid infusion of IV fluids, especially in the elderly
Sodium and water retention, increased aldosterone from:
  Decreased renal blood flow
    Congestive heart failure
    Renal failure
  Increased production of aldosterone
    Cushing's syndrome
  Aldosterone added to system
    Corticosteroid therapy
  Inability to destroy aldosterone
    Cirrhosis of liver

ONCOTIC PRESSURE
Decreased capillary oncotic pressure
Loss of serum protein
  Burns, draining wounds, fistulas
  Hemorrhage
  Nephrotic syndrome
  Chronic diarrhea
Decreased intake of protein
  Malnutrition
  Kwashiorkor
Decreased production of albumin
  Liver disease

Increased interstitial oncotic pressure
Increased capillary permeability to protein
  Burns
  Inflammatory reactions
    Trauma
    Infections
  Allergic reactions (hives)
Blocked lymphatics: decreased removal of tissue fluid and protein
  Malignant diseases
  Surgical removal of lymph nodes
  Elephantiasis

From Phipps, W.J., Long, B.C., and Woods, N.F.: Medical-surgical nursing: concepts and clinical practice, ed. 2, St. Louis, 1983, The C.V. Mosby Co.

NURSING MANAGEMENT OF PRIMARY FLUID IMBALANCES

Assessment
Factors to be assessed include the following:
Risk factors as presented in tables
Vital signs—orthostatic blood pressures
Weight
Skin turgor
Urine output—fluid intake and output balance
Urine specific gravity
Edema
Level of consciousness—changes in mental status

Nursing diagnoses
Fluid volume deficit related to disturbances in intake or failure of regulatory mechanisms
Fluid volume excess related to excessive fluid intake or failure of regulatory mechanisms
Potential for injury related to altered mental status
Alteration in peripheral and cerebral perfusion related to fluid loss
Potential impairment of skin integrity related to interstitial edema

Expected outcomes
Patient will return to a normal hydration status as evidenced by the alleviation of symptoms and restoration of normal laboratory values.
Patient will not experience injury during the period of altered mental status.
Patient will maintain intact skin.

Nursing interventions
Prevention and monitoring
Monitor IV fluid rates closely.
Monitor daily AM weights.
Monitor urine output, intake and output (I & O) balance, and urine specific gravity.
Assess vital signs, mental status, skin turgor, and mucous membranes.
Treatment
Administer drugs, give or restrict fluids as prescribed by physician.
Comfort and safety
Provide frequent mouth care.
Provide skin care, turning and positioning patient if edema present; avoid immobility.

TABLE 1-8 Signs and symptoms of sodium imbalance

Body System	Signs of Sodium Deficit	Signs of Sodium Excess
Skin	Poor turgor, may be cool and clammy if shock is incipient	Flushed, warm, dry, sticky mucous membranes; rubbery skin turgor
Cardiovascular	Orthostatic hypotension (severe cases lead to circulatory collapse, shock)	Hypotension, tachycardia
Central nervous system	Headache, apathy (severe cases lead to confusion and coma)	Irritability
Gastrointestinal	Anorexia, nausea, cramps	Thirst
Muscular	Muscle weakness, fatigue	Muscle weakness

Use side rails, supervise ambulation.

Orient patient to surroundings and treatment.

Patient teaching to prevent recurrence

Describe fluid needs during exercise and in hot weather.

Explain prescribed medications: diuretics.

Explain sodium restrictions in diet.

Evaluation

Electrolytes, intake and output, and serum osmolality are within normal ranges.

Patient maintains a stable weight.

Patient is free of accidental injury and skin breakdown.

Patient and family can describe medications and diet to be followed and can describe preventive measures to avoid recurrence of fluid imbalance.

ELECTROLYTE IMBALANCE

No single electrolyte can be out of balance without other electrolytes also being out of balance. Sodium, potassium, and calcium are all essential for the passage of nerve impulses. Whenever the balance of any of these electrolytes is disrupted, the imbalance is reflected in the nervous stimulation of muscles.

SODIUM IMBALANCE

Sodium is the primary extracellular cation and controls the osmotic pressure of the extracellular fluid compartment. Sodium is essential for neuromuscular function, for many intracellular chemical reactions, and for helping to maintain acid-base balance in the body. Sodium balance is largely controlled by aldosterone.

SODIUM DEFICIT (HYPONATREMIA)

Pathophysiology

A serum sodium level below 138 mEq/L can result from either a sodium loss or a water excess. As the sodium level in the extracellular fluid decreases, po-

RISK FACTORS AND CONDITIONS LEADING TO SODIUM DEFICIT

Sodium loss from gastrointestinal tract:
    Vomiting or diarrhea
    Gastrointestinal suction
    Gastrointestinal drainage: fistulas, biliary, ileostomy
Profuse perspiration:
    Fever
    Exercise
Excess diuretic effect
Shift of body fluids:
    Massive edema—ascites
    Burns
    Small bowel obstruction

tassium moves out of the intracellular fluid, causing subsequent disturbances in potassium balance. Even if there is no excess of body water, the decreasing osmolality creates a condition similar to water excess; water moves into the cell, leaving the extracellular compartment depleted. Both circulatory and cellular function are impaired. The box above lists risk factors and conditions that result in sodium deficit. Table 1-8 presents common signs and symptoms of both sodium deficit and sodium excess.

Medical Management

Lost sodium and water are replaced by administration of saline solution (0.9% NaCl) plus plasma expanders if patient is in shock. Other electrolytes are replaced as need is established by blood values. Salt or salty foods may be added to the diet.

SODIUM EXCESS (HYPERNATREMIA)

Pathophysiology

A serum sodium level greater than 145 mEq/L exists when there is an excess of sodium in relation to water in the extracellular fluid. Osmolality increases and water

TABLE 1-9 Signs and symptoms of potassium excess or deficit

Body System	Signs of Potassium Deficit	Signs of Potassium Excess
Cardiovascular	Arrhythmias ECG changes (flattened T waves) Cardiac arrest	Arrhythmias ECG changes (elevated T waves) Fibrillation/arrest
Gastrointestinal	Anorexia, nausea, vomiting Paralytic ileus	Nausea, vomiting Diarrhea
Central nervous	Lethargy, diminished deep tendon reflexes Mental depression	Numbness and tingling Irritability
Muscular	Muscle weakness Flaccid paralysis, respiratory arrest	Muscle irritability Muscle weakness Flaccid paralysis

RISK FACTORS AND CONDITIONS LEADING TO SODIUM EXCESS

Excessive ingestion of sodium:
    Normal saline infusions
    Oral intake of salt tablets
Loss of body water without proportional sodium loss
Inability to excrete sodium properly:
    Renal failure
    Increased aldosterone production
    Congestive heart failure

RISK FACTORS AND CONDITIONS LEADING TO POTASSIUM DEFICIT

Decreased potassium intake:
    NPO
    Severe dieting
    Failure to adequately replace losses
Increased potassium loss:
    Gastrointestinal losses
    Vomiting or diarrhea
    Draining fistulas
    Potassium wasting diuretics
        Thiazide diuretics
    Losses from cellular trauma, such as burns
Cellular shifts of potassium:
    Acidosis
    Alkalosis

leaves the cells to dilute the extracellular fluid, leaving the cells water-depleted and disrupting their function. The box above lists risk factors and conditions that result in sodium excess. Signs and symptoms were presented in Table 1-8.

Medical Management
A sodium excess is treated with liberal administration of water if cardiac and renal function are adequate. The patient may be given D_5W intravenously or water by mouth. Diuretics are used to facilitate sodium excretion.

POTASSIUM IMBALANCE
Potassium is the primary intracellular cation. It has a direct effect on muscle and nerve excitability, maintains intracellular osmotic pressure, and helps maintain acid-base balance. Potassium enters the cells during anabolism and glucose conversion to glycogen; potassium leaves the cell during cellular breakdown resulting from either trauma or catabolism.

POTASSIUM DEFICIT (HYPOKALEMIA)
Pathophysiology
A serum potassium below 3.5 mEq/L alters the polarization of cells, causing them to be less excitable. This loss of excitability can be life threatening when it occurs in cardiac muscle. The body conserves potassium less effectively than sodium and will excrete it through the kid-

neys even when it is needed. The box above lists risk factors and conditions that result in potassium deficit. Table 1-9 presents common signs and symptoms of both potassium deficit and potassium excess.

Medical Management
Medical management consists of prompt administration of potassium either orally or by IV. Oral administration may be by foods rich in potassium (see box on page 7), or by oral potassium preparations. Intravenous infusions of potassium ideally should not exceed 20 mEq per hour and should be extremely diluted (40 mEq/L) to control peripheral vein irritation.

POTASSIUM EXCESS (HYPERKALEMIA)
Pathophysiology
A serum potassium above 5.5 mEq/L rarely occurs in the presence of normal renal function. Excess potassium decreases the polarization of cells, causing them to become more excitable. Moderate excess causes nerve and muscle irritability, but severe hyperkalemia leads to weakness and paralysis. The box on p. 7 lists risk factors and con-

FOODS RICH IN POTASSIUM

FRUITS	VEGETABLES*	PROTEIN FOODS	BEVERAGES
Apricots	Asparagus	Beef	Cocoa
Bananas	Dried beans	Chicken	Cola drinks
Grapefruit	Broccoli	Liver	Dry instant tea and coffee
Melon	Cabbage	Pork	
Honeydew	Carrots	Veal	
Canteloupe	Celery	Turkey	
Dried fruits	Mushrooms	Milk	
Figs, dates, raisins	Dried peas	Nuts	
Oranges	Potatoes, white	Peanut butter	
	sweet		
	Spinach		
	Squash		

*Most raw vegetables contain potassium but it is frequently lost in cooking.

RISK FACTORS AND CONDITIONS LEADING TO POTASSIUM EXCESS

Decreased potassium loss
  Renal failure
  Adrenal insufficiency
  Potassium-sparing diuretics
Cellular shifts of potassium
  Trauma
  Metabolic acidosis
Excess potassium intake
  Dietary excess (in presence of renal insufficiency)
  Excessive IV administration

RISK FACTORS AND CONDITIONS LEADING TO CALCIUM DEFICIT

Inadequate calcium intake
  Dietary deficiency
Excess loss of calcium
  Kidney disease
  Draining intestinal fistula
Decreased absorption from GI tract
  Insufficient vitamin D
  Insufficient parathyroid hormone
  Pancreatic or intestinal disease—malabsorption
Excess binding of ionized calcium
  Transfusion with citrated blood
  Alkalosis

ditions that result in potassium excess. Signs and symptoms are presented in Table 1-9.

Medical Management
Medical management includes the following:
  Administration of cation exchange resins (Kayexalate) orally or by enema to bind the potassium and release sodium. Administration of sorbitol increases bowel motility to excrete excess potassium.
  Administration of 10% glucose with insulin to stimulate the movement of potassium into the cell.
  Bed rest with no oral food or fluid.
  Administration of IV calcium to antagonize the effect of excess potassium on the cardiac muscle.

CALCIUM IMBALANCE

Calcium is present in the blood in two forms: ionized and bound to plasma proteins. Only the ionized calcium is physiologically active. It functions to support blood clotting; smooth, skeletal, and cardiac muscle function; and nerve function. Both parathyroid hormone and vitamin D are necessary for normal absorption of calcium from the GI tract.

CALCIUM DEFICIT (HYPOCALCEMIA)

Pathophysiology
A serum calcium level below 4.5 mEq/L affects cell membrane chemistry. Calcium has a depressant effect on skeletal muscles. In hypocalcemia, depolarization takes place more easily, producing excitability of the nervous system and the skeletal, smooth, and cardiac muscles. The box above lists risk factors and conditions that result in calcium deficit. Table 1-10 presents common signs and symptoms of both calcium deficit and calcium excess.

Medical Management
Medical management includes administration of oral calcium salts and a high calcium diet. Slow administration of IV calcium gluconate may be ordered for severe deficits. Parathyroid hormone or vitamin D also may be administered if there are deficiencies in these substances.

CALCIUM EXCESS (HYPERCALCEMIA)

Pathophysiology
A serum calcium level above 5.8 mEq/L affects cell membrane chemistry by inhibiting depolarization and depress-

ing the function of nerves and skeletal, smooth, and cardiac muscles. Any condition causing immobility results in calcium leaving the bone and concentrating in the extracellular fluid. Excess calcium passing through the kidneys can cause precipitation and stone formation, especially in the presence of urine alkalinity. The box below lists risk factors and conditions that result in calcium excess. Common signs and symptoms are presented in Table 1-10.

Medical Management

The only definitive treatment of calcium excess is the removal of the cause. Administration of IV saline (physiologic flushing) followed by thiazide diuretic promotes calcium excretion with the sodium. Administration of inorganic phosphate, Mithiacin, or glucocorticoids increases calcium excretion. Acidification of urine by acid ash diet and increased fluid intake may be ordered to prevent formation of calcium stones by kidney.

RISK FACTORS AND CONDITIONS LEADING TO CALCIUM EXCESS

Calcium loss from bones
   Immobilization
   Carcinoma with bone metastasis
   Multiple melanoma
Excessive dietary intake
   High calcium diet, especially milk products
   Antacids containing calcium
Increased absorption or mobilization from bones
   Vitamin D therapy
   Increased parathyroid hormone
   Steroid therapy

NURSING MANAGEMENT OF ELECTROLYTE IMBALANCES

Assessment

Factors to be assessed include:
Risk factors as presented in tables
Vital signs:
   Orthostatic blood pressures
   ECG changes
Weight changes
Medication history and use
Skin turgor and mucous membranes
Urine:
   Intake and output balance
   Urine specific gravity and pH
Edema
Level of consciousness—changes in mental status
Subjective complaints
   Headache
   Muscle weakness
   Fatigue
   Anorexia, nausea
   Numbness or tingling
Hyperreflexia
Tetany: positive Chvostek's/Trousseau's signs
Vomiting
Diarrhea
Dietary intake

Nursing diagnoses

Fluid volume deficit related to disturbances in intake of electrolytes or failure of regulatory mechanisms
Fluid volume excess related to disturbances in intake of electrolytes or failure of regulatory mechanisms
Activity intolerance related to muscular weakness and fatigue

---

TABLE 1-10 Signs and symptoms of calcium imbalance

Body System	Signs of Calcium Deficit	Signs of Calcium Excess
Cardiovascular	Arrhythmias Cardiac arrest	Depressed activity Arrhythmias Cardiac arrest
Central nervous	Numbness, tingling, especially in fingertips and lips Twitching and convulsions in severe cases	Decreased deep tendon reflexes Lethargy, coma in severe cases
Muscular	Muscle spasm Tetany—positive Trousseau's and Chvostek's signs	Muscle fatigue and decreased tone
Gastrointestinal	Increased peristalsis—nausea, vomiting, diarrhea	Decreased gastrointestinal motility, anorexia, constipation
Skeletal	Osteoporosis and fractures	Bone pain Osteoporosis and fractures
Other	Abnormal calcium deposits in body tissue	Kidney stones Thirst, polyuria

Alteration in comfort related to neuromuscular and gastrointestinal symptoms

Potential for injury related to weakness and decreased mental status

Decreased cardiac output related to conduction disorders

Expected outcomes

Patient will return to a normal fluid and electrolyte balance as evidenced by alleviation of symptoms and restoration of normal laboratory values.

Patient will not experience injury during periods of altered mental status.

Patient will have sufficient energy and muscular strength to complete normal activities of daily living.

Patient will experience relief of symptoms of thirst, nausea, and diarrhea.

Patient will maintain an intake of nutrients adequate to meet body's need.

Nursing interventions

Record accurate intake and output
  Evaluate dietary intake.
  Evaluate balance of intake and output.
Assess vital signs frequently; skin turgor, status of mucous membranes, and level of consciousness.
Monitor laboratory values.
Check daily AM weights.
Administer IV fluids and medications as prescribed.
Provide comfort and safety measures.
  Administer mouth and skin care frequently.
  Use side rails, supervise ambulation.
Adjust patient activity level to energy level and tolerance.
Assist with activities of daily living as required.
Provide frequent position changes and skin massage.
Adjust meal content and schedule to include patient preferences.
Patient and family teaching (to prevent recurrence):
  Describe correct use of and compliance with medications.
  Explain diet or supplements if ordered—Na^+, K^+, Ca^{++}.
  Explain signs and symptoms indicative of imbalance.
  Describe measures to prevent imbalances during GI illnesses.

Evaluation

Electrolytes, intake and output, serum osmolality, urine specific gravity, and vital signs are within normal ranges.

Patient maintains a stable weight.

Patient is able to complete self-care safely in all activities of daily living.

Patient eats and digests a normal diet without occurrence of gastrointestinal symptoms.

Patient does not experience injury.

Patient and family can describe medications and diet to be followed at home and can describe preventive measures to avoid recurrence of electrolyte imbalance, if appropriate.

ACID-BASE IMBALANCES

The regulation of body pH is vital because even slight deviations from the normal range will cause significant changes in the rate of cellular chemical reactions. Acid-base balance is controlled by several regulatory mechanisms. The following values indicate normal acid-base parameters:

pH   7.35–7.45
P_{CO_2} 35–43 mm Hg
HCO_3 21–28 mEq/L

The body's three major mechanisms for controlling the acid-base balance include chemical buffers in the cells and extracellular fluid, respiratory retention or excretion of CO_2, and kidney regulation of the quantity of sodium bicarbonate. The buffers work continuously and instantaneously. Respiratory adjustments require minutes to hours in time while kidney adjustments require minutes to days. Together these mechanisms maintain the normal ratio of 20 parts of bicarbonate to one part of carbonic acid.

PATHOPHYSIOLOGY

Table 1-11 discusses the four major acid-base imbalances with their causative features, signs and symptoms, and method of compensation.

MEDICAL MANAGEMENT

Treatment depends on the specific imbalance.
Respiratory acidosis: improve alveolar exchange of O_2 and CO_2 by intermittent positive-pressure breathing (IPPB) and low flow O_2 administration.
Respiratory alkalosis: treat underlying condition; reduce respiration rate; counter tetany with calcium gluconate.
Metabolic acidosis: treat underlying cause; administer sodium bicarbonate either orally or by IV; monitor fluid and potassium levels as condition resolves.
Metabolic alkalosis: treat underlying condition; administer sodium, potassium, and ammonium chloride either orally or by IV as indicated by laboratory values.

TABLE 1-11 Common acid-base imbalances: causes, signs and symptoms, and mechanisms of compensation

Imbalance	Physiologic Causes	Signs and Symptoms	Mechanism of Compensation
Respiratory acidosis pH < 7.35 P_{CO_2} > 45 HCO_3 normal	Hypoventilation (lungs not removing sufficient amounts of CO_2), caused by: Respiratory infections CNS depression Paralysis of respiratory muscles Poor thoracic excursion—atelectasis Abdominal distention	Hypoventilation Decreased chest excursion Cyanosis Drowsiness Tachycardia	Kidneys retain and manufacture more bicarbonate. Hydrogen ions excreted in urine. Compensated values: pH 7.40 P_{CO_2} > 45 HCO_3 > 28
Respiratory alkalosis pH > 7.45 P_{CO_2} < 35 HCO_3 normal	Hyperventilation (lungs removing too much CO_2), caused by: Emotions: fear, hysteria Fever O_2 lack CNS stimulation	Hyperventilation Dizziness Light-headedness Tingling face and hands Convulsions	Kidneys excrete large amounts of bicarbonate. Compensated values: pH 7.40 P_{CO_2} < 35 HCO_3 < 21
Metabolic acidosis pH < 7.35 P_{CO_2} normal HCO_3 < 21	Bicarbonate loss Diarrhea Fistula drainage Acid gain or retention, caused by: Diabetic ketoacidosis Lactic acidosis Renal failure K^+ excess Salicylate poisoning	Headache, dizziness Kussmaul respiration Fruity breath odor Disorientation, coma Weakness High serum K^+	Lungs hyperventilate to excrete CO_2 and reduce serum carbonic acid levels. Compensated values: pH 7.40 P_{CO_2} < 35 HCO_3 < 21
Metabolic alkalosis pH > 7.45 P_{CO_2} normal HCO_3 > 28	Acid loss, caused by: Vomiting/GI suction Potassium depletion Steroids Bicarbonate retention, caused by: Excessive intake of baking soda Transfusion of citrated blood	Hypoventilation Numbness and tingling in extremities Bradycardia Confusion	Lungs hypoventilate to retain CO_2 and increase serum carbonic acid levels. Compensated values: pH 7.40 P_{CO_2} > 45 HCO_3 > 28

NURSING MANAGEMENT OF ACID-BASE IMBALANCES

Assessment
Both subjective and objective factors should be assessed.

Subjective complaints:
Numbness and tingling in face and extremities
Dizziness, light-headedness
Headache, weakness

Objective signs:
Rate and depth of respiration
Vital signs
Changes in mental status

Nursing diagnoses
Impaired gas exchange related to hyperventilation or hypoventilation
Alteration in comfort related to neuromuscular symptoms

Expected outcomes
Patient will return to an effective respiratory pattern.
Patient will experience relief of symptoms such as weakness, dizziness, numbness, and tingling.

Patient will return to a normal acid-base balance as evidenced by relief of symptoms and normal blood gas values.

Nursing interventions
Have the patient turn, cough, and deep breath every hour.
Clear airway—suction if needed, position in semi-Fowler's position.
Administer O_2 and medications as ordered.
Calm patient.
Use rebreather if needed to slow hyperventilation.
Monitor patient's vital signs and intake and output carefully.
Monitor blood gases and electrolyte values.
Assess effectiveness of prescribed interventions.

Evaluation
Patient is breathing room air with a respiratory rate of 12 to 18 breaths per minute. Lungs are clear to auscultation.
Patient's blood gases, electrolytes, and vital signs are within the normal range.
Patient is able to resume activity level and self-care activities.

BIBLIOGRAPHY

Cardin, S.: Acid-base balance in the patient with respiratory disease, Nurs. Clin. North Am. **15**(3):593-601, 1980.

Felver, L.: Understanding the electrolyte maze, Am. J. Nurs. **80**:1591-1599, 1980.

Friedman, F.B.: Clinical controversies: can we really trust those I & Os?, RN **45**(4):52-3, 118-120, 1982.

Goldberger, E.: A primer of water, electrolytes and acid-base syndromes, ed. 6, Philadelphia, 1980, Lea & Febiger.

Kee, J.L.: Fluids and electrolytes with clinical applications: a programmed approach, ed. 3, New York, 1982, John Wiley & Sons, Inc.

Menezel, L.K.: Clinical problems of electrolyte balance, Nurs. Clin. North Am. **15**(3):559-576, 1980.

Menezel, L.K.: Clinical problems of fluid balance, Nurs. Clin. North Am. **15**(3):549-558, 1980.

Rando, J.T.: Fluid and electrolyte management of the adult surgical patient, AANA J **50**:49-54, 1982.

Weldy, N.J.: Body fluids and electrolytes: a programmed instruction, ed. 3, St. Louis, 1980, The C.V. Mosby Co.

Zerwekh, J.V.: The dehydration question, Nursing 83 **13**(1):47-51, 1983.

Cancer

Few diseases evoke greater feelings of anxiety and fear than cancer. Its physiologic and psychologic impact on patients and families is profound. Despite significant progress in cancer care and control, the diagnosis still signifies pain, mutilation, and death to many. Nurses are products of their society and may share many of its negative attitudes toward the disease. Cancer nursing challenges every aspect of a nurse's creativity, skill, and commitment.

The incidence of cancer is 175 per 100,000 of the population. Despite significant success in treatment, cancer ranks second to heart disease as the leading cause of death in the United States. It is estimated that one out of every four Americans develops some form of cancer in his or her lifetime. Cancer occurs in both sexes and all ages. The incidence of all forms of cancer increases with age. Fig. 2-1 shows the incidence by involved organ for both cancer and cancer death for males and females. The box below lists the commonly identified risk or predisposing factors for the development of cancer. Current research indicates that the development of cancer is multicausal with some interplay of heredity; environment; exposure to viruses, pollutants, or radiation; and the individual's immune mechanisms.

TUMOR CLASSIFICATION SYSTEM

The extent of disease in each individual cancer patient is classifiable by the TNM (Tumor, Node, Metastases) quantification system shown in the box below. This

---

TNM STAGING CLASSIFICATION SYSTEM

TUMOR

TO	No evidence of primary tumor
TIS	Carcinoma in situ
T1, T2, T3, T4	Ascending degrees of tumor size and involvement

NODES

NO	No regional nodes demonstrably abnormal
N1a, N2a	Demonstrable regional lymph nodes, metastasis not suspected
N1b, N2b, N3	Demonstrable regional lymph nodes, metastasis suspected
Nx	Regional nodes cannot be assessed clinically

METASTASIS

MO	No evidence of distant metastasis
M1, M2, M3	Ascending degrees of metastatic involvement of host including distant nodes

From Phipps, W.J., Long, B.C., and Woods, N.F.: Medical-surgical nursing: concepts and clinical practice, ed. 2, St. Louis, 1983, The C.V. Mosby Co.

PREDISPOSING OR RISK FACTORS FOR THE DEVELOPMENT OF CANCER

ENVIRONMENTAL FACTORS	HOST SUSCEPTIBILITY	OTHER AREAS OF INTENSE INVESTIGATION
Air and water pollution	Inherited factors, such as cancer family syndrome, retinoblastoma	Diet
Excessive sun exposure	Hormonal factors, such as estrogens (DES)	Occupation
Chemical pollutants: tar, soot, asbestos, fuel oils, dyes	Immunologic factors, such as immunosuppression for any reason	Racial, cultural, geographic variabilities
Ionizing radiation	Chronic irritation to any body lesion	Physiologic and psychologic stress and coping patterns
Excess tobacco or alcohol use	Precancerous lesions	

classification system is used to provide a common basis for describing the extent of illness, to develop treatment protocols, and to identify prognosis.

PATHOPHYSIOLOGY OF CANCER

Cancer cells differ from normal cells in a variety of ways. Characteristics of cancer cells include:

Anaplasia: succeeding generations of cells increasingly lose their similarity to the parent tissue

Uncontrolled growth pattern: diminished or absent resting phase

Metastasis: ability to spread via blood or lymph system or directly extend into new locations and begin new growth

Larger and irregularly shaped nuclei

Disorderly growth: tumors are not encapsulated and may be necrotic at core because of poor vascular supply

Cancers produce symptoms in patients when they cause:

Obstruction of function

Pressure on surrounding tissue

Infiltration and destruction of surrounding tissue

Hemorrhage

Infection and ulceration

Pain

Cachexia syndrome: anorexia, weight loss, tissue, wasting, hypermetabolism

EARLY DETECTION AND PREVENTION

Primary prevention through the identification and control of carcinogens in the environment coupled with early detection of cancers offers the best approach to the reduction of the incidence of cancer deaths.

Table 2-1 lists the American Cancer Society's guidelines for cancer related checkups. Educating the public about the seven warning signs of cancer (*CAUTION*) is essential:

C hange in usual bowel or bladder function

A sore that does not heal

U nusual bleeding or discharge

T hickening or lump in the breast or elsewhere

I ndigestion or dysphagia

O bvious change in a wart or mole

N agging cough or hoarseness

MEDICAL MANAGEMENT OF CANCER

Medical management revolves around four major forms of intervention. These therapies are usually employed in

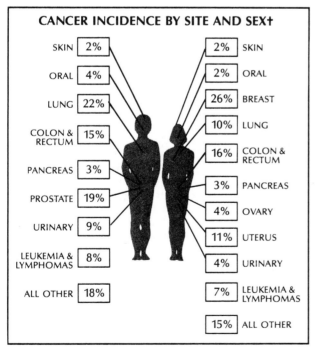

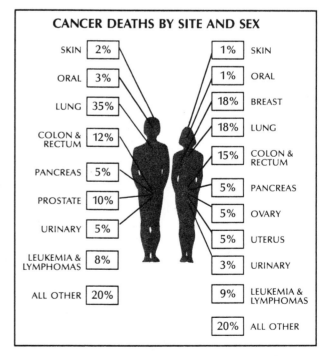

†Excluding non-melanoma skin cancer and carcinoma in situ.

FIGURE 2-1 Comparison of cancer incidence and deaths by site and sex (1984 estimates). (From American Cancer Society: 1984 Cancer facts and figures, New York, 1983, The Society.)

TABLE 2-1 Guidelines for cancer related checkups

Test or Examination	Sex	Age (yr)	Testing Intervals
Papanicolaou test (Pap test)	Female	Over 20; under 20 if sexually active	q 3 yr after two initial negative tests 1 yr apart
Pelvic examination	Female	20–40	q 3 yr
		Over 40 or at menopause	Yearly
Endometrial tissue sample	Female	At menopause if high risk	High risk: history of infertility, obesity, failure of ovulation, abnormal uterine bleeding, estrogen therapy
Breast self-examination	Female	Over 20	Monthly
Breast physical examination	Female	20–40	q 3 yr
		Over 40	Yearly
Mammogram	Female	35–40	One baseline mammogram
		Over 50	Yearly
Stool guaiac slide test	Male and female	Over 50	Yearly
Digital rectal examination	Male and female	Over 40	Yearly
Sigmoidoscopic examination	Male and female	Over 50	q 3–5 yr after two initial negative examinations 1 yr apart

From Phipps, W.J., Long, B.C., and Woods, N.F.: Medical-surgical nursing: concepts and clinical practice, ed. 2, St. Louis, 1983, The C.V. Mosby Co. American Cancer Society recommendations.

combination to strengthen the chances of destroying the malignant cells.

Surgery is the most common form of treatment and is used for cure, diagnosis and staging, palliation, ablative effects, control of pain, and reconstruction. Cancer surgery attempts to ensure a margin of healthy tissue and frequently results in significant loss of function as well as disturbance in body image.

Radiation is the use of ionizing radiation to cause damage and destruction to cancerous cells during their replicative cycles. Radiation can be delivered externally, by exposing the patient to rays, or internally, by placing radioactive material within the tissues or a body cavity. Radiation may be used for cure, palliation, reduction of tumor size, and elimination of pain or obstruction. The box on p. 14 lists basic radiation therapy information and principles of staff protection.

Chemotherapy includes the use of a wide variety of drugs that act to destroy rapidly dividing cells, both cancerous and noncancerous. It is used for both cure and palliation of symptoms. Table 2-2 lists the categories of chemotherapeutic drugs in common use and examples of each.

Immunotherapy is a research therapy in which researchers are attempting to stimulate the patient's own immune system to recognize cancer cells as "non-self" and destroy them. It includes approaches using nonspecific substances such as BCG and the antitumor effects of interferon. Table 2-3 lists the three major types of immunotherapy being utilized.

PRINCIPLES OF RADIATION THERAPY AND PROTECTION OF STAFF

- Radiation applied externally can cause injury only during the time the treatment is being administered. NOTE: Patient is never radioactive.
- Radiation with alpha or beta rays applied internally creates no hazard to staff, since these rays cannot pass through the patient's skin. Substances emitting gamma rays cause the patient to transmit gamma radiation.
- Each radiation substance has its own half-life: the period of time in which half its radioactivity is dissipated and the dangers of radiation are reduced.

To protect staff from the effects of radiation, these factors should be considered:
Amount of exposure to radiation sources
  Radiation doses are cumulative. Limit interactions with patients with internal radiation therapy to 15 minutes per visit; group activities to maximize use of time.
  Each nurse must wear his or her own film badge when in contact with source.
Strength of radiation substance
  Radiation safety officer can and should provide data about substance: its half-life, nature of rays, and ways it may be excreted from the body, for example, in urine, sweat, saliva, and so on.
Distance from radiation source
  Rays are more numerous and concentrated at close range.
Type and degree of shielding in use
  Lead-lined container and long-handled forceps must always be in room to contain source if dislodged.
  Proper receptacles for linens and excreta should be used if needed.
  Lead aprons for nursing staff if indicated.
Risk to staff
  Rotate nursing care among nurses who are at least risk from radiation hazard; pregnant nurses should not provide care.

TABLE 2-2 Drugs used in cancer chemotherapy

Agent	Mechanism of Action	Major Toxic Manifestations
Alkylating agents		
Chlorambucil (Leukeran) Melphalan (Alkeran) Cyclophosphamide (Cytoxan) Busulfan (Myleran) Thiophosphoramide (Thiotepa) Mechlorethamine (nitrogen mustard)	Interfere with DNA replication by attacking DNA synthesis throughout cell cycle (cell cycle nonspecific)	Bone marrow depression with leukopenia, thrombocytopenia, and bleeding; cyclophosphamide may cause alopecia and hemorrhagic cystitis
Antimetabolites		
Methotrexate (MTX) 6-Mercaptopurine (6-MP) 5-Fluorouracil (5-FU) Arabinocylcytosine (Cytosar) Cis-platinum (platinol)	Structural analogs of essential metabolites and therefore interfere with synthesis of these metabolites (cell cycle specific)	Bone marrow depression, oral and gastrointestinal ulceration
Antibiotics		
Doxorubicin (Adriamycin) Bleomycin (Blenoxane) Dactinomycin (Cosmegan) Cerubidine (Daunorubicin) Mithramycin (Mithracin) Mitomycin (Mutamycin)	Interfere with DNA or RNA synthesis, varying with the drug (cell cycle nonspecific)	Stomatitis, gastrointestinal disturbances, and bone marrow depression Doxorubicin causes cardiac toxicity at cumulative doses over 500 mg/m^2 Bleomycin can cause alopecia and pulmonary fibrosis, but only minimal bone marrow depression
Plant alkaloids		
Vinblastine (Velban)	Interfere with mitosis (cell cycle specific)	Alopecia, areflexia, bone marrow depression
Vincristine (Oncovin)		Neurotoxicity with ataxia and impaired fine motor skills, constipation and paralytic ileus
Steroid hormones		
Androgens (Neo-Hombreol) Estrogens (DES) Progestins (Depoprovera) Adrenocorticosteroids (Prednisone)	Alter the host environment for cell growth (cell cycle nonspecific)	Specific for the actions of the hormone

Adapted from Porth, C.: Pathophysiology: concepts of altered health states, Philadelphia, 1982, J.B. Lippincott Co.

TABLE 2-3 Types of immunotherapy

Type	Method	Substance Used
Nonspecific immunotherapy	Use of substances that increase the general immune capacity of the host	BCG *Corynebacterium parvum* Interferons
Specific immunotherapy	Use of substances antigenically related to the tumor or its products	1. Killed tumor cells from patient or patient with similar tumor 2. Altered tumor cells (more immunogenic) 3. Antigen extracted from tumor cells
Transfer of tumor immunity	Use of specific immune substances	1. Lymphocytes from another tumor patient 2. Immune RNA 3. Transfer factor

From Long, B.C., and Phipps, W.J.: Essentials of medical-surgical nursing: a nursing process approach, St. Louis, 1985, The C.V. Mosby Co.

NURSING MANAGEMENT OF THE PATIENT WITH CANCER

THE DIAGNOSTIC PERIOD

Assessment
The following subjective factors should be assessed:
Knowledge of diagnosis:
Establish what physician has told patient
Stage of grief
Coping skills of patient and family
Local/systemic effects of the tumor
General health state of patient

Nursing diagnoses
Alteration in comfort related to local or systemic effects of tumor
Ineffective individual or family coping related to the diagnosis of cancer
Fear related to the diagnosis of cancer or of death
Knowledge deficit related to the prognosis and treatment of cancer

Expected outcomes
Patient will experience decreased symptoms related to the local or systemic effects of tumor growth.
Patient and family will effectively cope with diagnosis.
Patient and family will be able to discuss advantages and disadvantages of various treatment options.
Patient will feel supported during the period of uncertainty associated with diagnostic workup.

Nursing interventions
Explore with patient feelings and concerns about diagnostic tests and outcomes.
Discuss patient and family's prior experiences with and feelings about cancer.
Avoid false reassurances and cliches that block honest communication.
Explain all tests and procedures thoroughly.
Include patient and family in all decisions about care.
Refer patient and family to the American Cancer Society and other community agencies.
Provide symptomatic relief where feasible.

Evaluation
Patient and family understand diagnosis and treatment plan.
Patient and family experience no more than moderate anxiety.
Patient and family maintain effective coping patterns.
Patient expresses an increased level of comfort.
Patient receives psychological support from family and nursing staff.

CANCER SURGERY

Assessment
Assessment for cancer surgery should include the following:
Standard preoperative assessment, risk factors
Patient's understanding of reason for surgery, nature of procedure, effects on body
Impact of surgery on patient's body image and role function

Nursing diagnoses
Variable diagnoses related to specific procedures plus:
Grieving related to loss of body part or function
Disturbance in self-concept related to altered body image
Spiritual distress related to dissemination of disease
Knowledge deficit related to self-care protocols

Expected outcomes
Patient will be prepared for surgery physically and psychologically.
Patient will recover from surgery without physiologic complications.
Patient will experience minimal discomfort.
Patient will appropriately grieve for physical loss.

Nursing interventions
Encourage patient to discuss feelings about surgical procedure and its effects on the body.
Assist patient and family to grieve over lost body part or function, or knowledge of widespread disease dissemination.
Provide teaching and reteaching as needed to keep patient informed about surgery and regimen of postsurgical care.
Teach patients skills and techniques needed to achieve self-care ability.
Ensure adequate postoperative pain relief.
Provide standard postoperative nursing interventions to identify complications and promote healing.
Refer patient to appropriate community support groups such as Reach to Recovery or Ostomy Club.

Evaluation
Patient recovers from surgery without complications and experiences only manageable pain.
Patient discusses surgical outcome and begins to display grief resolution.
Patient gradually assumes responsibility for self-care.

RADIATION

Assessment
Factors to be assessed include:
General physical status of patient, especially area to be irradiated.

Patient's understanding of nature and type of radiation
therapy, its goals, and its effects.
Patient's prior experiences with, and misconceptions
about, radiation therapy.

Nursing diagnoses
Diagnoses are variable depending on type of therapy, area
irradiated, and patient's health status. Common diagno-
ses include the following:
Impaired skin integrity related to effects of radiation
Alteration in comfort—nausea/vomiting related to ra-
diation syndrome
Alteration in nutrition—less than body requirements,
related to the anorexia of radiation syndrome
Activity intolerance related to the fatigue of radiation
syndrome
Potential for infection or injury related to immuno-
suppression
Social isolation related to radiation precautions
Knowledge deficit related to radiation therapy and ra-
diation precautions

Expected outcomes
Patient will maintain an intact skin.
Patient will have minimal discomfort.
Patient will not develop infection or bleeding.
Patient in isolation will not experience social or sensory
deprivation.
Patient will be knowledgeable about the sequence and
effects of radiation.
Patient will ingest an adequate balance of nutri-
ents.
Patient will complete self-care activities.

Nursing interventions
General
Teach patient about nature of radiation therapy and
expected side effects.
Encourage frequent rest periods.
Encourage patient to maintain usual self-care activi-
ties.
Teach patient about setting, equipment, and position-
ing used for therapy.
Skin care
Gently wash skin daily with tepid water and bland
soap. NURSING ALERT: Do not remove markings.
Consult radiologist concerning skin care. Vaseline,
A&D ointment, and corn starch are frequently em-
ployed. NURSING ALERT: Do not use cosmetics, lo-
tions, or powders that may contain heavy metal
base.
Teach patient to avoid constricting clothing or fric-
tion.
Teach patient to avoid prolonged exposure to sun,
wind, and extremes of temperature.

Nutrition
Prepare patient for likelihood of anorexia and nau-
sea.
Encourage small frequent meals throughout the
day.
Explore use of high protein, high carbohydrate, low
fat meals. Sweet foods are frequently better toler-
ated.
Encourage patient to rest after meals.
Avoid use of "empty calorie" foods. Offer enriched sup-
plements to meet nutritional needs.
Administer antiemetic medications as ordered.
Infection and injury
Monitor weekly blood tests.
Have patient avoid crowds and individuals with upper
respiratory infections.
Monitor vital signs.
Observe bleeding precautions if patient is thrombo-
cytopenic.

**Interventions for internal radiation therapy (See box on p.
14 for methods of staff protection.)**
Teach patient about rationale for therapy, side effects,
and reasons for required safety precautions.
Place patient in private room with signs that identify
nature and extent of radiation hazard.
Restrict visitors to 15-minute visits per day.
Counter effects of isolation by frequent visits from
doorway and encourage use of radio or television for
stimulation.
Promote comfort measures.
Teach patient to maintain bed rest, lying flat in bed
for cervical implants.
Use Foley catheter and low-residue diet to protect
against dislodgement of cervical implants.

Evaluation
Patient can state purpose of radiation therapy, nature
of the treatment and side effects, and actions to be
taken to manage side effects.
Patient has minimal discomfort from side effects—
does not vomit; maintains normal bowel elimination.
Patient's skin remains intact without evidence of
breakdown.
Patient remains afebrile and does not experience
bleeding or injury.
Patient maintains a normal body weight and eats a diet
that meets nutritional requirements.
Patient has sufficient energy to maintain self-care and
participate in usual activities.
Patient maintains orientation to reality and experiences minimal depression from isolation.

CHEMOTHERAPY

Assessment
Factors to be assessed include the following:
Patient's understanding of the nature and goals of chemotherapy—drugs used, expected side effects, and their management
General health status of patient
Patency of patient's veins and IV lines

Nursing diagnoses
Diagnoses are variable depending on type of drugs used, their specific side effects, and the patient's general health status. Common diagnoses include the following:
Knowledge deficit related to chemotherapy and its effects
Alteration in comfort related to stomatitis or vomiting
Alteration in nutrition—less than body requirements, related to anorexia, stomatitis, or vomiting
Potential impairment in skin integrity related to tissue sloughing
Altered self-concept (body image) related to alopecia
Potential for infection or injury related to immunosuppression
Alteration in oral mucous membranes related to cell destruction

Expected outcomes
Patient will be knowledgeable about drugs to be used and the management of their expected side effects.
Patient will maintain intact mucous membranes.
Patient will maintain an adequate and nutritious oral intake.
Patient will maintain intact veins.
Patient will maintain social interactions and make positive references to self.
Patients will be free of infection and not develop bleeding.

Nursing interventions
General
Teach patient names of drugs, expected side effects, and management of side effects.
Encourage patient to maintain self-care and usual activities, as tolerated.
Provide specific counseling about drug effects on fertility; include birth control and reproductive counseling as appropriate.
Infection and injury
Monitor daily or weekly blood counts. Be aware of expected nadir (low point).
Monitor vital signs and assess high risk sites regularly for early signs of infection, checking oral mucous membranes, lung sounds.
Teach importance of scrupulous personal hygiene; for

example, regular mouth care, perineal hygiene, short fingernails.
Use lubricants to prevent drying and cracking of skin.
Instruct family and friends with colds or flu not to visit.
Institute good hand washing, reverse isolation if prescribed.
Give no enemas or rectal medications; do not take rectal temperatures.
Institute bleeding precautions: no intramuscular injections, inspect for bruises, test stool and urine for blood.
Administer packed red blood cells and platelets as ordered.
Nutrition
Prepare patient for anorexia or nausea if expected with drug.
Administer emetics as prescribed. NURSING ALERT: Administer drugs *before* anticipated nausea so oral forms may be used.
Determine from patient best time for food and fluid intake in relation to treatment. Avoid food at time of treatment.
Avoid empty calorie foods. Offer enriched supplements to meet nutritional needs if they can be tolerated.
Experiment with food groups useful during periods of nausea: dry bulky foods, sweet foods, clear liquids. Avoid dairy products and red meats.
Keep environment clean and odor free.
Maintain fluid intake.
Teach relaxation techniques if appropriate.
Mucous membranes
Encourage frequent oral hygiene with mild mouth washes and soft toothbrush.
Assess frequently for *Candida* infection.
Use rinses and viscous lidocaine (Xylocaine) before meals for analgesia.
Adjust diet toward bland, mechanically soft foods.
Alopecia
Teach patient about hair loss—when it will occur and to what degree. NOTE: All body hair is affected. (Not all drugs cause hair loss.) NURSING ALERT: Reassure client that drug-induced hair loss is not permanent.
Plan with client in advance of hair loss the use and acquisition of wigs, scarves, and cosmetics.
Encourage patient to express feelings about hair loss.
Employ ice caps if prescribed and patient desires.
NOTE: Ice caps are not employed for patients with leukemia or other blood-borne cancers because cancer cells are sequestered from effects of drugs.
Vein integrity
Monitor all infusions carefully. Ensure that IV is patent before beginning drug administration.
Know which drugs cause widespread tissue necrosis, for example, nitrogen mustard and doxorubicin.

Monitor these infusions continuously.

If extravasation occurs, immediately discontinue infusion and apply ice to site.

Encourage patient to use and exercise arms between treatments if possible.

Evaluation

Patient can state purpose of chemotherapy, drugs to be used, expected side effects, and their management.

Patient has minimal discomfort from side effects—does not vomit, maintains normal bowel elimination.

Patient's mucous membranes and veins are intact.

Patient is afebrile, does not experience bleeding or injury.

Patient maintains a stable body weight and eats sufficient nutrients to meet basic body needs.

Patient maintains normal social interactions and chooses method to deal with alopecia.

PAIN

Assessment

Factors to be assessed include the following:

Nature of pain experience—location, quantity, severity, duration, influencing factors

Patient's prior experience with pain and pain tolerance

Nursing diagnosis

Alteration in comfort: mild to severe pain related to local and systemic effects of cancer cell growth

Expected outcomes

Patient will experience relief of pain.

Patient will be in control of the pain experience and be able to participate in normal daily activities.

Nursing interventions

Administer narcotics and analgesics promptly and as ordered.

Medications should be given routinely, not prn (as needed).

Administer drugs by mouth if possible; avoid intramuscular (IM) route.

Psychological addiction is not a major concern.

Inadequate pain control increases anxiety and intensifies the pain experience.

Aspirin remains the most effective single medication for mild to moderate pain.

Explore use of oral morphine solutions, patient-controlled analgesia, or IV morphine drips for chronic severe pain.

Observe, record, and report the patient's responses to both the pain and the analgesia.

Augment analgesia with other measures, such as relaxation, distraction, and nursing comfort measures including massage, heat, or cold.

Prevent the side effects of high dose narcotics, particularly constipation.

Evaluation

Patient experiences a decreased level of pain.

Patient is able to participate in activities of daily living.

SUPPORTIVE CARE FOR PATIENT AND FAMILY

Assessment

Factors to be assessed include:

Family interaction patterns

Support systems and resources available in the community

Family and patient's knowledge about disease, its progression, and outcome

Nursing diagnoses

Ineffective family coping related to terminal illness of family member.

Alteration in family processes related to care for family member with advanced cancer

Anticipatory or dysfunctional grieving related to terminal illness of family member

Expected outcomes

Patient and family will be accurately informed about the progress and prognosis of patient's condition.

Patient and family will maintain supportive interaction.

Patient and family will resolve guilt feelings and begin appropriate disengagement.

Patient and family will utilize resources and supports in community.

Nursing interventions

Support and strengthen patient's and family's coping methods unless dysfunctional.

Involve patient and family in all decision making about care.

Provide accurate information to patient concerning symptoms and prognosis.

Encourage all efforts by patient to maintain independence in self-care.

Facilitate family participation in patient's care.

Assist in planning alternatives to terminal hospitalization—hospice or home care—if family desires such help.

Provide and encourage time for patient and family to be alone together and talk about disease and impending death: encourage verbalization of feelings about death.

Initiate contact with community agencies that may be of assistance to family.

Realize that patient and family will need extra support from nurses during periods when symptoms return or worsen.

Evaluation

Patient and family experience ongoing support from nursing staff.

Family has approached and is receiving support from community agencies.

Patient and families maintain normal activities and role relationships as long as symptoms permit.

Patient and family communicate openly about disease progress and incipient separation through death.

BIBLIOGRAPHY

Bersani, G., and Carl, W.: Oral care for cancer patients, Am. J. Nurs. **83:**533-536, 1983.

Blumberg, F., Flaherty, M., and Lewis, J.: Cancer in the adult. In coping with cancer, Bethesda, MD, 1980, National Cancer Institute.

Bouchard-Kurtz, R.E., and Speese-Owens, N.F.: Nursing care of the cancer patient, ed. 4, St. Louis, 1981, The C.V. Mosby Co.

DeVita, V., Jr., Hellman, S., and Rosenberg, S.A.: Cancer principles and practice of oncology, Philadelphia, 1981, J.B. Lippincott Co.

Haskell, C.: Cancer treatment, Philadelphia, 1980, W.B. Saunders Co.

Holland, J.: Understanding the cancer patient, CA **30:**135-139, 1980.

Kelly, P.P., and Tinsley, C.: Planning care for the patient receiving external radiation, Am. J. Nurs. **81:**338-342, 1981.

Kennedy, M., et al.: Chemotherapy related nausea and vomiting: a survey to identify problems and interventions, Oncol. Nurs. Forum **8:**19-22, 1981.

Koren, M.E.: Cancer immunotherapy: what, why, when, how? Nursing 81 **11**(1):34-41, 1981.

Kripman, A.G.: Drug therapy and cancer pain, Ca. Nurs. **3:**39-46, 1980.

McAdams, C.W.: Interferon: the penicillin of the future, Am. J. Nurs. **80:**714-718, 1980.

McKhann, C.: Cancer immunotherapy: a realistic appraisal, CA **30:**286-293, 1980.

Rosembaum, E.H.: Living with cancer, St. Louis, 1982, The C.V. Mosby Co.

Varricchio, C.G.: The patient on radiation therapy, Am. J. Nurs. **81:**334-337, 1981.

Vredevoe, D., et al.: Concepts of oncology nursing, Englewood Cliffs, NJ, 1981, Prentice-Hall, Inc.

NURSING CARE PLAN

CANCER OF LARYNX FOLLOWING LARYNGECTOMY

Nursing Diagnoses	Expected Patient Outcomes	Nursing Interventions
Anxiety related to surgery and loss of ability to communicate	Patient does not exhibit signs of severe anxiety	1. Maintain a calm, unhurried environment. 2. Assure patient that airway will be suctioned to facilitate breathing. 3. Provide simple explanations of activities and events. 4. Provide for some type of patient communication system. 5. Give family opportunities to share their concerns; provide them with information about patient's progress and how they can support patient. 6. Encourage self-care as soon as feasible. 7. Suggest visit by laryngectomee, if desirable. 8. Suggest patient and partner participate in special organization, such as Lost Chord Club, after hospital discharge.

Ineffective airway clearance related to copious postoperative secretions	Patient's airway is clear to auscultation	1. Place patient in semi-Fowler's position.
		2. Monitor for noisy respirations, increased pulse and respiratory rate, and restlessness, indicating need for suctioning.
		3. Suction laryngectomy tube or stoma as needed (may be every 5 min initially).
		4. Provide tracheostomy care, if a tube is used.
		5. Provide air humidification.
		6. Encourage deep breathing and coughing.
		7. Minimize use of respiratory depressants (narcotics).
		8. Teach patient to protect stoma after discharge by:
		  a. Light covering (especially when shaving face)
		  b. Protection from water
		  c. Avoidance of dusty or smoky environment
		  d. Avoidance of talcum powder after bath

Alteration in comfort, related to postoperative pain and dry mouth	Patient experiences only manageable postoperative discomfort	1. Provide mouth care while N/G tube is in place. 2. Encourage patient to spit out saliva rather than swallowing when N/G tube is in place 3. Give prescribed analgesics (aspirin, acetaminophen, or codeine preferred). 4. Encourage other pain-relieving measures. 5. Encourage ambulation when permitted.

NURSING CARE PLAN

CANCER OF LARYNX FOLLOWING LARYNGECTOMY—cont'd

Nursing Diagnoses	Expected Patient Outcomes	Nursing Interventions
Potential alteration in nutrition; less than body requirements. Related to altered ability to swallow after operation	Patient maintains normal weight	1. Give prescribed tube feedings. 2. When N/G tube is removed, give fluids initially and stay with patient for initial meals until swallowing is tolerated. 3. Encourage optimum food intake as tolerated. 4. Stop oral feedings if tracheal secretions show food particles. 5. Monitor weight 2 to 3 times/week.

Impaired verbal communications related to effects of surgery	Patient communicates with others; patient begins speech rehabilitation	1. Assist patient to communicate by hand signals or by writing during initial phase.
		2. Anticipate patient needs so requests are minimized.
		3. Support activities of speech therapist.
		4. For patient learning esophageal speech:
		  a. Encourage patient to practice burping
		  b. Monitor for gastric flatus or discomfort from swallowed air
		5. For patient with tracheal-esophageal prosthesis, teach patient:
		  a. How to remove, clean, and reinsert prosthesis
		  b. How to cover stoma when speaking
		  c. Avoidance of "sticky" foods that may clog prosthesis (such as cheese, pasta, beans)
		6. Discuss availability of mechanical devices for speech aid or for telephone use.

Knowledge deficit related to self-care needs	Patient understands self-care and can demonstrate appropriate stoma care	1. Teach patient:
		  a. Description of anatomical changes
		  b. Care of stoma, including self-suctioning
		  c. Methods to protect stoma
		  d. Availability of community resources
		  e. Symptoms requiring medical follow-up

Disorders of the Musculoskeletal System

Disorders and injuries of the musculoskeletal system range from those that cause the client only minor discomfort and inconvenience to those that are life threatening. Included here are musculoskeletal disorders that commonly require hospitalization.

Regardless of the precipitating factors, patients with musculoskeletal disorders need to be assessed in a variety of areas before care for them can be effectively planned. Areas include:

Subjective

Patient's current health status

History of present illness and dysfunction

Pain assessment—nature, location, duration, and severity

Impact of dysfunction on activities of daily living

Presence and degree of weakness

Diet and activity patterns

Objective

Presence of obvious deformities

Posture, gait, and balance

Joint range of motion

Muscle strength

Peripheral pulses

Use of assistive devices

Figure 3-1 shows the anatomical structure of the musculoskeletal system. The following are common terms used in describing musculoskeletal function and disorders.

adduction Movement toward the midline of the body

abduction Movement away from the midline of the body

flexion Joint movement that decreases the angle between the two bones

extension Joint movement that widens the angle between the two bones

internal rotation Movement along the longitudinal axis in the direction of the midline of the body

external rotation Movement along the longitudinal axis away from the midline of the body

subluxation Partial dislocation of a joint

scoliosis Lateral curvature of the spine

kyphosis Curvature of the spine in which the convexity of the curve is posterior, usually in the thoracic region

valgus deformity The distal arm of the angle of the joint points away from the midline of the body

varus deformity The distal arm of the angle of the joint points toward the midline of the body

ulnar deviation Condition in which fingers deviate at the metacarpophalangeal joints toward the ulnar aspect of the hand

swan neck deformity Combination deformity in which there is flexion contracture of the metacarpophalangeal joint, hyperextension of the proximal interphalangeal joint, and flexion of the distal interphalangeal joint

FRACTURES

Fractures represent one of the most common problems of the musculoskeletal system. A fracture is a traumatic injury to a bone in which the continuity of the tissue of the bone is interrupted. There are a number of ways to classify or describe fractures, some of which are presented in Table 3-1.

Pathophysiology

Problems with fractures result from the direct loss of function of the part as well as corresponding damage to the surrounding muscles, nerves, ligaments and tendons, blood vessels, and soft tissue. Other problems emerge from the immobility necessary for healing of the tissue and bone.

Bone healing occurs by a process known as callus, or new bone, formation. This is a multistage process that begins with hematoma formation at the fractured bone ends. Gradually this hematoma transforms into a fibrous network with calcium deposits, new bone formation, and destruction of dead bone.

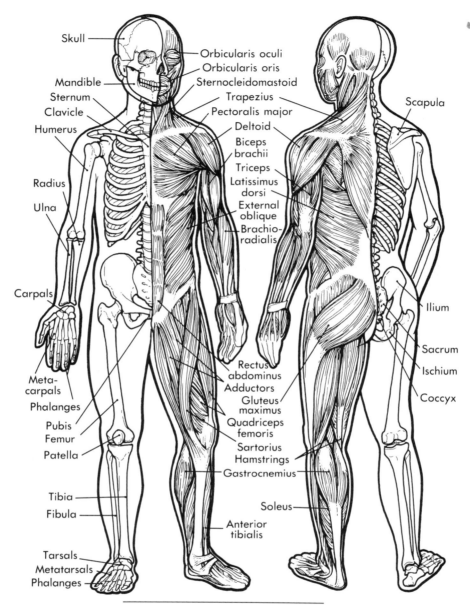

FIGURE 3-1 Musculoskeletal system.

Medical Management

Immobilization to hold bone fragments together so healing can occur is the cornerstone of any medical treatment. Depending on the severity and the location of the fracture, medical management may involve reduction and realignment with treatment either by cast or traction.

Fixation may be external or internal. External fixation (closed reduction) involves blind realignment of fractured bone parts, which is verified by x-ray film. Internal fixation (open reduction) uses direct operative visualization and realignment of the bone parts.

Traction involves the use of continuous pull on a bone and surrounding tissue to reduce and immobilize the fracture, overcome muscle spasm, and correct deformi-

ties. There are numerous forms of traction. Most fit into one of the following categories:

skin traction traction is applied to the skin through moleskin or adhesive and the traction weight is applied indirectly to the bone through the skin (examples: Buck's, Russell, pelvic)

skeletal traction traction is applied directly to the bone through the insertion of wires or pins usually positioned distally to the fracture site (examples: overhead arm, balanced suspension)

running traction direct pull without support of the part (examples: Buck's, cervical)

balanced traction direct pull on the part with extremity supported in a splint and held in place with balanced counterweights (examples: Thomas splint with Pearson attachment)

TABLE 3-1 Types of fractures

Type	Description
Complete	Complete separation of the bone, producing two fragments.
Incomplete	Partial break in the bone without separation.
Simple or closed	Bone is broken; skin is intact.
Compound or open	Fracture parts extend through the skin.
Fracture without displacement	Bone is broken; bone fragments are in alignment in normal position.
Fracture with displacement	Bone fragments have separated at the point of fracture.
Comminuted	Bone has broken into several fragments.
Impacted (telescoped)	One bone fragment is forcibly driven into another.
Greenstick	Fracture is limited to splintering of one side of the bone (occurs most often in children with soft bones).
Transverse	Break is across the bone.
Oblique	Line of fracture is at an oblique angle to the bone shaft.
Spiral	Line of fracture encircles the bone.

From Long, B.C., and Phipps, W.J., Essentials of medical-surgical nursing: a nursing process approach, St. Louis, 1985, The C.V. Mosby Co.

Nursing Management
  Assessment
  Subjective
  History of trauma
  Health history for conditions that may influence healing and treatment
  Degree of pain, weakness
  Usual diet and activity patterns
  Objective
  Loss of function, obvious deformity
  Swelling and discoloration
  Presence of bleeding or tissue damage
  Baseline vital signs, neurocirculatory data

Nursing diagnoses
Nursing diagnoses are variable based on the location and extent of the injury as well as the type of treatment. Commonly encountered diagnoses include the following:
  Alteration in comfort—pain related to bone displacement and muscle spasm
  Impaired physical mobility related to either cast or traction
  Actual or potential impairment of skin integrity related to trauma, cast irritation, skeletal traction, or immobility

Altered tissue perfusion related to edema and cast constriction
Alteration in bowel elimination—constipation related to immobility
Alteration in nutrition—more than body requirements related to immobility and decreased energy expenditure
Self-care deficit in feeding, bathing/hygiene, dressing/grooming, or toileting related to casts or traction
Knowledge deficit related to the correct use of ambulatory assistive devices

Expected outcomes
Patient will experience minimal discomfort from fracture once reduction and realignment have been completed.
Patient will continue maximal activity level permitted by treatment.
Patient's skin will remain intact; infection will not develop at pin sites; tissue injuries will heal without infection or complications.
Patient will maintain adequate circulation and nerve conduction to areas distal to cast or traction setup.
Patient will pass soft stool daily or every other day.
Patient will maintain desired body weight.
Patient will participate in self-care to the extent allowed by injury, cast, or traction.
Patient will learn the correct use of canes, crutches, walkers or other self-help devices.

Nursing interventions
Care of casts

Immediate
Position patient on firm mattress with overbed trapeze.
Support fresh cast on pillows until dry.
Use flat of hand to move cast if necessary—do not embed fingers. Support at normal joint positions.
Allow free air circulation for drying; do not use heat lamps or hot hair dryers. Drying casts generate heat.
Institute neurocirculatory checks hourly—observe color, temperature, swelling, circulation, sensation, movement, pain. See Table 3-2 for detailed signs and symptoms of neurocirculatory impairment.
Medicate as prescribed. NOTE: Pain should decrease after realignment and resolution of tissue damage.
Assess bleeding through cast and monitor systemic signs.
Apply ice pack to reduce swelling.

Ongoing
Maintain neurocirculatory checks each shift.
Do not tightly cover cast with any substance because skin breathes through porous plaster.

TABLE 3-2 Signs and symptoms of neurocirculatory impairment

Observation	Interpretation
Tissue color white	Decreased arterial blood supply
Tissue color blue	Venous stasis and poorly oxygenated tissue
Color slow to return to nail bed after application of moderate pressure	Decreased arterial blood supply
Edema	Fluid accumulating in tissues; poor venous return
Tissue cold or cool to touch	Decreased arterial blood supply
Patient unable to move parts distal to cast	Pressure on nerves innervating parts distal to cast
Patient complaint of heightened or decreased sensation or paresthesia in part underlying or distal to cast	Pressure on nerves innervating parts underlying or distal to cast
Patient complaint of extreme pain unrelieved by elevation, analgesic, or repositioning	Pressure on nerve endings in parts underlying or distal to cast

Note: Compare opposite side to determine extent of deviation from normal.
From Phipps, W.J., Long, B.C., and Woods, N.F.: Medical-surgical nursing: concepts and clinical practice, ed. 2, St. Louis, 1983, The C.V. Mosby Co.

Clean cast application debris from skin and petal cast margins with stockinette to prevent skin irritation.

Protect casts exposed to body excretions with waterproof material around perineal area. Remove soiling with scouring powder on a damp cloth.

Provide regular skin care to skin around cast and that affected by decreased mobility.

Note any odor that may indicate necrotic tissue or infection.

Patient Teaching

Teach patient who will recover at home the signs and symptoms indicative of complications.

Teach patient to keep cast clean and dry, and not put foreign objects into the cast for scratching.

Teach patient to adjust fluids and diet to prevent constipation, urinary calculi, and weight gain.

Instruct patient in range of motion and isometric exercise as appropriate.

Teach patient how to ambulate safely using crutches or walker. The box above describes the common crutch walking gaits.

Teach patient exercises to increase triceps strength if crutch walking will be used: wheelchair or bed push-ups.

COMMON CRUTCH WALKING GAITS

WEIGHT BEARING

Two-point gait—crutch on one side moves forward simultaneously with opposite leg; same motion is repeated on other side.

Four-point gait—two-point gait is broken down and performed more slowly. Crutch is placed and then followed by the opposite leg. Both motions are then repeated with the opposite side.

Swing-through gait—both crutches are moved forward together, then both legs are swung past the crutches by lifting both lower limbs.

NON-WEIGHT BEARING

Three-point gait—both crutches are moved forward together. Then the body swings forward to that position by lifting placed leg. Second limb is held off the ground at all times.

Patient in traction

Do not release or alter traction weights. Traction weights and pulley ropes must hang freely.

Teach patient limitations of movement necessitated by type of injury and kind of traction.

Prevent complications of immobility:

Increase fluids.

Decrease calories and increase roughage in diet; offer stool softeners.

Provide regular, thorough skin care, inspect all areas in contact with traction apparatus; use sheepskin or alternating pressure matress.

Provide patient with age-appropriate diversions.

Promote circulation by use of range of motion and isometric exercises as permissible.

Teach patient to cough and deep breathe.

Monitor patient for incidence of fat emboli: dyspnea, pallor, alteration in mental status, petechiae in neck and shoulder region.

Provide pin care as ordered:

Inspect pin insertion sites carefully every shift per routines.

Cleanse sites with saline, peroxide, or Betadine solutions.

Use antibiotic ointments and dry sterile dressings if ordered.

Evaluation

Patient states that pain is minimal or absent.

Patient maintains maximal allowable activity and participates in self-care activities.

Patient's skin is intact; pin sites and soft tissue injuries heal without infection.

Patient maintains adequate circulation and nerve conduction to areas treated by cast or traction.

Patient maintains a normal elimination pattern.

Patient's weight remains stable.

Patient can demonstrate correct use of cane, crutches, walker, or other self-help device.

Patient can state exercise, diet, or activity restrictions to be followed at home and has made plans for follow-up care.

FRACTURED HIP

Fractures of the hip generally fall into two categories. Intracapsular fractures occur within the hip joint and capsule. Extracapsular fractures occur outside the capsule to an area below the lesser trochanter. Fractured hips occur most frequently in older adults when they fall. They occur more commonly in women because of the osteoporotic and degenerative changes of the postmenopausal period.

Pathophysiology
The clinical signs of a hip fracture include pain, loss of movement, shortening of the leg on the affected side, abduction and external rotation. Displaced fractures may cause serious disruption to the blood supply of the hip and result in avascular necrosis.

Medical Management
The treatment of choice is surgical repair, which allows for early mobilization of the patient. Pinning with screws, nails, and pins or prosthetic replacement of the femoral head and neck are the usual approaches. The site of the fracture, condition of the bone, and adequacy of the blood supply to the hip will dictate the approach and device used. Patient management for both treatments is similar. Surgery may be delayed while the patient's overall health status is evaluated. Buck's traction is frequently employed to relieve pain and muscle spasm prior to surgery.

Nursing Management
Assessment
Preoperative
Circumstances of injury
Current health and mental status
Degree of pain and muscle spasm
Patient's ability to urinate
Traction setup
Postoperative
Routine surgical assessment: vital signs, respiratory, circulatory, wound
Position of operative leg and condition of dressing
Family support available for rehabilitation period
Orientation and alertness

Nursing diagnoses
Diagnoses are variable depending on the general health status of patients and their responses to surgery.

Diagnoses that are common with and specific to the fractured hip procedure include the following:
Preoperative
Alteration in comfort—pain related to displaced fracture
Impaired physical mobility related to fracture and traction
Alteration in urinary elimination related to swelling in pelvic region.
Altered thought processes related to shock and pain of trauma
Knowledge deficit related to surgical repair and postoperative interventions
Postoperative
Impaired physical mobility related to non-weight bearing
Self-care deficit related to positioning and immobility
Knowledge deficit related to correct use of walker or crutches
Disordered family functioning related to postdischarge care of patient

Expected outcomes
Preoperative
Patient will have pain and spasm decrease to a tolerable level.
Patient will follow activity restrictions before surgery and be free of early complications of immobility.
Patient will establish an adequate urinary output.
Patient will remain oriented to circumstances and surroundings.
Patient will be able to explain the nature of proposed surgery and the associated requirements for positioning and activity.
Postoperative
Patient will be free of the complications of immobility.
Patient will successfully manage activities of daily living.
Patient will demonstrate correct use of walker or crutches.
Patient and family will make safe and satisfactory plans for care after discharge.

Nursing interventions
Preoperative
Maintain patient on bed rest in Buck's traction if ordered.
Administer analgesics as ordered.
Keep head of bed lower than 45 degrees.
Turn only slightly to unaffected side.
Use fracture pan for voiding or place Foley catheter if patient is unable to void.
Encourage deep breathing and coughing; use TED's; assess for cardiac and respiratory complications.

Teach patient about surgery and position requirements in the postoperative period.

Postoperative: position

Maintain abduction of affected leg with splints or pillows.

Use trochanter rolls to prevent external rotation.

Avoid hip flexion by keeping head of bed low.

Turn every two hours to unaffected side, supporting the operative leg in an abducted position.

Postoperative: activity

Begin getting patient out of bed according to physician's order.

Teach non-weight bearing or partial weight bearing techniques.

Teach patient quadriceps and gluteal set exercises for strengthening.

Work with physical therapy plan to teach safe ambulation, transfer techniques, and range of motion.

General

Aggressively employ standard interventions to combat effects of immobility. Observe patient for signs of atelectasis, wound infection, skin breakdown, thrombophlebitis, or pulmonary embolus.

Encourage patient to remain active in self-care.

Provide meaningful stimuli to keep patient oriented and hopeful about the future.

Assist patient and family to explore alternatives available in community for postdischarge care.

Evaluation

Preoperative

Patient has minimal pain.

Patient maintains bed rest with affected leg in abduction.

Patient exhibits no early signs of the complications of immobility.

Patient maintains an adequate urinary output.

Patient remains oriented to time, place, and person.

Patient can explain the proposed surgery and the postoperative care.

Postoperative

Patient is free of the complications of immobility.

Patient resumes responsibility for self-care and completes activities of daily living.

Patient demonstrates the correct use of crutches or walker.

Patient and family have made satisfactory arrangements for the patient's postdischarge care.

ARTHRITIS

Rheumatic diseases include a wide range of clinical conditions. The term *arthritis* means inflammation of a joint. It is a condition that exists in a number of specific diseases but the term is frequently used to describe any condition involving pain and stiffness of the musculoskeletal system. It is estimated that arthritis affects some 20 million people in the United States. The three most common forms of arthritis are rheumatoid arthritis, osteoarthritis, and gouty arthritis.

Rheumatoid arthritis is a chronic, systemic inflammatory disease characterized by recurrent inflammation in joints and related structures that can result in crippling deformities. It is more prevalent in women than men by a 2:1 to 3:1 ratio, and usually appears during the young adult years. Possibly autoimmune in nature, it follows a pattern of exacerbation and remission. Rheumatoid arthritis primarily affects proximal joints, although virtually all joints can become involved. Involvement is usually bilaterally symmetric.

Osteoarthritis is a slow, progressive, noninflammatory, chronic disease primarily of the weight bearing joints. It is characterized by pain, stiffness, and limitation of motion. Severity ranges from the annoying to the disabling. Most prevalent in the 50- to 70-year-old group, it is believed to be a degenerative process that accompanies aging but can occur secondary to trauma or excess strain. Table 3-3 compares major characteristics of rheumatoid arthritis and osteoarthritis.

Gouty arthritis is a metabolic disorder of purine metabolism in which excess uric acid leads to the formation of

TABLE 3-3 Differential characteristics between rheumatoid arthritis and osteoarthritis

Rheumatoid Arthritis	Osteoarthritis
Systemic disease; people are sick with malaise, fever, fatigue	Local joint disease; people have no systemic symptoms
Signs of inflammation present both locally in joints and systemically as pain, fever, soreness, malaise	Inflammatory signs are less prominent and are local (not systemic) when present
Fingers and proximal interphalangeal joints are involved more commonly	Distal interphalangeal joints are involved more commonly
Subcutaneous, extra-articular (rheumatoid) nodules are present in tissues around (not in) the joints in 20% of clients	No periarticular or subcutaneous nodes are present; Heberden's nodes are bony enlargements within the joints
Bony ankylosis and osteoporosis are common	Ankylosis and osteoporosis are uncommon
Elevated sedimentation rate; elevated serum rheumatoid factors	Normal sedimentation rate and blood chemistries
Young adults to older adults are affected (25–50 years of age)	Adults are affected during later years (from 45 years of age)

From Mourad, L.: Nursing care of adults with orthopedic conditions, New York, 1980, John Wiley & Sons.

urate crystals in the synovial tissue, producing intense inflammation. It is an inherited disorder affecting men eight to nine times more often than women. The peak age of onset is the fifth decade, but it can occur at any age. The great toe is most commonly involved. Patients may develop tophi, deposits of monosodium urate, in the tissues.

Pathophysiology
Rheumatoid arthritis
The disease process of rheumatoid arthritis begins with synovial inflammation with edema, congestion, and fibrin exudate. Continued inflammation produces synovial thickening and formation of pannus where it joins the articular cartilage. Gradual erosion of the articular cartilage eventually results in ankylosis and fusion, immobilizing the joint. The destruction of cartilage and bone, and the weakening of tendons and ligaments lead to joint subluxation and dislocation. Rheumatoid arthritis is accompanied by elevated erythrocyte sedimentation rate, decreased red blood cells, and mild elevation in white blood cells; 50% to 90% of patients exhibit a positive rheumatoid factor.

Osteoarthritis
In osteoarthritis the articular cartilage becomes yellow and opaque. It softens and the surfaces become roughened, frayed, or cracked. Cartilage may be destroyed and underlying bone altered. New bone (Heberden's nodes and Bouchard's nodes) appears at joint margins and may even break off. Serologic and synovial fluid examinations have essentially normal outcomes.

Gouty arthritis
In gouty arthritis uric acid deposits trigger intense inflammation and pain. Deposits and tophi cause gradual destruction of joints and bone. If unchecked, the disease can produce renal damage. It is accompanied by elevated uric acid levels, and urate crystals in the synovial fluid.

Medical Management
Rheumatoid arthritis and osteoarthritis
Treatment for rheumatoid arthritis and osteoarthritis involves drug intervention with salicylates, and nonsteroidal and steroid antiinflammatory agents. See Table 3-4. Other methods of management include physical therapy aimed at maintaining joint range of motion, balancing of rest and activity, maintenance of good general health status, and surgical intervention to prevent or correct deformities and increase functional usage. See Table 3-5 for descriptions of commonly used surgical procedures.

Gouty arthritis
Acute gouty arthritis attacks can be controlled and recurrent attacks can be prevented through administration of antiinflammatory drugs and reduction of the body pool of urates and uric acid. Colchicine is the drug of choice for treatment of acute attack. Allopurinol (Zyloprim), probenicid (Benemid), and sulfinpyrazone (Anturane) are used to decrease uric acid levels. An augment to therapy is diet regulation. Reducing purine intake and increasing fluid intake prevents crystallization. Purines are particularly high in red meats and legumes.

Nursing Management
Assessment
Both subjective and objective factors should be assessed.
Rheumatoid arthritis and osteoarthritis—subjective
History and management of disorder
Diet and medication history
Patient and family coping patterns
Complaints of pain, weakness, and stiffness
Effects of disease on usual patterns of activities
Rheumatoid arthritis and osteoarthritis—objective
Current health status
Joint range of motion, muscle strength/atrophy, swelling
Presence of obvious deformities—swan neck, ulnar deviation
Functional abilities for self-care—gait and ambulation, bathing, feeding, toileting activities
Presence of bony protuberance, such as Heberden's or Bouchard's nodes (osteoarthritis only)
Systemic symptoms of fever, tachycardia, weight loss, anemia (rheumatoid only)

Nursing diagnoses
Diagnoses are variable according to extent and severity of the disease process. Common diagnoses encountered with rheumatoid and osteoarthritis include:
Alteration in comfort—pain in joints related to inflammation or degeneration
Activity intolerance related to weakened muscles, pain, or anemia
Potential for injury related to decreased muscle strength, balance, and coordination
Impaired physical mobility related to joint destruction and decreased muscle strength
Self-care deficit in feeding, bathing/hygiene, dressing/grooming or toileting related to pain and limitation of movement
Disturbance in self-concept—body image and role performance related to deformed joints and impaired mobility
Knowledge deficit related to the control and management of arthritis and its complications.

Expected outcomes
Patient will experience a decrease in pain and stiffness.

TABLE 3-4 Medications prescribed in the treatment of rheumatoid arthritis

Medication	Action	Side Effects/Toxic Effects	Precautions
Salicylates			
Examples: acetylsalicyclic acid, choline salicylates	Analgesic, antipyretic, antiinflammatory	Gastric irritation; dose-related salicylism; skin rash; hypersensitivity	Take with food, milk, or antacid; space every 4 to 6 hr to maintain antiinflammatory effect
Nonsteroidal antiinflammatory agents			
Indomethacin (Indocin)	Analgesic, antiinflammatory	Headache; dizziness; insomnia; confusion; gastrointestinal irritation	Take with food, milk, or antacid; discontinue if CNS symptoms develop and notify physician
Ibuprofen (Motrin)	Same as indomethacin	Same as indomethacin but believed less irritating to gastrointestinal tract	Delayed absorption if taken with food
Tolmetin sodium (Tolectin)	Same as indomethacin	Same as indomethacin	Take with food or milk
Naproxen (Naprosyn)	Same as indomethacin	Same as indomethacin; also drowsiness	Take with food, milk, or antacid; avoid driving until dosage effect established
Fenoprofen calcium (Nalfon)	Same as indomethacin	Same as naproxen	Delayed absorption if taken with food; avoid driving until dosage effect established
Sulindac (Clinoril)	Same as indomethacin	Same as indomethacin; plus skin rash	Take with food, milk, or antacid; not to be used with acetylsalicylic acid
Potent antiinflammatory agents			
Adrenocorticosteroids (e.g., prednisone)	Interfere with body's normal inflammatory response	Fluid retention; sodium retention; potassium depletion; hypertension; decreased healing potential; increased susceptibility to infection; gastrointestinal irritation; hirsutism, osteoporosis, fat deposits; diabetes mellitus; myopathy; adrenal insufficiency or adrenal crisis if abruptly withdrawn	Take with food, milk, or antacid; dosage not to be increased or decreased without physician's supervision; take in morning if taken on once-a-day basis
Phenylbutazone (Butazolidin)	Antiinflammatory; analgesic at subcortical site in brain	Gastrointestinal irritation; hematologic toxicity; hypertension, impaired renal function	Used for a short term (7–10 days); take with food or milk

From Phipps, W.J., Long, B.C., and Woods, N.F.: Medical-surgical nursing: concepts and clinical practice, ed. 2, St. Louis, 1983, The C.V. Mosby Co.

Patient will demonstrate increased energy through involvement in self-care activities.

Patient will not fall or experience injury.

Patient will have increased joint mobility and muscle strength.

Patient will increase self-concept by participating more in personal and family activities.

Patient will understand disease process and the management of symptoms.

Nursing interventions
Pain

Teach patient to balance rest and activity.

Teach patient about medications and their side effects.

Caution about gastrointestinal effects.

Tell patient to avoid PRN usage.

Apply heat or cold to joints for comfort and muscle relaxation.

During acute attack, rheumatoid arthritis patient should be on bed rest with joints held in position of function.

Mobility

Encourage patient to perform prescribed exercises.

Patient should avoid AM exercise when stiffness is acute.

Teach patient to exercise only to the point of pain.

Assist patient with range of motion exercises as needed.

Focus on exercise directed at increasing functional capacities.

TABLE 3-4 Medications prescribed in the treatment of rheumatoid arthritis—cont'd

Medication	Action	Side Effects/Toxic Effects	Precautions
Slow acting antiinflammatory agents			
Antimalarials			
Hydroxy-chloroquine (Plaquenil)	Antiinflammatory (mechanism unknown); effect not expected to be noted for 6–12 mo after beginning therapy	Gastrointestinal disturbances; retinal edema that may result in blindness	Eye examination before beginning therapy and every 6 mo thereafter
Chloroquine (Aralen)	Same as hydroxychloroquine	Same as hydroxychloroquine	Same as hydroxychloroquine
Quinacrine (Atabrine)	Same as hydroxychloroquine	Same as hydroxychloroquine but may be better tolerated; yellow discoloration of the skin	May be stopped periodically to prevent deepening of skin discoloration
Gold salts (Myochrysine, Solganol)	Antiinflammatory	Renal and hepatic damage; corneal deposits; dermatitis; ulcerations in mouth; hematologic changes	Urinalysis and CBC before each injection; report dermatitis, metallic taste in mouth, or lesions in mouth to physician
Penicillamine (Cuprimine)	Antiinflammatory (mechanism unclear); effect not expected to be noted until several months after beginning treatment	Fever; rash; nephrotic syndrome; hematologic changes; gastrointestinal irritation; lupuslike syndromes; allergic reactions (33% probability if allergic to penicillin); retarded wound healing	Urinalysis, CBC, differential, hemoglobin and platelet count at least weekly for 3 mo, then monthly; report skin rash, fever to physician; food interferes with absorption—take on empty stomach between meals

TABLE 3-5 Surgical interventions for arthritis

Procedure	Description	Expected Outcome
Synovectomy	Removal of synovial tissue to arrest the arthritic process in a particular joint	Maintains joint function Prevents recurrent inflammation
Arthrotomy	Exploration of a joint	Drains Removes damaged tissue
Arthroplasty	Joint reconstruction by reshaping bones, replacement of all or part of a joint with prosthetic parts	Restores motion and function Relieves pain Corrects deformity

Adjustment

Encourage use of basic nutritious diet to foster optimal general health.

Encourage weight loss if indicated.

Encourage patient to express fears and frustration about chronic progressive nature of the disease.

Teach environmental modifications for safety and comfort such as supportive shoes, hand rails in bathtub, and raised toilet seats.

Explore use of self-help devices to foster independence in activities of daily living.

Teach patient and family to maintain regular medical supervision and avoid quack therapies.

Evaluation

Patient reports a decrease in pain and stiffness.

Patient has sufficient energy to participate in self-care and social activities of daily living.

Patient reports increased range of motion and muscle strength.

Patient states improved feelings about self.

Patient can describe purpose and side effects of medications, select appropriate foods for healthy diet, and demonstrate prescribed exercise program.

Patient and family modify environment to improve safety.

TABLE 3-6 Nursing interventions for the patient with a total hip or total knee replacement

Procedure	Preoperative Interventions	Postoperative Interventions	General Surgical Interventions
Total hip replacement	Scrupulously clean skin and prepare patient as per surgeon's routine. Administer prophylactic antibiotics. Teach patient and family about surgical procedure and postoperative restrictions concerning movement and positioning.	Position according to surgeon's practice and preference: usually hip is kept in wide abduction with slings or pillows. Avoid external rotation by using sandbags or rolls. Keep head of bed elevated 45 to 60 degrees for meals only to avoid hip flexion. Turn to unaffected side with operative leg maintained in abduction. Encourage patient to do bed exercises (quadriceps and gluteal sets exercises) to strengthen muscles for ambulation. Assist with ambulation and progressive weight bearing as ordered—usually begins 2 to 4 days after surgery. Patient should use walker for support. Teach patient in preparation for discharge to: avoid hip flexion greater than 90 degrees, use raised toilet seat for at least two months, observe activity and weight bearing restrictions, use self-help devices to avoid bending and stooping.	Maintain drainage system; note type and amount of drainage. Keep operative area free from contamination: Assess site regularly. Change dressing as needed. Administer antibiotics as ordered. Administer anticoagulant if prescribed for risk of thrombus.
Total knee replacement	Scrupulously clean skin and prepare patient per surgeon's routine Teach patient and family about surgical procedure and exercises to be employed in postoperative period (quadriceps sets and straight leg lifts).	Provide sufficient analgesia to allow patient to perform exercises. Begin active flexion exercises after dressing removal. Assist with ambulation (partial weight bearing) once patient demonstrates quadriceps muscle control.	Maintain drainage system; note type and amount of drainage. Keep operative area free from contamination: Assess site regularly. Change dressing as needed. Administer antibiotics as ordered.

TABLE 3-7 Nonarticular rheumatic diseases

Disorder	Description	Signs and Symptoms	Medical Management
Bursitis	Inflammation of the bursa, acute or chronic, caused by trauma, strain or overuse of the joint. Shoulder bursa is most commonly affected.	Severe pain, especially on joint movement	Rest for involved area Antiinflammatory analgesic agents Application of cold during acute period
Carpal tunnel syndrome	Pressure is exerted by the flexion tendon sheaths on the median nerve at the wrist. Condition usually localized.	Disorders in sensation (burning, tingling) in the middle three fingers—especially during prolonged flexion Referred pain to upper extremity	Rest Splinting of wrist Surgical release of carpal ligament
Dupuytren's contracture	Palmar fascia on ulnar side of one or both hands becomes thickened and shortened.	Progressive inability to extend fourth and fifth fingers; painless Palmar skin is tense with puckers and nodules	As condition worsens, surgical intervention to remove involved palmar fascia and release contracture
Fibrositis and fibromyositis	Commonly occurring self-limiting symptom complex	Pain and stiffness in neck, shoulder girdle, and extremities Pain worsens with activity and subsides with rest	Management directed at specific symptoms Rest, analgesics, and physical therapy

TOTAL JOINT REPLACEMENT

Total joint replacement is increasingly being used to correct deformities and maintain functional capacities. Table 3-6 discusses the pre- and postoperative care involved in the two most common procedures, total hip replacement and total knee replacement.

Table 3-7 presents characteristics of some common nonarticular rheumatic diseases. They include rheumatic diseases involving supportive structures near the joints but not the joints themselves.

COLLAGEN DISEASE

Collagen disorders are a group of diseases involving the connective tissue of the body. These diseases share some pathological features. The cause of these diseases is unknown and they are grouped together largely on the basis of signs and symptoms. Management is largely treating symptoms and providing support. The category includes systemic lupus erythematosus, polymyositis, progressive systemic sclerosis (scleroderma), necrotizing arteritis, and Sjögren's syndrome.

The management of systemic lupus is presented below. See Table 3-8 for the major characteristics of SLE and the other disorders.

TABLE 3-8 Collagen disorders: pathophysiology, signs and symptoms, and medical management

Disorder	Pathophysiology	Signs and Symptoms	Medical Management
Systemic lupus erythematosus (SLE) (chronic inflammatory disease)	Severe vasculitis with necrosis of walls of small arteries Thickening of glomerular basement membrane Lymph node necrosis Fibrous villous synovitis Lesions in nervous system	Arthritis symptoms Weakness, fatigue Sun sensitivity—rash reaction Erythema in butterfly pattern over nose and cheeks Specific organ symptoms Positive LE cell reaction	High-dose glucocorticosteroids Salicylates General supportive care
Polymyositis (dermatomyositis) (inflammatory disease involving striated, voluntary muscle)	Primary degeneration of muscle fibers Necrosis of parts or entire groups of muscle fibers Interstitial fibrosis	Muscle weakness and fatigue especially in pelvic and shoulder muscles Muscle pain or tenderness Eventual contractures and atrophy Dusky red skin rash if dermatomyositis form EMG, muscle biopsy results Elevated serum enzymes	High-dose glucocorticosteroids Physical therapy and occupational therapy for exercise regimen
Progressive systemic sclerosis (PSS, scleroderma) (sclerosis involving connective tissue throughout the body)	Involved tissue becomes fibrotic Changes may be accompanied by vascular lesions	Gradual thickening and tightening of the skin on face and body Telangiectasis on lips, tongue, face Pain and stiffness, muscle weakness Fibrosis of vital organs produces local effects	Glucocorticosteroids for those with myositis symptoms Salicylates Range of motion exercise
Necrotizing arteritis (inflammation of the blood vessels)	Inflammation and necrosis of arterial wall Body attempts to clear necrosis cause fibrosis and intimal proliferation Partial or complete vessel occlusion, infarction, or aneurysm	Involvement of vessels anywhere in body—angina, MI, hypertension, peripheral neuropathy, intractable headaches Elevated white blood count (WBC) and erythrocyte sedimentation rate (ESR). Angiography results show vessel destruction	High-dose glucocorticosteroids Rest
Sjögren's syndrome (chronic inflammation of lacrimal and parotid glands)	Infiltration of lacrimal and parotid glands by lymphocytes and plasma cells Decrease in flow of tears and saliva	Dry gritty sensation in eyes—redness and itching Difficulty in chewing or swallowing or with speech Corneal, tongue, and lip ulceration	Symptomatic care with eye drops, increased fluids, and hard candy to stimulate saliva

SYSTEMIC LUPUS ERYTHEMATOSUS (SLE)

SLE is a chronic inflammatory disease of unknown etiology that affects women, particularly adolescents and young adults, four times more often than men. It was named for the characteristic rash that accompanies it.

Pathophysiology

Common pathologic manifestations include the following:

Severe vasculitis with necrosis of small arterial walls

Thickening of glomerular basement membrane and necrosis of glomerular capillaries

Lymph node necrosis

Fibrous villous synovitis

It is suspected that a disorder of immunity may cause immune complexes to be deposited in the tissue. A second possibility is the presence of a viral infection resulting from an immunologic abnormality. Depending on the organ involved, the patient may have findings of glomerulonephritis, pleuritis, pericarditis, peritonitis, neuritis, or anemia.

Medical Management

The use of adrenocorticosteroids is the cornerstone of medical intervention. Joint pain may be treated by salicylates. Other care is aimed at dealing with the specific symptoms confronting a patient.

Nursing Management

Assessment

Factors to be assessed include:

History, symptoms, and course of the disease

Patient's medication regimen and compliance

Side effects of high dose steroids

Patient response to chronic progressive disorder

Presence of arthritic-like symptoms or skin rashes

Other specific system assessments as suggested by symptoms

Nursing diagnoses

Diagnoses will be variable based on the patient's disease course and current symptoms. Common diagnoses include the following:

Alteration in comfort—pain related to joint inflammation

Activity intolerance related to fatigue and weakness

Disturbance in self-concept (body image) related to skin rashes and side effects of adrenocorticosteroids

Knowledge deficit related to use of adrenocorticosteroids and the management of side effects

Expected outcomes

Patient will experience less pain, increased comfort.

Patient will have sufficient energy to complete self-care and normal social activities.

Patient will incorporate body changes into a satisfactory body image.

Patient will be knowledgeable about prescribed medications, side effects, and their management.

Nursing interventions

Administer prescribed medications.

Discuss the management of side effects through diet modification and fluid balance.

Plan with patient a balanced program of rest and exercise.

Teach patient to avoid excessive sun exposure by covering body surfaces, wearing a wide brimmed hat, and using a sunscreen when exposed to direct sunlight.

Provide symptomatic and supportive care as indicated by patient symptoms.

Encourage patient to verbalize feelings about chronic progressive disease.

Evaluation

Patient reports increased comfort and is able to participate in self-care activities.

Patient reports an increased energy level and resumes normal patterns of work and social activities.

Patient remains involved socially and makes positive references to self.

Patient and family can discuss prescribed medications and activities to control and manage their side effects.

HERNIATED NUCLEUS PULPOSUS

Herniated nucleus pulposus is a condition in which the gelatinous intravertebral disc protrudes through the surrounding cartilage, causing pressure on the spinal nerve roots.

Pathophysiology

Herniation may be triggered by a sudden strain from improper lifting or trauma in spinal region. The condition may be predisposed by damage of rheumatoid arthritis or osteoarthritis. Nerve pressure produces low back pain radiating down path of sciatic nerve in posterior thigh. There will frequently be paresthesias in leg and foot, muscle weakness, and muscle spasm. The most common sites of herniation are at L3–4, L4–5, and L5–S1. A myelogram may be used to confirm the diagnosis.

Medical Management

Conservative medical management includes bed rest with a firm mattress, antispasmodics (diazepam) and analgesics, physical therapy for deep heat and massage, and pelvic traction to relieve spasms.

Surgical intervention includes discectomy, laminectomy, or spinal fusions if multiple vertebrae are involved or spine is unstable.

Nursing Management
Assessment
Factors to be assessed include the following:
Pain pattern and extent, duration, and severity
Presence of paresthesias or muscle weakness
History of trauma or degenerative disease
Actions that relieve or improve pain
Patient's normal activities of daily living, occupation, and leisure
Patient's knowledge of surgery or therapy prescribed

Nursing diagnoses
Diagnoses will vary slightly depending on patient's symptoms, treatment, and general health status. Common diagnoses include the following:
Alteration in comfort—pain related to herniated disc
Activity intolerance related to pain and muscle spasm
Impaired physical mobility related to pain and weakness
Knowledge deficit related to therapy, surgery, postoperative positioning, normal body mechanics, or back strengthening exercises.

Expected outcomes
Patient will experience decreased pain and muscle spasm.
Patient will be able to resume normal activity patterns.
Patient will demonstrate understanding of therapy, surgical procedure, body mechanics, and exercises to strengthen back.

Nursing interventions
Conservative
Encourage patient to maintain bed rest with head of bed low, knees slightly flexed.
Establish and maintain pelvic traction if ordered.
Administer analgesics and muscle relaxants as ordered.
Use nursing measures to augment pain relief, such as diversion, heat, back rubs.
Monitor for and prevent complications of immobility by increasing roughage and fluids, giving frequent skin care and position changes, encouraging deep breathing and range of motion exercises, observing for Homans' sign, calf tenderness.

Surgical
Teach patient about procedure and restrictions for postoperative positioning.
Teach patient about log rolling, coughing, deep breathing.
Obtain baseline preoperative neurologic assessment.
Check movement and sensation in lower extremities frequently in postoperative period.
Encourage ambulation—patient should avoid sitting.
Administer stool softeners to prevent straining.
Teach patient principles of good body mechanics. Patient should:
Maintain broad base of support
Use large groups of muscles
Maintain good posture
Squat, not bend
Pull objects rather than pushing
Teach patient back-strengthening exercises.
NOTE: If patient undergoes spinal fusion, he or she may be ordered to have prolonged bed rest and have a second surgical incision from bone graft. Meticulous attention to monitoring and preventing the complications of immobility is required.

Evaluation
Patient is free of pain and muscle spasm.
Patient gradually resumes normal activity pattern and experiences no residual weakness.
Patient demonstrates good posture and the principles of body mechanics in moving. Patient regularly practices back-strengthening exercises.

BIBLIOGRAPHY
Cohen, S., and Viellion, G.: Nursing care of a patient in traction, Am. J. Nurs. **79**:1771-1798, 1979.
Dickinson, G.R., and Gorman, T.K.: Adult arthritis: the assessment, Am. J. Nurs. **83**:262-265, 1983.
Hay, B.K., *et al.*: External fixation: option for fractures, AORN J. **34**:417-423, Sept. 1981.
Meyers, M.H., McNell, D.V., and Nelson, K.: Total hip replacement—a team effort, Am. J. Nurs. **78**:1485-1488, 1978.
Mourad, L.: Nursing care of adults with orthopedic conditions, New York, 1980, John Wiley & Sons.
Richards, M.: Osteoporosis . . . bane of the elderly, Geriatric Nurs. **3**:98-102, Mar.-Apr. 1982.
Simpson, C.F., and Dickson, G.R.: Adult arthritis: exercise, Am. J. Nurs. **83**:273-274, 1983.
Strand, C.V., and Clark, S.R.: Adult arthritis: drugs and remedies, Am. J. Nurs. **83**:266-270, 1983.
Turner, P.: Caring for emotional needs of orthopedic trauma patients, AORN J. **36**:566-570, Oct. 1982.
White, J.: Teaching patients to manage systemic lupus erythematosus, Nursing 78 **8**:26-35, 1978.

NURSING CARE PLAN

FRACTURED HIP AND PROSTHETIC IMPLANT

Nursing Diagnoses	Expected Patient Outcomes	Nursing Interventions
Alteration in comfort, pain related to surgical procedure	Patient is comfortable	1. Give prescribed analgesics at timely intervals during initial period. 2. Teach relaxation techniques, as appropriate. 3. Use other pertinent pain-relieving techniques. 4. As pain decreases, use milder analgesics.
Impaired physical mobility related to pain and weight-bearing restrictions	Patient is active within prescribed limitations and remains free of the complications of immobility	1. Determine from physician the limits of motion and weight bearing permitted. 2. Encourage activity within the prescribed limits. 3. Encourage isometric exercises. 4. Assist patient to ambulate, when permitted, using the appropriate ambulatory aid.
Potential for injury related to surgical procedure and decreased mobility	Patient does not experience neurocirculatory or respiratory complications. Hip remains in alignment	1. Perform neurocirculatory checks once an hour for first 24 to 48 hours. 2. Notify physician for any changes from preoperative status. 3. Encourage active range of motion and exercises of unaffected limbs. 4. Encourage deep breathing and coughing exercises. 5. Avoid hip flexion and adduction: 　a. Assist patient to turn by supporting leg in abduction. 　b. Use pillows to maintain abduction when patient is lying in bed. 　c. Patient should avoid sitting initially; when sitting is permitted, elevate sitting surface with pillows to keep angle of hip within prescribed limits. 　d. Patient should avoid elevating leg when sitting. 6. Avoid positioning patient on operative side.
Potential impairment of skin integrity related to immobility and surgical incisions	Patient's skin remains intact; infection does not occur	1. Monitor pressure areas for signs of pressure. 2. Massage reddened areas gently. 3. Use heel pads and other protective pads as necessary. 4. Use aseptic technique for any dressing changes.
Potential for alteration in bowel elimination; constipation related to decreased mobility	Stools are soft, occur at usual frequency	1. Encourage fluid intake of 2000 to 3000 ml/day. 2. Encourage activity within prescribed limits. 3. Encourage high fiber foods in diet. 4. Give prescribed stool softeners, suppositories, or laxatives.
Knowledge deficit related to treatment regimen and restrictions	Patient understands treatment regimen, follows positioning and weight-bearing restrictions	1. Teach patient: 　a. Rationale for activity restrictions. 　b. No flexion of affected hip beyond 60 degrees for 10 days or 90 degrees from tenth day to 2 months. 　c. No adduction of affected leg beyond midline for 2 months. 　d. Maintenance of partial weight bearing status for approximately 2 months. 　e. No elevation of leg when sitting. 　f. Need for follow-up care until fracture is fully healed.

NURSING CARE PLAN

RHEUMATOID ARTHRITIS

Nursing Diagnoses	Expected Patient Outcomes	Nursing Interventions
Alteration in comfort: joint pain related to inflammation	Patient experiences decreased pain and stiffness	1. Assess pain characteristics. 2. Provide prescribed medications on time. 3. Apply heat or cold, as appropriate, especially prior to exercise or at bedtime. 4. Encourage patient to change position frequently. 5. Provide rest periods. 6. Encourage use of resting splints.
Impaired physical mobility related to joint destruction and decreased muscle strength	Patient demonstrates improved active range of motion and muscle strength	1. Encourage regular active range of motion exercises of joints to greatest degree possible. 2. Encourage patient to assist with ADL to greatest degree possible. 3. Give analgesic or heat/cold treatments prior to exercise. 4. Provide support and assistance to patient during exercise prescribed by physician or physical therapist. 5. Avoid exercises if joint is acutely inflamed.
Potential for injury related to impaired mobility and weakness	Patient uses assistive devices effectively to avoid injury Patient does not experience joint deformity	1. Position joints to promote joint function; avoid positions such as knee or neck flexion. 2. Encourage active range of motion exercises. 3. Encourage other prescribed exercises and ambulation alternated with rest periods. 4. Encourage isometric exercises when joints are acutely inflamed. 5. Provide appropriate ambulatory devices (walker, cane). 6. Encourage use of shoes rather than slippers when ambulating. 7. Teach joint protective techniques. 8. Teach use of safety devices as appropriate (such as safety arms on toilets or grab bars on tubs or showers).
Self-care deficit in personal hygiene and feeding related to pain and limitation of movement	Patient demonstrates ability to perform self-care activities	1. Encourage patient to participate in ADL to greatest degree possible. 2. Give patient sufficient time for ADL. 3. Use comfort measures as needed before required activities. 4. Use assistive devices for dressing and feeding as appropriate.
Self-concept disturbance in body image and role performance related to deformed joints and impaired mobility	Patient has a more positive self-concept	1. Provide patient with opportunities to discuss feelings about body changes and increased dependence on others. 2. Help patient identify personal strengths. 3. Allow patient maximum independence possible within physical limitations. 4. Anticipate patient needs for assistance and provide help as necessary. 5. Assist family to participate in patient's care so they can see what patient can do and thus provide positive encouragement and help patient maintain optimal independence.

Continued.

NURSING CARE PLAN

RHEUMATOID ARTHRITIS—cont'd

Nursing Diagnoses	Expected Patient Outcomes	Nursing Interventions
Knowledge deficit related to the control and management of arthritis and its complications	Patient describes disease process and therapeutic regimen	1. Teach patient: a. Nature of disorder. b. Medication program. c. Exercise program. d. Balance of activity with rest. e. Correct use of heat/cold packs and assistive devices. f. Measures to prevent injury. g. Basics of good nutrition and importance of avoiding overweight. h. Community resources.

Neurologic Disorders

The nervous system functions as the coordinator and regulator of all body activity, collecting and processing sensory information and transmitting information along motor pathways to effector muscles and glands for action. Neurologic problems may be related to trauma, infection, neoplasm, vascular impairment, or degenerative processes. The effects of neurologic disorders range from decreased or absent function to excessive uncontrolled function. Nursing care for common neurologic disorders is described in this chapter. Figure 4-1 shows the anatomic structure of the nervous system.

CHRONIC/DEGENERATIVE NEUROLOGIC DISORDERS

Neurologic disorders require individuals to make multiple adjustments in their life style. Diseases that are chronic or degenerative add additional stress and create the need for comprehensive and creative nursing management.

CONVULSIVE DISORDERS (EPILEPSY)

Seizures may be defined as transitory disturbances in consciousness and motor, sensory, or autonomic functions resulting from uncontrolled electrical discharges in the brain. They are a symptom of a wide variety of disorders including:

Cerebral anoxia
Hypoglycemia
Infections with high temperature
Neoplasms
Trauma and scar tissue
Metabolic disturbances
Electrolyte imbalances
Drugs and poisons
Inflammation and abscess
Increased intracranial pressure

Epilepsy is a chronic brain dysfunction characterized by recurrent seizures. In many cases the etiology is unknown although heredity is frequently implicated. Table 4-1 describes the common types of seizures.

Pathophysiology

Seizures represent sudden, excessive, disorderly discharges of the neurons of the brain. The process may last from a few seconds to as long as 5 minutes. Fatigue of the precipitating neurons is believed to help end the seizure. The seizure is usually followed by a period of inhibition of cerebral function, usually incomplete.

Medical Management

If no correctable cause can be uncovered, medical management focuses on the control of seizures through anticonvulsant medication. Table 4-2 presents some of the common medications used to control seizures. EEGs are used extensively to diagnose and localize seizures.

Nursing Management

Assessment—subjective

History of seizure disorder and manifestations
Patient's knowledge of seizure disorder
Patient's knowledge of prescribed medications, side effects; degree of compliance
Patient's description of aura experience, if any, and postictal feelings
Patient's social adjustment to seizure disorder

Assessment—objective

Sequence and duration of seizure if observed (see Table 4-3)
Observed behavior before seizure
Side effects of medications

Nursing diagnoses

Potential for injury related to loss of consciousness and tonic clonic muscle movements

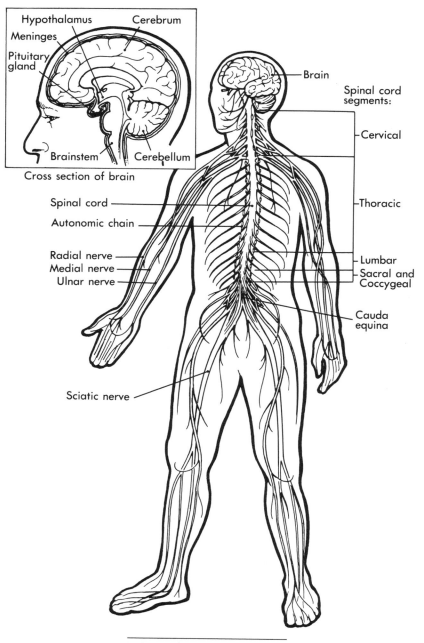

FIGURE 4-1 Nervous system.

Knowledge deficit related to optimal seizure management

Disturbance in self-concept, self-esteem, and role performance related to socially stigmatizing aspects of seizures

Ineffective individual coping related to the diagnosis of epilepsy and its treatment restrictions

Ineffective airway clearance related to the glottal obstruction occurring during grand mal seizure

Expected outcomes

Patient will not experience injury during seizures.

Patient will be knowledgeable about medications and life-style adaptations related to seizure management.

Patient will develop increased self-esteem and fulfill developmental tasks appropriate to age group.

Patient will voluntarily comply with treatment regimen.

TABLE 4-1 Common types of seizures

Type	Characteristics

I. Generalized
  A. Grand mal
	Bilaterally symmetrical, with no local onset
	Most common and dramatic type of seizure
	Progression:
	  1. Aura—change in sensation or affect that precedes seizure and occurs in about 50% of all patients. It may include numbness, odors, lights, dizziness.
	  2. Cry—caused by spasms of thorax expelling air through glottis or abrupt inspiratory effort.
	  3. Loss of consciousness—sudden and profound, and variable in duration.
	  4. Tonic clonic contractions—immediate bilateral tonic contraction with cessation of respiration and cyanosis, followed by clonic rhythmic contractions of increasing strength. Shallow respiration returns. Urinary and fecal incontinence may occur.
	  5. Postictal condition—patient experiences partial return of consciousness to a groggy confused state. Headache, muscle pain, and need for deep sleep frequently follow.

B. Petit mal	Most common during childhood.
	Progression:
	  1. Sudden impairment or loss of consciousness with little or no motor movement.
	  2. Duration is usually not more than 10 to 20 seconds, but may occur many times in a day.

II. Partial seizures
  A. Psychomotor—
    Temporal lobe
    Complex partial
	Have a localized onset
	Complex seizures may occur at any age
	  1. Sudden change in awareness or consciousness—patient may have complex hallucination aura.
	  2. Patient may behave as if partially conscious or intoxicated and engage in antisocial behavior such as exposing self or perform repetitive meaningless acts such as buttoning and unbuttoning.
	  3. Patient may have autonomic complaints—chest pain, dyspnea, etc.
	  4. End of seizure—patient may be confused, amnesiac, and groggy.

B. Focal seizures
    Jacksonian
	Arise in any localized motor or sensory portion of cortex
	  1. Symptoms depend on site of occurrence.
	  2. Progressive involvement of adjacent motor or sensory areas may exist.
	  3. Consciousness is usually maintained unless seizure progresses to full grand mal seizure.

TABLE 4-2 Drugs used to prevent seizures

Drug	Seizure Type	Toxic Effects
Phenytoin sodium (Dilantin)	Grand mal, focal, psychomotor	Ataxia, vomiting, nystagmus, drowsiness, rash, fever, gum hypertrophy, lymphadenopathy
Phenobarbital (Luminal)	Grand mal, focal, psychomotor	Drowsiness, rash
Primidone (Mysoline)	Grand mal, focal, psychomotor	Drowsiness, ataxia
Mephenytoin (Mesantoin)	Grand mal, focal, psychomotor	Ataxia, nystagmus, pancytopenia, rash
Ethosuximide (Zarontin)	Petit mal, psychomotor, myoclonic, akinetic	Drowsiness, nausea, agranulocytosis
Trimethadione (Tridione)	Petit mal	Rash, photophobia, agranulocytosis, nephrosis
Diazepam (Valium)	Status epilepticus, mixed	Drowsiness, ataxia
Carbamazepine (Tegretol)	Grand mal, psychomotor	Rash, drowsiness, ataxia
Valproic acid (Depakene)	Petit mal	Nausea, vomiting, indigestion, sedation, emotional disturbance, weakness, altered blood coagulation
Clonazepam (Clonopin)	Petit mal	Drowsiness, ataxia, hypotension, respiratory depression

Modified from Phipps, W.J., Long, B.C., and Woods, N.F.: Medical-surgical nursing: concepts and clinical practice, ed. 2, St. Louis, 1983, The C.V. Mosby Co.

Patient will maintain adequate cerebral oxygenation during grand mal seizure.

Nursing interventions

Employ seizure precautions for any patient with seizure history:

Keep padded tongue blade or oral airway at bedside.
Use padded side rails.
Supervise ambulation.
Have ready access to oxygen, suction, and anticonvulsant medications.

TABLE 4-3 Observations to be made about a person having a seizure

Aura	Presence or absence; nature if present; ability of patient to describe it (somatic, visceral, psychic)
Cry	Presence or absence
Onset	Site of initial body movements; deviation of head and eyes; chewing and salivation; posture of body; sensory changes
Tonic and clonic phases	Movements of body as to progression; skin color and airway; pupillary changes; incontinence; duration of each phase
Relaxation (sleep)	Duration and behavior
Postictal phase	Duration; general behavior; ability to remember anything about the seizure; orientation; pupillary changes; headache; injuries present
Duration of entire seizure	Measure by clock
Level of consciousness	Length of unconsciousness if present

From Phipps, W.J., Long, B.C., and Woods, N.F.: Medical-surgical nursing: concepts and clinical practice, ed. 2, St. Louis, 1983, The C.V. Mosby Co.

Protect patient from injury. The box on p. 42 outlines specific nursing interventions during a seizure.

Record nature and progression of seizure (see Table 4-3).

Encourage patient to verbalize feelings about seizures and problems encountered in social settings.

Teach patient about prescribed medications and expected side effects.

Encourage good mouth care if patient is receiving Dilantin.

Encourage life-style modifications:
  Nutritious diet
  Balance of rest and activity
  Avoidance of alcohol and acute stress

Discuss restrictions on employment, driving, and leisure mandated by seizure activity.

Encourage patient and family to make contact with local epilepsy society for support.

Evaluation

Patient is free of physical injury related to seizures.

Patient with grand mal seizures does not experience cerebral anoxia.

Patient and family can discuss prescribed medications, side effects, and life-style modifications that will enhance seizure control.

Patient successfully engages in tasks appropriate for age and speaks positively of self.

Patient expresses desire and motivation to maintain treatment regimen and gain control of seizures.

NURSING CARE DURING A SEIZURE

Never leave patient alone during seizure.

If patient is upright, lower to bed or floor and clear immediate environment to prevent injury.

Loosen constrictive clothing, especially around the neck.

Turn head to side if feasible to help keep airway open. Cushion head.

Provide privacy.

No effort should be made to restrain the individual during the seizure.

A padded tongue blade or oral airway may be inserted to protect tongue and mouth if jaws are not already clenched. *Never attempt to pry open the mouth once jaws are clenched.*

Record sequence and progression of seizure accurately.

Gently reorient patient at end of seizure, and provide for postictal rest and sleep.

PARKINSON'S DISEASE, PARKINSONISM

One of the more common nervous system disorders, Parkinsonism basically involves a cluster of symptoms whose cause is unknown in most cases, but which can be induced by use of certain drugs, arteriosclerosis, or some viral disorders. Symptoms commonly occur after age 50, and there is no known cure for the disorder.

Pathophysiology

The pathologic process involves a gradual degeneration of the nerve cells of the basal ganglia with depletion of the available dopamine (a neurotransmitter essential for proper muscle movement). The result is impairment in the centers of coordination; in control of muscle tone; and in the control of the initiation and inhibition of movements.

Medical Management

Care of Parkinsonism involves treating symptoms and providing support. Drug therapy is the cornerstone of medical care, and includes:

  Anticholinergic drugs (Artane, Cogenten, and Akineton)

  Dopamine precursor drugs (Levodopa)

  Antiviral agents that have anti-Parkinsonian activity (Symmetrol)

  Combination of Levodopa and a drug limiting its peripheral metabolism (Sinemet)

Drug therapy is supplemented by appropriate diet and exercise prescriptions.

Nursing Management

  Assessment—subjective

  History and course of the disease

  Patient's knowledge of disease process, medication and side effects

  Patient's complaints of fatigue, incoordination

Assessment—objective
Presence of "classic triad" of symptoms:
   tremor (pillrolling type—more prominent at rest)
   rigidity (jerky movements)
   bradykinesia (slow or retarded movements)
Absence of automatic associated body movements—stooped posture, deadpan expression, shuffling gait, difficulty initiating movement, drooling saliva
Signs of complications—dysphagia, constipation, movement "freezing," incontinence, general debilitation, depression
General nutritional status
Elimination patterns and control

Nursing Diagnoses
Diagnoses associated with Parkinsonism will vary depending on the stage of disease and severity of symptoms. Common diagnoses include the following:
   Alteration in bowel elimination—constipation related to decreased mobility, food and fluid intake
   Alterations in comfort—pain and soreness related to muscle flexion and rigidity
   Impaired physical mobility related to muscle rigidity and bradykinesia
   Self-care deficit in feeding, bathing/hygiene, dressing/grooming, and toileting related to muscle rigidity and bradykinesia
   Alteration in nutrition—less than body requirements related to dysphagia
   Knowledge deficit related to medications and activities that will promote muscle function and control symptoms
   Impaired verbal communication related to rigid facial muscles and decreased voice volume
   Potential for injury related to posture defects, muscle rigidity, and propulsive gait
   Potential for social isolation related to impaired mobility, communication disorders, and lack of affect

Expected outcomes
Patient will maintain sufficient muscle strength and flexibility to maintain independence.
Patient will maintain a regular pattern of bowel elimination.
Patient will experience minimal discomfort from sore muscles.
Patient will eat a diet that maintains appropriate weight and meets body's baseline nutritional needs.
Patient and family will be knowledgeable about prescribed medications and their side effects as well as exercises and activities to decrease symptoms.
Patient will be able to communicate verbally and maintain active social interaction.
Patient will not experience injury related to disease symptoms.

Nursing interventions
Rigidity
Administer medications as prescribed; teach about side effects (nausea, hypotension, palpitations, arrhythmias, confusion, and hallucinations are all common effects of dopaminergic drugs).
Promote regular exercise and ambulation, particularly muscle stretching.
Explore use of hot packs and massage.
Encourage active or passive range of motion every 4 hours.
Encourage patient to hold hands behind back to improve gait and posture.
Bradykinesia
Teach patient to use upright straight chair—placing back chair legs on blocks makes it easier to get up.
Remove scatter rugs and clutter furniture—provide hand rails.
Suggest that patient modify clothing with wide zippers or Velcro closures as needed.
Teach patient to consciously think about lifting feet over imaginary lines on floor.
Nutrition
Plan nutritious meals high in roughage, easily chewed.
   Cut all food into safe sizes.
   Keep fluid intake high.
Provide smaller, more frequent meals to prevent exhaustion.
Allow sufficient time for eating.
Monitor weight.
Communication
Allow enough time and be patient.
Listen carefully.
Encourage patient to do breathing and vocal exercises to increase voice volume and strength.

Evaluation
Patient engages in regular planned exercise and has sufficient strength and flexibility to remain independent in activities of daily living.
Patient maintains regular bowel elimination.
Patient expresses absence of pain.
Patient maintains desired weight.
Patient and family are knowledgeable about disease, complications, medications and side effects, and plan of treatment.
Patient communicates verbally and maintains social contacts and interactions.
Patient and family plan together for home modifications to increase safety.

MULTIPLE SCLEROSIS

Multiple sclerosis is a degenerative disease that occurs primarily in northern temperate climates and typically affects young adults between ages 20 and 40. The disease usually follows a downhill course toward progressive disability over a period of about 20 years.

Pathophysiology

Despite significant research, the cause of multiple sclerosis remains unknown, although viruses and autoimmunity are most strongly suspected. Multiple sclerosis produces random patches of demyelination of the white matter of the spinal cord and brain. Impulses are slowed or blocked. It follows a pattern of exacerbation and remission and produces a great variety of signs and symptoms.

Medical Management

There is no definitive diagnosis or treatment for multiple sclerosis. Diagnosis is established from course of clinical symptoms. Treatment is directed at symptom management through ACTH treatment during exacerbations, maintenance corticosteroid therapy, physical therapy for muscle strengthening, and patient education and support to maintain optimal health.

Nursing Management

Assessment—subjective

History and course of the disease (early symptoms are usually transitory)

Patient's knowledge of disease process, treatment, and medication

Patient's complaints of weakness, numbness, fatigue, double vision, spots before eyes

Patient's response to chronic progressive nature of the disease

Assessment—objective

Bowel or bladder problems—frequency, urgency, incontinence

Presence of tremor, muscle spasm, spastic ataxia, loss of coordination

Nystagmus (rapid oscillation of eyeballs), speech disorders (scanning speech)

Behavior, including euphoria and crying spells

Nursing diagnosis

Diagnoses associated with multiple sclerosis are highly variable depending on the individual patient's symptoms and stage of the disease. Common diagnoses include the following:

Alteration in bowel elimination—constipation or incontinence related to interruption of motor impulses

Alteration in patterns of urinary elimination—frequency, urgency, and incontinence related to irregular nervous stimulation

Impaired physical mobility related to tremor, muscle spasticity, and incoordination

Self-care deficit in feeding, bathing/hygiene, dressing/grooming, and toileting related to muscle weakness, spasticity, and incoordination

Alteration in visual sensory perception related to interruption of optic nerve pathways

Disturbance in self-concept (body image, self-esteem, or role performance) related to impaired mobility and loss of control over self-care

Ineffective individual or family coping related to the chronic progressive nature of the disease

Expected outcomes

Patient will maintain control over bowel and bladder function.

Patient will maintain sufficient muscular function and control to remain independent in the activities of daily living.

Patient will not be injured during periods of disordered vision.

Patient will maintain a positive self-concept through continued involvement in family and occupational activities.

Patient and family will work together to cope adequately with condition of decreasing function.

Nursing interventions

Administer prescribed medications; teach patient and family about drugs and side effects.

Mobility

Stretching and range of motion exercises every shift; provide gait training.

Encourage ambulation; teach use of assistive devices as indicated.

Teach patient and family routine interventions to prevent the complications of immobility.

Good general health. Good general health is thought to decrease likelihood of exacerbations

Teach patient to eat nutritious high-protein diet and take supplemental vitamins.

Encourage patient to balance rest and activity and avoid fatigue.

Encourage patient to avoid extremes of heat and cold and exposure to infection.

Treat all infection immediately.

Elimination

Follow intermittent catheterization program or bladder retraining program.

Keep fluid intake high.

Protect patient against soiling and leaking.

Initiate bowel program with stool softeners and suppositories.

Adjustment

Encourage patient to verbalize feelings and concerns.

Calmly assist patient to deal with mood swings.

Refer patient to support groups in community.

TABLE 4-4 Infrequently occurring degenerative disorders of the nervous system

Disorder	Description	Signs and Symptoms	Management
Myasthenia gravis	Disease affecting young adults in which nerve impulses fail to pass the myoneural junction to the muscle: Inadequate secretion of acetylcholine Excessive amounts of cholinesterase Nonresponse of muscle fibers	Muscle weakness, generalized severe fatigue of rapid onset that disappears with rest. Primarily affects head, neck, and upper body: Weakness in arm and hand Drooping facial muscles, ptosis Inability to chew or swallow Failure of muscles of respiration	Administration of anticholinesterase drugs—neostigmine (Prostigmin), pyridostigmine (Mestinon)—in rigid, carefully spaced schedules. Life-style with a balance of rest and activity—spacing activities and maintenance of optimal health.
Amyotrophic lateral sclerosis (ALS, or Lou Gehrig's disease)	Motor neuron disease in which myelin sheaths are replaced by scar tissue. Affects nerves in brain, spinal cord, or both, distorts or blocks impulses.	Early signs are fatigue, awkwardness, and dysphagia. Progresses to muscle weakness, atrophy, tremor, and spasticity of flexor muscles. No sensory loss occurs. Death is frequently from respiratory failure, usually within 5 years.	Treatment is aimed at relieving symptoms: Assistance with daily activities Prosthesis or assistive devices for weakened muscles Feeding tubes Emotional support
Syringomyelia	Cavities or cysts form and progressively destroy spinal cord or lower brainstem. Destruction starts in gray matter and works outward. Cysts fill with cerebrospinal fluid (CSF), further disrupting function.	Early signs are segmental loss of sense of pain and temperature, weakness and atrophy of hands and arms. Flaccid paralysis alters to spastic when upper neurons are involved. Death may occur from paralysis of muscles for breathing and swallowing.	Decompression spinal surgery may provide temporary relief from symptoms Prevention of injury from sensory loss Supportive care for daily activities Feeding tubes, respiratory support
Alzheimer's disease	Cells of brain show plaque deposits and disruption of neurofibrils with interference with function.	Stage 1—mild mental impairment, forgetfulness, impairment of judgment Stage 2—confusion, irritation, restlessness, fecal and urinary incontinence Stage 3—complete incapacity	No available treatment Nursing measures aimed at maintaining good general health, environmental safety, and continence Supportive help for family

Evaluation

Patient will follow a bowel and bladder program that supports regular elimination and a minimum number of accidents.

Patient maintains self-care independence, engages in regular range of motion exercise, and ambulates effectively with assistive devices.

Patient modifies environment and visual stimuli appropriately to maintain safe, independent ambulation.

Patient maintains stable weight, plans and eats nutritious meals, and is free of frequent infection.

Patient and family verbalize their fears and concerns about the future and work together for realistic planning.

Table 4-4 presents basic information about less common degenerative neurologic disorders for which the care is largely treating symptoms and providing support.

CEREBROVASCULAR DISEASE

Cerebrovascular disease is a broad category that includes any disturbance involving the blood supply to the brain. It includes arteriosclerosis/atherosclerosis, aneurysms, arteriovenous malformation, emboli, and hypertension. Cerebrovascular accident is the most common clinical outcome of cerebrovascular disease.

CEREBROVASCULAR ACCIDENT (CVA)

CVA is a severe sudden interruption of the blood supply to the brain that produces focal neurologic signs and symptoms from cerebral anoxia and interruption of cerebral metabolism. It is the third leading cause of death in the United States. CVAs are usually classified as being either thrombotic or hemorrhagic. The box on p. 46 lists common conditions causing CVA.

CONDITIONS CAUSING CVA

THROMBUS:

Atherosclerosis in intracranial and extracranial arteries
Adjacency to intracerebral hemorrhage
Arteritis caused by collagen (autoimmune) disease or bacterial arteritis
Hypercoagulability such as in polycythemia
Cerebral venous thromboses

EMBOLI:

Valves damaged by rheumatic heart disease
Myocardial infarction
Atrial fibrillation (this arrhythmia causes variable emptying of left ventricle, blood pools and small clots form and then at times the ventricle will be emptied completely with release of small emboli)
Bacterial endocarditis and nonbacterial endocarditis causing clots to form on endocardium

HEMORRHAGE:

Hypertensive intracerebral hemorrhage
Subarachnoid hemorrhage
Rupture of aneurysm
Arteriovenous malformation
Hypocoagulation (as in patients with blood dyscrasias)

GENERALIZED HYPOXIA:

Severe hypotension, cardiopulmonary arrest, or severe depression in cardiac output caused by arrhythmias

LOCALIZED HYPOXIA:

Cerebral artery spasms associated with subarachnoid hemorrhage
Cerebral artery vasoconstriction associated with migraine headaches

From Phipps, W.J., Long, B.C., and Woods, N.F.: Medical-surgical nursing: concepts and clinical practice, ed. 2, St. Louis, 1983, The C.V. Mosby Co.

Pathophysiology

Any condition causing altered perfusion can lead to cerebral hypoxia. Brain cell responses vary according to the degree and duration of decreased oxygen. Prolonged hypoxia leads to infarction and permanent damage. Cerebral edema accompanies the hypoxia and worsens the initial deficits.

The two vessels most frequently affected are the middle cerebral and internal carotid arteries. Symptoms will vary widely based on the location and extent of injury.

Medical Management

Early treatment differs for thrombotic (92%) and hemorrhagic (8%) strokes.

Patients with thrombotic strokes may be given anticoagulants or vasodilators to prevent further damage. Remaining care consists of support of vital functions and prompt initiation of active rehabilitation.

Patients with hemorrhagic strokes are placed on absolute bed rest to prevent additional bleeding. Meticulous monitoring of vital functions is necessary until their con-

TRANSIENT ISCHEMIC ATTACKS (TIAs)

Definition: Transient episodes of reversible cerebral ischemia accompanied by temporary occurrences of neurologic dysfunction

Cause: May be produced by any of the conditions that cause CVA. Most commonly they precede a thrombotic stroke and may result from vessel spasm. Attacks may occur many times over the course of weeks or months or years. They warn of an underlying pathologic condition.

Symptoms: Focal deficits are quite varied depending on the site of ischemia. Some of the more common deficits include:

One-sided weakness of the lower face, hands and fingers, arm, or leg
Transient dysphasia
Some sensory impairment
Moment of clumsiness or incoordination

Treatment: Resolve associated risk factors and health conditions.
Vasodilators, anticoagulants, and aspirin may be used to decrease platelet aggregation and prevent clotting.
Surgical correction may be needed if cause is an isolated extracranial lesion.

ditions stabilize. Surgery may be attempted if an aneurysm is the cause of the bleeding. Patients will gradually begin active rehabilitation.

Nursing Management

Assessment—subjective

Onset and sequence of symptoms
Co-existing health problems
History of transient ischemic attacks (TIAs) (see the box above)
Patient's complaints of headaches and sensory disturbances: visual, touch, hearing
Emotional response, patient and family

Assessment—objective

Level of consciousness—cognitive functioning
Vital signs
Presence of motor deficits—hemiparesis or hemiplegia
Expressive or receptive aphasia
Bowel and bladder function
Signs of increased intracranial pressure (see box on page 50)
Seizure activity

Nursing diagnoses

Diagnoses will be variable dependent on the precipitating cause and degree of severity of the CVA. Common diagnoses encountered in the thrombotic stroke patient during the rehabilitation phase include:

Impaired physical mobility related to hemiplegia
Self-care deficit in feeding, bathing/hygiene, dressing/

grooming, or toileting related to hemiplegia and altered thought processes

Impaired verbal communication related to expressive or receptive aphasia

Alteration in bowel elimination—constipation or incontinence related to interruption of voluntary motor control

Alteration in patterns of urinary elimination—retention or incontinence related to interruption of voluntary motor control

Sensory perceptual alteration (visual, kinesthetic) related to cerebral hypoxia

Alteration in thought processes related to cerebral hypoxia

Potential for ineffective individual and family coping related to the physical and mental changes resulting from the CVA

Expected outcomes (for rehabilitative phase)

Patient will become independent in the activities of daily living.

Patient will ambulate independently using appropriate assistive devices.

Patient will successfully communicate needs to nursing staff and family.

Patient will reestablish a normal pattern of bowel and bladder elimination and be free of accidents.

Patient will learn to compensate for sensory perceptual deficits and function safely in the environment.

Patient will participate in decision making and not experience significant mood disorder.

Patient and family will adjust to nature of residual disabilities and plan appropriately for postdischarge care.

Nursing interventions

Acute phase

Maintain an open airway:
  Keep patient in side-lying position.
  Use oral airway and have suction ready.
  Initiate deep breathing and gentle coughing.

Assess and record vital signs, level of consciousness, and do neurologic checks frequently.

Monitor fluid balance accurately:
  Keep careful records of intake and output.
  Regulate IV carefully.
  Maintain fluid intake at 1000 ml/day if ordered.

Turn and position every 2 hours.

Administer passive range of motion exercises each shift.

Examine and massage skin every 2 hours:
  Keep skin clean and dry.
  Use pressure relief devices.
  Apply TED stockings.

Begin oral feedings as ordered—put patient in high Fowler's position.
  Check for gag reflex.

Offer easily swallowed foods (pureed)—avoid liquids.

Record bowel elimination.
  Institute use of stool softeners and suppositories as needed.

Avoid prolonged use of Foley catheter.
  Increase fluids as allowed and offer use of bedpan/urinal frequently.

Support patient and family.
  Establish effective means of communication.

NOTE: These same basic interventions are appropriate for patients experiencing decreased consciousness from other causes.

Rehabilitative phase

Mobility

Implement exercise program designed by physical therapy department.

Initiate balance exercise at bedside.

Teach technique for transfer to wheelchair or toilet.

Teach use of assistive device for ambulation.

Explore need for sling to prevent shoulder subluxation.

Nutrition

Teach patient to use unaffected side for feeding.
  Provide self-help devices such as rocker knife and plate guards.
  Increase fluids and roughage as swallowing improves.
  Remind patient to empty paralyzed side of mouth.

Elimination

Continue bowel and bladder retraining programs.

Communication

Establish nature, extent of communication disorder.

Work with speech therapy department to plan appropriate therapy.

Apply basic principles for aphasic patients (see boxes on p. 48)

Share appropriate techniques with family.

Psychological

Be alert to spatial perceptual difficulties associated with right hemisphere stroke. Patient may have trouble judging position and distance.

Patient may behave and act impulsively.

Patient may deny left side.

Provide full mirror to assist patient with posture.

Assist patient to reestablish control over emotion and behavior and set limits.

Assist family to assess patient's capabilities and plan for post-discharge care.

Initiate referrals to appropriate community agencies.

Evaluation

Patient has switched self-care activities to unaffected side and is independent in the activities of daily living using appropriate self-help devices.

Patient can make safe transfers and ambulate with the use of assistive devices.

BASIC TYPES OF APHASIA

Motor (Expressive): Inability to use the symbols of speech to speak or write words. Muscles of speech are not paralyzed.

Sensory (Receptive): Inability to comprehend the spoken or written word.

Global aphasia: Presence of both motor and sensory problems at the same time.

Dysarthria: Weakness in the muscles of speech, creates difficulties in pronouncing words or swallowing.

NURSING INTERVENTIONS FOR APHASIA

GENERAL:
Establish a relaxed environment.
Encourage persistence and the desire to communicate.
Control and limit the amount of stimuli in environment.

SENSORY (RECEPTIVE):
Sit down and establish eye contact.
Face patient and speak simply and slowly.
Reword the message if misunderstood.
Use appropriate gestures to supplement words.
Allow sufficient time for patient to process words.
Use a normal tone of voice.

MOTOR (EXPRESSIVE):
Avoid interrupting and rushing patient.
Emphasize simple concrete words used for daily care.
Discuss topics of interest to patient.
Encourage use of other means of communication.
Convey acceptance and encourage patient to talk.
Don't speak for the patient.

NURSING CARE FOR THE PATIENT WITH AN INTRACRANIAL HEMORRHAGE DURING THE ACUTE STAGE

Keep patient absolutely quiet to prevent additional bleeding.
Provide strict bed rest with head of bed elevated 30 degrees.
Keep room quiet, darkened.
Minimize stimulation—avoid use of TV, radio, loud noises, extensive conversation.
Minimize vagal stimulation—no rectal temperatures, no ice water, no straining for bowel movement.
Avoid coughing and abrupt turning or position changes.
Perform complete and accurate vital signs with neurochecks as ordered once an hour or more frequently; report changes immediately.
Monitor intake and output and IV flow rates carefully.
Administer Amicar as ordered to promote clot formation.

Patient is free of complications of immobility.
Patient is able to communicate needs and desires successfully.
Patient has reestablished bowel and bladder control.
Patient is aware of sensory perceptual deficits and practices methods to compensate for them.
Patient is able to solve problems effectively in self-care and has only mild mood swings.
Patient and family have discussed and planned appropriate post-discharge care.

NOTE: The patient who has experienced a hemorrhagic stroke, especially one related to bleeding from a cerebral aneurysm, is at special risk during the initial care period. The box on p. 48 details some specific nursing interventions for this period.

INFECTIONS OF CENTRAL NERVOUS SYSTEM

The nervous system may be attacked by a variety of organisms and viruses as well as suffer from toxic reactions to bacterial and viral disease. The meninges or the brain itself may be affected. If an infection becomes walled off, it may cause an abscess.

MENINGITIS

Meningitis is an acute infection of the meninges that may be caused by a variety of bacteria and viruses. Children are affected more often because of their frequent upper respiratory infections.

Pathophysiology
Organisms that reach the brain disseminate quickly through the meninges and into the ventricles. This dissemination produces the following:
Congestion of the meningeal vessels
Edema of brain tissue
Increased intracranial pressure
Generalized inflammation with white blood cell exudate formation
Hydrocephalus if exudate blocks ventricular passages
Diagnosis is confirmed by isolation and identification of organism from the cerebrospinal fluid (CSF).

Medical Management
Medical management consists of the following:
Massive doses of antibiotic specific for the causative organism
Steroids and osmotic diuretics to reduce cerebral edema
Anticonvulsants to control seizures
Respiratory isolation for 24 to 48 hours after antibiotics begin

Nursing Management
Assessment-Subjective
History of respiratory infection

History and severity of symptoms: headache, vomiting, stiff neck, fever

Assessment-Objective
Vital signs (high fever)

Change in level of consciousness and orientation

Signs of meningeal irritation:

Positive Kernig's sign—inability to completely extend the legs without pain

Positive Brudzinski's sign—patient flexes hips and knees when neck is passively flexed

Nursing diagnoses
Diagnoses will depend on the severity and stage of the disease. The patient initially may be critically ill and completely prostrated. Basic diagnoses include the following:

Alteration in comfort—pain related to pronounced headache and stiff neck

Fluid volume deficit related to high fever

Potential for injury related to decreased cerebral tissue perfusion

Alteration in nutrition—less than body needs related to severe nausea and vomiting

Expected outcomes
Patient will experience decreased pain.

Patient will maintain an adequate fluid balance; elevated temperature will be decreased.

Patient will not experience injury.

Patient's nutritional needs will be met and a stable weight is maintained

Nursing interventions
Administer prescribed medications and fluids.

Monitor accurate intake and output; assess skin turgor, mucous membranes.

Offer nutritious semi-liquid diet as tolerated.

Keep room darkened; keep sensory stimuli to a minimum.

Keep side rails up; do not abruptly move or jar patient.

Maintain accurate records of vital signs and neurological checks.

Maintain appropriate isolation procedures.

Evaluation
Patient is comfortable, participates actively in self-care.

Patient is well hydrated, has an adequate urinary output.

Patient does not sustain injury or complications of immobility.

Patient returns to normal diet and is not losing weight.

NOTE: Encephalitis, an inflammation of the brain tissue, is a relatively rare, very serious disease with a high mortality. Treatment is basically supportive and follows that generally outlined above.

HEAD TRAUMA

Craniocerebral trauma causes about 80,000 deaths yearly. It is the major cause of death in individuals aged 1 to 35, but causes death and serious disability in people of all ages. Table 4-5 describes the common types of brain injuries caused by head trauma. The degree of external damage is not necessarily indicative of the extent of brain injury, but compound and depressed skull fractures are associated with serious brain damage.

TABLE 4-5 Damage of brain tissue due to trauma

Type of Injury	Characteristics	Structural Alteration	Effects
Concussion	Immediate and transitory impairment of neurologic function caused by the mechanical force	No	Possible loss of consciousness may be instantaneous or delayed—usually is reversible.
Contusion	Likened to bruising with extravasation of blood cells	Yes	Injury may be at site of impact or at opposite site. Often cortex is damaged.
Laceration	Tearing of tissues caused by sharp fragment or a shearing force	Yes	Hemorrhage is a serious complication.
Intracranial hemorrhage	Bleeding into the epidural, subdural, subarachnoid spaces, or into the brain or ventricles	Yes	Effects depend on the site of injury and degree of bleeding
Epidural hematoma	Rupture of a large vessel that lies above the dura mater; tear is usually in an artery (middle meningeal is the most common site)		Signs of rising intracranial pressure develop rapidly with rapid deterioration into full coma.
Subdural hematoma	Usually results from venous bleeding below the dura mater; bleeding may produce acute, subacute or chronic hematoma formation		Signs of rising intracranial pressure may develop within days, weeks or even months after the injury.

Pathophysiology

Head injuries all create concern over rising intracranial pressure. The rigid skull leaves little room for expansion. Any alteration in brain mass, blood volume, CSF volume, or pressure can create hypoxia. The box below reviews the pathologic sequence that occurs as intracranial pressure rises.

Medical Management

Management involves measures to identify and correct the underlying cause of increasing intracranial pressure and cerebral edema. These measures include:

Corticosteroids (dexamethasone) to reduce inflammation

Osmotic diuretics (mannitol) to reduce cerebral edema

Fluid restriction and systemic diuretics (Lasix)

Anticonvulsants (Dilantin) to control seizures

Barbiturates (Nembutal) to decrease pressure

Surgical repair of fracture or laceration

Airway management with endotracheal tube or tracheostomy

Nursing Management

Assessment—subjective

History of the trauma and sequence of symptoms

Patient's complaints of headache, double vision

Assessment—objective

Vital signs

Level of consciousness

Respiratory status

Signs of rising intracranial pressure (see box at right)

Motor strength and equality

Speech difficulties

Bleeding or CSF drainage from ears or nose

Vomiting

PATHOLOGIC SEQUENCE OF INCREASING INTRACRANIAL PRESSURE

An increase in brain tissue, vascular tissue and volume, or cerebral spinal fluid volume from any cause increases pressure within the cranial cavity. After the brain's compensatory mechanisms have been utilized, the following sequence occurs:

1. Cerebral blood flow decreases, resulting in inadequate perfusion.
2. Inadequate perfusion leads to increasing pCO_2 and decreasing pO_2 values.
3. Oxygenation changes trigger vasodilation and cerebral edema.
4. Edema further increases intracranial pressure, resulting in a downward spiral of tissue compression and displacement that may be irreversible and fatal.

Nursing diagnoses

The diagnoses associated with head injury will depend on the severity and type of the injury. Common diagnoses include the following:

Alteration in cerebral tissue perfusion related to increased intracranial pressure

Alteration in thought processes related to decreasing level of consciousness

Impaired physical mobility related to decreasing level of consciousness and interruption of motor impulses

Potential for injury and infection related to decreasing level of consciousness and head trauma

Alteration in urinary and bowel elimination patterns related to interruption of motor control

Alteration in comfort—pain related to head trauma

Ineffective airway clearance related to increasing intracranial pressure

Expected outcomes

Patient will not experience undetected increase in intracranial pressure.

Patient will remain alert and appropriately oriented to the environment and treatment regimen.

Patient will not experience common complications of immobility during period of bed rest and treatment.

SIGNS OF INCREASING INTRACRANIAL PRESSURE (ICP)

1. Change in level of consciousness
   ALERT: One of the earliest and most sensitive signs of rising ICP is restlessness.
2. Pupillary signs
   Pressure on the oculomotor nerve
   Slower response, pupil inequality, or fixed dilated pupils
3. Blood pressure and pulse
   Increasing systolic pressure with stable or falling diastolic pressure
   Widening pulse pressure
   Slowing of the pulse rate from pressure on the vagus nerve
4. Respirations
   Changes are usually quite late
   Slowing of rate and an irregular breathing pattern
5. Temperature
   Failure of thermoregulatory center occurs late
   High uncontrolled temperature
6. Focal signs
   Muscle weakness or paralysis
   Decreasing response to pain stimulus in comatose patients
   Positive Babinski's sign
   Decerebrate or decorticate posture
7. Visceral
   Decreasing visual acuity
   Papilledema
8. Headache and vomiting

Patient will not experience environmental injury or develop preventable infection.

Patient will maintain regular patterns of urinary and bowel elimination.

Patient will experience manageable levels of discomfort.

Patient will maintain a clear airway for optimal oxygen and carbon dioxide exchange.

Nursing interventions

Perform accurate neurological checks at frequent intervals including:

Vital signs

Level of consciousness using either Glasgow coma scale or hospital-developed continuum (see box below)

Oculomotor nerve function

Motor and sensory status—hand grips, voluntary movement, sensation.

Administer medications as ordered to reduce or stabilize intracranial pressure.

Maintain bed rest with head of bed slightly elevated as ordered (15 to 30 degrees). Keep environmental stimuli to a minimum.

Use side rails, seizure precautions; avoid neck flexion, sudden movements.

Institute nursing measures or cooling blanket to control temperature. *Note:* Increased temperature dramatically increases brain's metabolic demands.

Observe for signs of hypoxia, such as cyanosis, color changes in nail beds and mucous membranes, restlessness, altered respiratory rate.

Monitor arterial blood gas results.

Observe for bloody or serous drainage from nose or ears.

ALERT: Drainage may indicate tearing of meninges and escape of CSF and precede meningitis. If present:

Do not clean, pack, or obstruct in any way.

Promote gravity drainage onto sterile towel or dressing.

Determine whether serous fluid is CSF or mucus (CSF tests positive for sugar and produces a halo when blotted and dried on gauze).

Change dressings frequently.

Administer antibiotics as ordered.

Do not suction through the nose.

Monitor intake and output carefully. Check specific gravity hourly, maintain fluid restrictions. Diabetes insipidus increases urine output while inappropriate ADH syndrome decreases it.

Employ bulk cathartics and stool softeners to prevent straining at elimination.

Teach patient to avoid coughing and sneezing if possible. Avoid all isometric contraction.

Institute standard nursing measures for passive range of motion, turning, skin care, and TED stockings to prevent complications of immobility.

Offer support to patient and family to deal with high anxiety situation with uncertain outcome.

NOTE: Many individuals who experience minor head

LEVEL OF CONSCIOUSNESS RATING SCALES

I. FIVE-POINT LEVEL OF CONSCIOUSNESS SCALE

1. Alert—normal mental activity, aware, mentally functional.
2. Obtunded/Drowsy—sleepy, very short attention span, can respond appropriately if aroused.
3. Stupor—apathetic, slow moving, expression blank, staring; aroused only by vigorous stimuli.
4. Light coma—not oriented to time, place, or person. Aroused only by painful stimuli—response is only grunt or grimace or withdrawal from pain.
5. Deep coma—no response except decerebrate or decorticate posture.

II. GLASGOW COMA SCALE SCORING

Eyes open	4	spontaneously
	3	to speech
	2	to pain
	1	none
Best verbal response	5	oriented
	4	confused
	3	inappropriate words
	2	incomprehensible sounds
	1	none
Best motor response	5	obeys commands
	4	localizes pain
	3	flexion to pain
	2	extension to pain
	1	none

TEACHING INSTRUCTIONS FOR HEAD INJURY PATIENTS AND FAMILIES

Patient should be awakened periodically through the first 24 hours to ensure patient is arousable.

During first 24 to 48 hours, patient and family should watch carefully for the following warning signs:
1. Vomiting—often with force behind it
2. Unusual sleepiness, dizziness, loss of balance, or falling
3. Complaint of double vision, blurring, or jerky eye movements
4. A slight headache is expected—worsening headache or complaints of feeling worse when moving about should be reported
5. Bleeding or discharge from nose or ears
6. Seizures: any twitching or movement of arms or legs that patient cannot stop
7. Any behavior or symptom not normal for the individual

A physician should be called at once if any of these signs are observed. If a physician is unavailable, emergency services should be contacted immediately.

SPECIFIC NURSING INTERVENTIONS FOR THE CRANIOTOMY PATIENT

PREOPERATIVE PERIOD:

Assess baseline neurologic status.

Encourage patient and family to verbalize fears and concerns.

Provide detailed teaching about procedures; postoperative care; movement and activity restrictions; and equipment to be used.

Prepare family for patient's appearance after the operation:
Head dressing, shaved scalp
Edema and bruising
Temporary decrease in mental status

POSTOPERATIVE PERIOD:

Complete or perform nursing interventions for monitoring neurologic status, dealing with rising intracranial pressure; and preventing complications of immobility. In addition:
Positioning:
Supratentorial surgery—head of bed elevated 45 degrees. Patient turned only between back and unaffected side if tumor was large to prevent shift of brain tissue. Infratentorial surgery—head of bed flat, avoid positioning patient on back, to prevent shift of brain tissue downward. Avoid neck flexion.
Observe for the following side effects of high-dose glucocorticosteroid therapy:
Elevated blood glucose, glycosuria
Stress ulcer (guaiac test all stools)
Check urinary output and specific gravity for the following:
Diabetes insipidus: increased output; decreased specific gravity
Inappropriate ADH syndrome: decreased output
Assist and support patient and family in dealing with residual effects of the tumor or surgery.

TYPES OF BRAIN TUMORS

Gliomas: Account for about one-half of all brain tumors; arise from the brain connective tissue. They tend to be infiltrative, difficult to excise completely, and grow rapidly. Glioblastomas and medulloblastomas are the most highly malignant and are usually fatal within a matter of months. Astrocytomas and oligodendrogliomas are slower growing, but still frequently fatal in less than a year.

Meningiomas: Account for 13% to 18% of all primary intracranial tumors; arise from the meningeal coverings of the brain. They vary widely in histologic features and size and are usually benign. They are frequently encapsulated and surgical cure is possible.

Acoustic Neuromas: Account for about 8% of all primary intracranial tumors; may arise from any of the cranial nerves. When the acoustic nerve is affected, the tumor grows from nerve sheath but usually extends to affect the nerve fibers. They are slow growing.

Pituitary Adenoma: May arise from a variety of pituitary tissue types. They are successfully treated by surgery, using either the standard craniotomy or the transsphenoidal approach.

injury are sent home after the initial evaluation. The box on p. 52 lists specific teaching instructions that should be provided to patients and families.

Evaluation

Patient is free of the effects of increased intracranial pressure.

Patient is alert and oriented and functions at pre-injury cognitive level.

Patient has optimal oxygen and carbon dioxide exchange.

Patient maintains full range of motion, recovers muscle strength, and maintains an intact skin.

Patient is free of injury.

Patient resumes pre-injury patterns of urinary and bowel elimination.

Patient is free of pain.

INTRACRANIAL SURGERY

Cranial surgery may be required for debriding or repairing effects of head trauma, repairing aneurysms, treating abscesses, or excising brain tumors.

BRAIN TUMOR

The box on p. 52 presents the commonly occurring forms of brain tumor. Symptoms may vary significantly depending on the tumor's location and speed of growth. Surgical intervention is the treatment of choice.

Nursing interventions following craniotomy surgery closely follow those discussed for head injury. The box on p. 52 describes interventions that relate specifically to

TABLE 4-6 Functional level of spinal cord disruption with rehabilitation potential

Cord Segment	Autonomic	Movement Remaining	Rehabilitation Potential
Quadriplegia			
C1-C3	Usually fatal. Vagus domination of heart, respiration, blood vessels, all organs below	Neck and above. Innervation to diaphragm lost, no independent respiratory function.	Drive electric wheelchair equipped with portable respirator by using chin control or mouth stick. No bowel or bladder control.
C4	Vagus domination of heart, respirations, and all vessels and organs below	Sensation and movement above neck.	Drive electric wheelchair by using chin control or mouth stick. No bowel or bladder control.
C5	Vagus domination as C4	Full neck, partial shoulder, back, biceps. Gross elbow—cannot roll over or use hands. Decreased respiratory reserve.	Drive electric wheelchair with mobile hand supports. Some can utilize powered hand splints. No bowel or bladder control.
C6	Vagus domination as C4	Shoulder and upper back—abduction and rotation at shoulder, full biceps-elbow flexion. Wrist extension. Thumb—weak grasp. Decreased respiratory reserve.	Assist with transfer and some self-care. Feed self with hand devices. Push wheelchair on smooth, flat surface. No bowel or bladder control.
C7-C8	Vagus domination as C4	All triceps-elbow extension. Finger extensors and flexors. Good grasp though still decreased strength. Can roll over and sit up in bed. Decreased respiratory reserve.	Transfer self to wheelchair, push self on most surfaces, most self-care. Wheelchair-independent. Some can drive car with powered hand controls. No bowel or bladder control.
Paraplegia			
T1-T6	Sympathetic innervation to heart, vagus domination of rest	Full innervation of upper extremities and back plus essential intrinsic muscles of hand. Full strength and dexterity of grasp. Decreased trunk stability and decreased respiratory reserve.	Fully independent in self-care and in wheelchair. Most can drive car with hand controls. Full body brace for exercise but not for functional ambulation. No bladder or bowel control.
T6-T12	Vagus domination only of leg vessels, GI-GU organs	Full, stable thoracic muscles and upper back. Intercostals functional so increased respiratory reserve.	Wheelchair-independent. Can stand erect with full body brace; can ambulate on crutches, with swing-through gait difficult. Cannot climb stairs. No bladder or bowel control.
L1-L2	Vagus domination of leg vessels as above	Varying control of legs and pelvis. Low back instability.	Good sitting balance. Full use of wheelchair.
L3-L4	Partial domination of leg vessels and organs as T6	Quadriceps and hip flexors, no hamstrings. Flail ankles.	Completely independent ambulation with short leg braces and canes. Cannot stand for long periods. Bladder and bowel continence.

From Lewis, Sharon and Collier, Idola, Medical surgical nursing, McGraw-Hill, 1983.

the care of the craniotomy patient beyond those previously discussed.

SPINAL CORD INJURY

Spinal cord injury from accidents is a significant cause of serious disability and death in the United States. Approximately 6000 to 8000 new cases occur annually. Injury may occur from fracture or displacement of one or more vertebrae with damage to the underlying spinal cord and nerve roots or from pressure and destruction resulting from intramedullary lesions.

Pathophysiology
Even relatively minor compression or displacement of the spinal column can result in serious cord compression. Edema occurs, which worsens the compression.

Complete cord injury involves a total transection of the spinal cord accompanied by complete loss of voluntary movement or sensation below the level of injury. An incomplete cord injury involves a partial transection or injury to the spinal cord which results in loss of voluntary movement or sensation below the level of injury according to the degree of damage.

Spinal shock is a period of flaccid paralysis and complete loss of reflexes that initially follows almost all spinal cord injury. It is accompanied by cardiovascular instability, urinary retention, and paralytic ileus, and may persist for a few days to several months. Table 4-6 details the functions lost at various levels of cord injury.

Medical Management
Initial interventions are aimed at supporting vital functions and preventing further cord damage. Early surgery

may be indicated to decompress or fuse the spinal column or to insert rods to stabilize the spine and correct deformities. Drug intervention with analgesics, anticholinergics, steroids, and sympathomimetics is also employed. Long term stabilization of the spine may be accomplished by the use of Crutchfield tongs with traction and turning frames or halo traction devices.

Nursing Management (Initial care and rehabilitation)
Assessment—subjective
Description of the accident or injury
History of loss of consciousness
Presence or absence and level of sensation
Sensory disturbances: pain, paresthesias

Assessment—objective
Respiratory status and quality of respirations
Level of consciousness
Degree and level of motor ability and strength
Baseline vital signs
Body position and alignment

Nursing diagnoses
Nursing diagnoses will vary depending on the level and severity of the injury and the stage of rehabilitation. Some common diagnoses include the following:

Ineffective breathing pattern or ineffective airway clearance related to weakness or paralysis of intercostal muscles
Alteration in bowel elimination—incontinence or constipation related to loss of voluntary muscle control and immobility
Impaired physical mobility related to loss of spinal nerve innervation
Self-care deficit in feeding, bathing/hygiene, dressing/grooming, or toileting related to loss of voluntary muscle control
Disturbance in self-concept (body image, self-esteem, role performance, or personal identity) related to loss of self-care abilities
Sensory perceptual tactile alteration related to loss of sensory innervation
Sexual dysfunction related to effects of spinal cord injury.
Potential impairment of skin integrity related to decreased sensory perception and immobility
Alteration in peripheral tissue perfusion related to vasomotor instability
Alteration in patterns of urinary elimination related to loss of voluntary bladder control
Ineffective individual or family coping related to irreversible effects of spinal cord injury and disability
Knowledge deficit related to nature and treatment of spinal cord injury

Expected outcomes
Patient will maintain adequate oxygen and carbon dioxide exchange and not develop atelectasis or pneumonia.
Patient will reestablish a regular pattern of bowel elimination through a bowel training program.
Patient will not develop complications related to decreased mobility.
Patient will be independent in the activities of daily living to the extent possible with level of injury, using appropriate assistive devices.
Patient will integrate body changes resulting from injury into an altered but positive view of self and have appropriate life goals.
Patient will receive sufficient meaningful stimuli to compensate for sensory perceptual losses of the injury.
Patient will not experience skin breakdown.
Patient will receive counseling concerning sexual gratification within limitations of the injury.
Patient will achieve vascular stability with adequate peripheral tissue perfusion.
Patient will establish a pattern of urinary elimination consistent with the level of spinal damage.
Patient and family will be assisted to develop effective patterns of communicating their fears and frustrations and effectively plan for the future.
Patient and family will be knowledgeable about skills and equipment necessary to handle postdischarge care effectively.

Nursing interventions
Immediate period
Maintain realignment and stabilization of the spinal column, using halo traction, Crutchfield tongs, or other devices.
Avoid any head flexion if cervical injury exists.
Log roll patient to prevent twisting of spine.
Assess respiratory adequacy frequently: provide appropriate care for intubated patient requiring respiratory assistance.
Administer medications as prescribed.
Observe for vasomotor instability (spinal shock):
  Assess vital signs frequently.
Change positions slowly.
Assess for resolution paralytic ileus.
Begin intermittent catheterization routine and institute bowel program.
Record accurate intake and output.
Observe for signs of stress ulcer.
Initiate meticulous skin care program.
Begin range of motion exercise if permitted.
Rehabilitation
Avoid complications of decreased mobility.
  Put TED stockings on patient
  Teach patient pressure release exercises (wheel-

chair push-ups) and importance of frequent skin inspection.

Encourage participation in physical therapy exercise program.

Encourage deep breathing, use incentive spirometer for patients with thoracic and cervical injuries.

Institute bowel program.

Provide adequate or increased fluid and roughage in diet.

Use stool softeners, suppositories, digital stimulation

Maintain schedule and keep accurate records.

Institute bladder retraining if possible.

Use Credé maneuver and massage.

Teach catheterization techniques to patient or family member.

Teach importance of maintaining an acid urine, high fluid intake, and acting promptly if appearance or smell of urine changes.

Assist patient to improve self-care capacities.

Teach use of appropriate assistive devices.

Teach transfer techniques and wheelchair safety.

Encourage family involvement in techniques of care.

Be alert to occurrence of autonomic dysreflexia in patients with cervical injury (see box on this page).

Provide patient with accurate information about sexual capacities and fertility specific to level of injury.

Encourage expression of feelings.

Encourage and support all efforts by patient and family to cope with injury and communicate effectively about needs for today and planning for the future.

Support grief resolution.

Initiate contact with appropriate community services.

Evaluation

Patient is free of atelectasis or pneumonia, practices deep breathing and coughing regularly.

Patient maintains a pattern of regular bowel elimination, can insert suppositories, and demonstrates correct digital stimulation.

Patient maintains full range of motion in all joints.

Patient has achieved maximal ability in self-care possible with level of injury.

Patient has integrated body and life-style changes of injury and speaks positively of self and the future.

Patient compensates appropriately for absent sensory stimuli.

Patient maintains an intact skin and can demonstrate appropriate pressure release exercises and inspection.

Patient possesses factual data about the impact of the injury on sexual gratification and is able to ventilate feelings.

Patient has stable peripheral perfusion and knows how to recognize and correct autonomic dysreflexia.

Patient maintains regular urinary elimination through intermittent catheterization or Credé emptying methods.

AUTONOMIC DYSREFLEXIA

Autonomic dysreflexia occurs in patients with injuries above T_6, most commonly with cervical damage. It represents a condition in which there are grossly exaggerated autonomic responses to simple visceral stimuli.

SIGNS AND SYMPTOMS

Paroxysmal hypertension to malignant levels
Bradycardia
Severe throbbing headache
Diaphoresis
Gooseflesh

INTERVENTIONS

The most effective intervention is to decrease the stimuli: A full bowel or bladder is the most common stimulus.

Place patient in sitting position if permitted.

Check catheter for patency.

Catheterize if a prolonged interval.

Check rectum for impaction.

If interventions are ineffective, it may be necessary to administer potent vasodilator or ganglionic blocking agent to reduce blood pressure.

Patient and family are able to express feelings and fears honestly and are making appropriate plans together for future care.

Patient and family are knowledgeable about equipment and skills needed for care and are in touch with appropriate community services.

BIBLIOGRAPHY

Carlson, C.: Psychological aspects of neurologic disability, Nurs. Clin. North Am. **15:**309-320, 1980.

Connolly, R., *et al.:* Update: head injury, J. Neurosurg. Nurs. **13:**195-201, 1981.

Garrett, E.: Parkinsonism: forgotten considerations in medical treatment and nursing care, J. Neurosurg. Nurs. **14:**13-18, 1982.

Hollans, N., *et al.:* Overview of multiple sclerosis and nursing care of the multiple sclerosis patient, J. Neurosurg. Nurs. **14:**28-33, 1982.

Johnson, L.: If your patient has increased intracranial pressure; your goal should be no surprises, Nursing 83 **15:**58-64, 1983.

Jones, C.: Glasgow coma scale, Am. J. Nurs. **79:**1551-1553, 1979.

Loen, M., and Snyder, M.: Psychosocial aspects of care of the long-term comatose patient, J. Neurosurg. Nurs. **11:**235-237, 1979.

Martin, N., *et al.:* Comprehensive rehabilitation nursing, New York, 1981, McGraw-Hill Book Co.

Mauss-Clum, N.: Bringing the unconscious patient back safely—nursing makes the critical difference, J. Neurosurg. Nurs. **14:**32-43, 1982.

Monson, R.: Autonomic dysreflexia: a nursing challenge, Rehabil. Nurs. **6:**18-19, 1981.

Norman, E., *et al.:* Seizure disorders, Am. J. Nurs. **81:**983-1000, 1981.

Polhopek, M.: Stroke: an update on vascular disease, J. Neurosurg. Nurs. **12:**81-87, 1980.

Woodward, E.: The total patient: implications for nursing care of the epileptic, J. Neurosurg. Nurs. **14:**166-169, 1982.

Young, M.: A bedside guide to understanding the signs of increased intracranial pressure, Nursing 81 **11:**59-62, 1981.

NURSING CARE PLAN

CEREBROVASCULAR ACCIDENT

Nursing Diagnoses	Expected Patient Outcomes	Nursing Interventions
Alteration in cerebral tissue perfusion related to vascular thromboses or hemorrhage	Patient will experience increased blood flow to the brain and will not develop further damage	1. Assess vital signs and level of consciousness at frequent intervals during first 2 days; report increased temperature, slowing of pulse and respiration, and deepening of coma. 2. Maintain patent airway and administer prescribed oxygen. 3. Maintain fluid intake at prescribed level; avoid overhydration which may lead to cerebral edema. 4. Give prescribed medications to prevent further cerebral thromboses, hemorrhage or edema or to prevent seizures. 5. Provide rest and a quiet environment initially.
Potential for injury related to diminished or absent protective reflexes	Patient's eyes remain moist and unscratched Patient maintains full range of motion in all joints Patient's lung fields are clear to auscultation	1. Protect eye on affected side, if necessary, by keeping cornea moist (such as with artificial tears) and covering with eye shield; give eye care every 2 to 4 hours as necessary. 2. Position patient with limbs in normal anatomic position; use counterpositioning: shoulder abducted, elbow slightly flexed, hand and foot in dorsiflexion, leg and knee in neutral position with hip in slight internal rotation. 3. Change patient's position every 2 hours; turn onto the unaffected side, and into prone position, if possible. 4. Keep head flat or slightly elevated. 5. Perform passive or active ROM to all extremities several times a day. 6. Apply elastic stockings and keep legs elevated when patient sits up in a chair.
Potential impairment of skin integrity related to decreased mobility	Patient's skin remains intact	1. Monitor pressure areas for signs of skin breakdown. 2. Use turning sheet when changing patient's position every 2 hours to prevent shearing effect on skin. 3. Encourage patient to assist in turning self as able. 4. Use preventive measures for pressure areas. 5. If patient is incontinent, monitor frequently and keep bed pads clean and dry at all times; wash and dry perineal area as needed.
Alteration in nutrition less than body requirements related to decreased swallowing and self-care abilities	Patient takes in required nutrients and maintains stable weight	1. Provide intravenous fluids and tube feedings as prescribed during initial period. 2. Assess ability to swallow before initiating oral feedings. 3. Position patient with head elevated and turned to unaffected side when feeding patient. 4. Provide foods initially that are easier to swallow (soft or pureed foods, except for mashed potatoes). Avoid clear liquids.

NURSING CARE PLAN

CEREBROVASCULAR ACCIDENT—cont'd

Nursing Diagnoses	Expected Patient Outcomes	Nursing Interventions
Alteration in nutrition—cont'd		5. Use training cup or feeding syringe for fluids, as necessary. 6. Inspect mouth for food trapped in cheek pockets. Teach patient to use tongue to clear food from paralyzed side of mouth. 7. Be patient when feeding patient and provide directions for swallowing, as needed. 8. Encourage wearing of dentures. 9. Encourage patient to feed self as soon as able; provide self-help devices as necessary. 10. Assess food/fluid intake and offer supplementary feedings as needed.
Impaired physical mobility related to muscle weakness or paralysis	Patient maintains adequate muscle tone and achieves maximal independence in ambulation	1. Encourage active range of motion exercises, including exercise of unaffected limbs. 2. Encourage patient to move self in bed as able. 3. Teach patient how to sit up on side of bed and to transfer to chair when permitted. 4. Support activities initiated by physical therapy. 5. Encourage ambulation when possible and provide support. 6. Provide good shoe support for transfer and ambulation.
Self-care deficit in hygiene, dressing, and grooming related to muscle weakness and paralysis	Patient achieves independence in the activities of daily living	1. Provide basic ADL needs as necessary during initial period but encourage patient to begin to participate at ability level. 2. Transfer all self-care activities to unaffected side. 3. Provide sufficient time for ADL. 4. Meet with physical therapist and occupational therapist to optimize patient's learning needs. 5. Facilitate use of self-help devices, as needed.
Alteration in patterns of urinary elimination related to disruption of normal voluntary control	Patient will achieve urinary continence	1. Monitor urinary output and signs of retention or incontinence. 2. Assure patient that urinary problems will probably improve. 3. Provide catheter care if retention catheter is needed initially. 4. Offer bedpan or urinal after meals and at regular intervals. 5. Provide fluids to maximum amount prescribed; provide greater amounts before 4:00 P.M. 6. Use disposable pants or external urinary system as indicated.
Alteration in bowel elimination—constipation related to interruption of voluntary motor control	Patient will establish a regular pattern of bowel elimination	1. Monitor frequency and characteristics of stool; note time of defecation. 2. Monitor for fecal impaction every 3 to 4 days. 3. Assure patient that control of defecation may be achieved. 4. Give prescribed stool softener or suppositories. 5. Place patient on bedpan or commode after meals and at times noted for incontinence. 6. Caution patient not to strain at defecation.

Continued.

NURSING CARE PLAN

CEREBROVASCULAR ACCIDENT—cont'd

Nursing Diagnoses	Expected Patient Outcomes	Nursing Interventions
Impaired verbal communication related to expressive or receptive aphasia	Patient will successfully communicate with staff and family	1. Speak slowly and distinctly. 2. Phrase questions that can be answered by yes or no (or by appropriate signals). 3. Try to anticipate patient needs. 4. Provide call signal within reach of unaffected hand. 5. Begin speech therapy as soon as possible. 6. Encourage patient to verbalize and practice speech.
Sensory perceptual alteration (visual, kinesthetic) related to cerebral hypoxia	Patient will gradually compensate for sensory perceptual deficits	1. Place patient in multibed environment. 2. Suggest family bring some familiar objects, such as pictures. Keep objects within patient's visual field. 3. Place patient's bed so that people approach from side of intact vision. 4. Provide a constant routine. 5. Provide diversional activities. 6. Assist patient to maintain correct posture.
Potential for ineffective individual and family coping related to the physical and mental changes from the CVA	Patient and family will adjust to the residual disabilities and make appropriate plans for care after discharge	1. Provide information about condition and probable progress toward increased function. 2. Explain that emotional lability is part of the disorder and that improvement will be noted. 3. Explain patient's behavior to family/friends and encourage them to visit and interact with patient. 4. Give family/friends opportunities to share their concerns to be more supportive of patient. 5. Encourage family to maintain previous role relationships, as possible. 6. Identify patient's strengths and resources. 7. Explore need for assistance from community services.

CHAPTER 5

Disorders of the Eyes and Ears

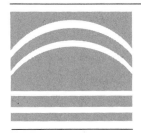

Vision and hearing contribute immeasurably to our understanding and enjoyment of the environment. When the eyes or ears are threatened or impaired, nursing care is directed toward preserving function, helping people meet their basic needs, strengthening support systems, and encouraging effective coping.

The major disorders of the eye affecting adults are infections, glaucoma, cataracts, and retinal detachment. Disorders of the ear are usually classified according to outer, middle, or inner ear problems. Figure 5-1 shows a horizontal section through the left eyeball.

EYE INFECTION/INFLAMMATION

Infection and inflammation can occur in any of the eye structures and may be caused by microorganisms, mechanical irritation, or sensitivity. There are more than 1 million cases of eye inflammation annually, two thirds of which are conjunctivitis. Table 5-1 describes common inflammations involving the eye.

Pathophysiology
Most eye inflammations are relatively benign, self-limiting disorders that respond promptly to local therapy and antibiotics. They create discomfort and minor interruption of function from the inflammatory response, but resolve without permanent effect. Refer to Table 5-1 for common signs and symptoms.

Medical Management
Standard medical interventions include warm compresses, topical or systemic antibiotics, and patching if eye rest is needed. Refer to Table 5-1 for specific therapies. Table 5-2 lists commonly prescribed ophthalmic drugs and their uses.

Nursing Management
Assessment—subjective
History and progression of symptoms
Patient's complaints of itching, tearing, pain, or photophobia (light sensitivity)

Assessment—objective
Presence of redness or discharge, crusts
Blepharospasm (spasmodic blinking)
Eyelid edema

Nursing diagnoses
Diagnoses vary slightly based on nature and severity of inflammation but will usually include the following:
Alteration in comfort—pain and itching related to infectious process
Actual or potential alteration in visual sensory perception related to presence of infection
Knowledge deficit related to development of infection and proper treatment techniques

Expected outcomes
Patient will experience decreased discomfort.
Inflammation will heal without complications.
Patient's visual perception will return to preinflammation levels.
Patient will institute proper treatment and follow measures to prevent reinfection.

Nursing interventions
Apply warm or cold compresses as prescribed:
　Warm: comforts, cleanses eye, and promotes healing
　Cold: controls itching and edema
The box on p. 62 lists guidelines for the use of eye compresses
Provide eye pads if ordered to relieve photophobia and protect the eye.

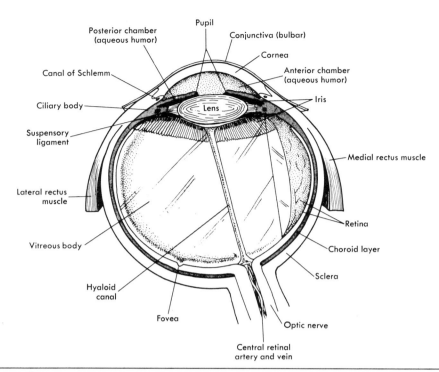

FIGURE 5-1 Horizontal section through left eyeball. (From Long, B.C., and Phipps, W.J.: Essentials of medical-surgical nursing: a nursing process approach, St. Louis, 1985, The C.V. Mosby Co.)

TABLE 5-1 Inflammations of the eye

Disorder	Description	Signs and Symptoms	Medical Therapy
Hordeolum (sty)	Staphylococcus infection of gland at eyelid margin	Localized abscess at base of eyelash, edema of lid, pain	Hot compresses to hasten pointing of abscess, topical antibiotic
Chalazion	Cyst from obstruction of sebaceous gland at eyelid margin	Initially, edema and discomfort; later, painless mass in lid	Warm compresses and topical antibiotic initially; surgical removal if cyst becomes large and presses on cornea
Blepharitis	Inflammation of lid margins, usually by staphylococci	Itching, redness, pain of lid, lacrimation, photophobia; crusting ulceration; lids become glued together during sleep	Warm compresses followed by erythromycin or bacitracin eye ointment; steroid eye drops may be prescribed
Conjunctivitis (pink eye)	Inflammation of conjunctiva by viruses, bacteria (highly infectious), allergy, trauma (sunburn)	Redness of conjunctiva, lid edema, crusting discharge on lids and cornea of eye; itching with allergies	Cleansing of lids and lashes, warm compresses; topical antibiotics; steroid eye drops for allergies (contraindicated for herpes simplex virus); no eye patch
Keratitis	Inflammation of cornea by bacteria, herpes simplex virus, allergies, vitamin A deficiency	Severe eye pain, photophobia, tearing, blepharospasm, loss of vision if uncontrolled	Warm compresses; topical antibiotics for bacterial infections; atropine sulfate; Idoxuridine for herpes simplex; eye patch, rest; corneal grafting if cornea injured
Corneal ulcer	Necrosis of corneal tissue from trauma, inflammation; may be superficial or may penetrate deeper tissue	Pain and blepharospasm may occur; ulcer may be outlined by fluorescein dye	Superficial ulcer: antibiotic eye drops, eye patch. Deep ulcer: topical and systemic antibiotics, atropine sulfate, warm compresses, eye patch; cautery; corneal transplant if necessary

From Long, B.C., and Phipps, W.J.: Essentials of medical-surgical nursing: a nursing process approach, St. Louis, 1985, The C.V. Mosby Co.

TABLE 5-2 Commonly used ophthalmic drugs

Drug	Action	Uses
Mydriatics		
Phenylephrine (Neo-Synephrine)	Dilate pupil	Examination of interior of eye
Epinephrine bitartrate (Epitrate)		Prevent adhesions of iris with cornea in eye inflammations
Cycloplegics		
Atropine sulfate (Atropisol, Isopto-Atropine)	Dilate pupil	Decrease pain and photophobia and provide rest for inflammations of iris and ciliary body and for diseases of cornea
Cyclopentolate (Cyclogyl)	Paralyze ciliary muscle and iris	
Homatropine (Isopto-Homatropine)		
Scopolamine hydrobromide		Eye examinations
Tropicamide (Mydriacyl)		
Miotics		
Pilocarpine (Pilocel, Ocusert)	Constrict pupil	Treat glaucoma
Carbachol (Carbacel)	Permit better drainage of intra-ocular fluid	
Physostigmine (Eserine)		
Demecarium bromide (Humorsol)		
Osmotic Agents		
Mannitol (Osmitrol) (IV)	Decrease intraocular pressure	Treat acute glaucoma
Glycerin (Glyrol, Osmoglyn) (PO)		Eye surgery
Urea (Urevert, Ureaphil) (IV)		
Topical Anesthetics		
Proparacaine (Ophthaine, Ophthetic, Alcaine)	Decrease sensation (pain)	Surgery, treatments
Lidocaine (Xylocaine)		Treat eye inflammations
Topical Antibiotics		
Polysporin (Polymyxin B, bacitracin)	Anti-infective	Treat eye inflammations
Neosporin (Polymyxin B, neomycin, bacitracin)		
Bacitracin		
Idoxuridine (IDU)		
Gentamicin sulfate (Garamycin)		
Chloramphenicol (Chloromycetin, Chloroptic)		
Steroids		
Prednisone	Anti-inflammatory	Treat eye inflammations and allergic reactions
Prednisolone		
Methylprednisolone (Depo-Medrol)		
Triamcinolone (Aristocort)		
Dexamethasone (Decadron)		
Fluorometholone		

Modified from Long, B.C., and Phipps, W.J.: Essentials of medical-surgical nursing: a nursing process approach, St. Louis, 1985, The C.V. Mosby Co. and Phipps, W.J., Long, B.C., and Woods, N.F.: Medical-surgical nursing: concepts and clinical practice, ed. 2, St. Louis, 1983, The C.V. Mosby Co.

ALERT: Eye pads must not be used if bacterial infection is present as they enhance bacterial growth.

Administer prescribed eye medications.

Each patient must have and use own eye drops and ointments to prevent cross-infection; use separate bottles for each eye. The box on p. 62 describes the proper instillation of eye drops and ointments.

Administer eye irrigations if prescribed to remove secretions or foreign body. The box on p. 62 describes proper sequence for eye irrigation.

Teach patient to avoid touching either eye while infection is present.

Evaluation

Patient's infection resolves without complication or loss of vision.

Patient's discomfort has resolved.

Patient can demonstrate proper technique for applying compresses, irrigating the eye, or instilling eye medications.

GUIDELINES FOR APPLICATION OF MOIST EYE COMPRESSES

GENERAL PRINCIPLES
Use aeseptic technique if infection is present.
If bilateral infection, use separate equipment for each.
Wash hands thoroughly before and after soaks.
If bilateral infection, wash hands between treatments of eyes.

WARM COMPRESSES
Temperature should not exceed 120° F (49° C).
A clean, fresh washcloth is effective for use in the house.
Never reuse cloth for a second treatment.
Carefully handle and dispose of infected materials.

COLD COMPRESSES
Rubber glove or plastic bag packed with ice chips may be used as disposable compress.

GUIDELINES FOR INSTILLING EYE MEDICATIONS

EYEDROPS
1. Wash hands before touching eyes.
2. Clean eyes before instilling eye drops if crusting or discharge is present.
3. Ask patient to tilt head back and look up.
4. Evert lower lid by pulling down gently on skin below eye.
5. Approach eye by bringing dropper tip in from side, not directly from front.
6. Place drops on *center* of conjunctival sac of lower lid: Avoid touching eye.
7. Ask patient not to squeeze eye shut (to prevent loss of medication down cheek).
8. Provide patient with a tissue.

OINTMENT
1. Follow steps 1 through 4 above.
2. Place the ointment from tube directly onto exposed conjunctival sac.
3. Avoid touching eye with tube.

GUIDELINES FOR EYE IRRIGATIONS

1. Place patient lying toward one side to prevent fluid from flowing into other eye.
2. Direct the irrigating fluid along the conjunctiva from the *inner* to the outer canthus.
3. Avoid directing a forceful stream onto eyeball or touching any eye structure.
4. A piece of gauze may be wrapped around index finger to raise upper lid for better cleaning if heavy discharge exists.

GLAUCOMA

The term *glaucoma* refers to an eye disease characterized by increased intraocular pressure associated with progressive loss of peripheral vision. Permanent vision loss is preventable with early detection. Glaucoma occurs in middle-aged and older adults and accounts for 12% to 15% of all blindness in the United States.

Pathophysiology
In the normal eye there is a balance between the production and drainage of aqueous humor, permitting a stable intraocular pressure. In glaucoma, obstruction to the drainage of aqueous humor increases the intraocular pressure and produces damage to the optic nerve.

Chronic simple (wide angle) glaucoma, a common form of the disease, takes a slow and insidious course, resulting from degenerative changes.

Acute (narrow angle) glaucoma is the result of an abrupt change in the angle of the iris and causes dramatic symptoms and rapid loss of vision.

Medical Management
Acute glaucoma is a medical emergency since irreversible blindness may occur in 24 to 36 hours. Treatment includes the following:
Miotics to constrict pupil and facilitate drainage
Carbonic anhydrase inhibitors (Diamox) to decrease production of fluid
Surgery to correct iris obstruction (iridectomy)
Chronic simple glaucoma is treated by early detection and lowering of intraocular pressure through the use of:
Miotics
Carbonic anhydrase inhibitors
Surgery is performed in some cases to provide a permanent filtration pathway for aqueous humor (trabeculectomy, sclerotomy)
Table 5-3 lists drugs used in the treatment of glaucoma.

Nursing Management
Assessment—subjective (chronic glaucoma)
Patient's complaints of
Loss of peripheral vision (tunnel vision)
Dull eye pain, especially in morning
Difficulty adjusting to darkness
Halos seen around lights

Assessment—objective
Need for frequent eyeglass prescription changes
Elevated intraocular pressure

TABLE 5-3 Drugs used in treatment of glaucoma

Drug	Form
Cholinergic Drugs (Miotics)	
Pilocarpine (Pilocel, Ocusert)	0.5%–3% solution
Carbachol (Carbacel)	0.25%–3% solution
Cholinesterase Inhibitors (Miotics)	
Physostigmine (Eserine)	0.25%–1% solution or ointment
Isoflurophate (DFP) (Floropryl)	0.01%–0.1% solution
Demecarium bromide (Humorsol)	0.125%–0.25% solution
Echothiophate iodide (Phospho-line iodide)	0.06%–0.125% solution
Adrenergic Agents	
Epinephryl borate (Eppy)	0.5%–1% solution
Epinephrine hydrochloride (Glaucon)	0.5%–2% solution
Epinephrine bitartrate (Epitrate)	2% solution
Carbonic Anhydrase Inhibitors	
Acetazolamide (Diamox)	125–250 mg tablets 500 mg capsules, sequential 500 mg vials for IM or IV use
Erthoxyzolamide (Cardrase)	125–250 mg tablets
Dichlorphenamide (Daranide)	25–50 mg tablets
Methazolamide (Neptazane)	25–50 mg tablets
Osmotic Agents	
Glycerin (glycerin, Osmoglyn, Ophthalgan)	Mix with equal amount of orange juice (oral)
Mannitol (Osmitrol)	10%–20% solution for IV use
Urea (Ureaphil, Urevert)	30% solution for IV use
Beta-Adrenergic Blocker	
Timolol maleate (Timoptic)	0.25%–0.5% solution

From Phipps, W.J., Long, B.C., and Woods, N.F.: Medical-surgical nursing: concepts and clinical practice, ed. 2, St. Louis, 1983, The C.V. Mosby Co.

Assessment—acute

Patient's complaints of
    Severe eye pain
    Nausea and vomiting
    Blurred vision
    Acutely increased intraocular pressure

Nursing diagnoses

Diagnoses will depend on the stage and acuity of the disease but commonly include the following:

Alteration in comfort—eye pain related to elevated intraocular pressure

Alteration in visual sensory perception related to decreasing peripheral vision

Knowledge deficit related to the disease process of glaucoma and the drugs used to control it

Expected outcomes

Patient will be free of eye pain.

Patient will experience no further loss of visual sensory perception.

Patient will understand the disease process of glaucoma and be able to describe drugs used in its treatment and how to administer them.

Nursing interventions

Administer prescribed medications.

Teach patient safe and correct use of eye drops (refer to box on p. 62).

If surgery is performed, provide standard postoperative eye surgery care and teaching.

(Acute glaucoma) Apply cold compresses and administer analgesics as prescribed.

Teach patient need for regular eye drop administration and need for regular medical follow up.

Evaluation

Patient reports no eye pain.

Patient's visual status has stabilized; patient practices safety measures to compensate for diminished peripheral vision.

Patient can discuss long term irreversible nature of the disease; can discuss purpose and side effects of medications ordered; can demonstrate safe and correct eye drop administration.

CATARACT

A cataract is a clouding or opacity of the lens that leads to gradual painless blurring of vision and loss of sight. The most common cause of cataracts is aging; 85% of persons over age 80 have some lens clouding. Cataracts are also associated with injury. They can be present at birth, and can be secondary to other eye disease.

Pathophysiology

Cataracts develop as the result of alterations in metabolism and the movement of nutrients within the lens. Persons with diabetes tend to develop cataracts at an earlier age because of an accumulation of sorbitol.

Light rays are unable to pass through the opaque lens to the retina.

Medical Management

Operative treatment is the only effective management of cataracts. Surgeons no longer wait for cataracts to ripen but intervene when visual loss interferes with activities of daily living. There are numerous approaches to cataract removal. The box below lists some of the current procedures.

Nursing Management

Assessment—subjective

Patient's report of painless loss of vision occurring over a period of years

Assessment—objective

Visible opacity of the lens, unilateral or bilateral

Nursing diagnoses

Alteration in visual sensory perception related to decreased stimulus access to the retina

Potential for injury related to decreasing vision

Expected outcomes

Patient will not experience injury during period of failing vision.

Patient will experience improved vision following surgery.

Patient will not suffer postoperative complications.

Nursing interventions

Preoperative

Assess patient's vision in unaffected eye.

Ensure that patient understands nature of procedure and use of local anesthesia, and any postoperative care routines.

Encourage patient to discuss fears related to eye surgery.

APPROACHES TO CATARACT REMOVAL

TYPES

Intracapsular extraction—removal of the entire lens
Extracapsular extraction—removal of lens material without disturbing the membrane capsule

TECHNIQUES

Phacoemulsification—insertion of an instrument that uses ultrasonic vibration to break up lens material for removal by irrigation
Cryoextraction—cataract lifted out by adhering lens to a sub-zero probe

---

Postoperative

Avoid activities that increase intraocular pressure:
Squeezing shut the eyelids
Bending over at the waist
Straining for lifting, coughing, defecation
NOTE: Surgeons vary on strictness of activity restrictions.
Maintain a safe environment:
Encourage patient to lie on back or unaffected side.
Use eye shield at night.
Organize self-care articles on unaffected side.
Be alert to complaints of severe pain or pressure that may indicate complications.
Assist with activities of daily living as needed.
Teach patient about corrective lenses to be used during rehabilitation and associated safety concerns:
Cataract lenses magnify objects by about 20% to 25%, distance is distorted, which affects reaching for objects and using stairs
Cataract lenses distort peripheral vision: patient has clear vision straight ahead and must turn head from side to side to compensate.
Cataract lenses are heavy (plastic much less so), pressure sores can occur on nose and ears.
Colors may appear distorted.
Contact lenses improve the degree of vision correction.
NOTE: If an intraocular lens is implanted during surgery, glasses or contact lenses may not be required after surgery.

Evaluation

Patient has not been injured during postoperative period.
Patient experiences gradual improvement of vision.
Patient makes successful adaptation to the distortions of cataract lenses and moves about safely in the environment.

RETINAL DETACHMENT

Retinal detachment occurs when the two retinal layers separate because of either fluid accumulation or contraction of the vitreous body. Usually there is no apparent cause but detachment can be caused by sudden severe physical exertion, lens loss (as after cataract surgery), degenerative changes of myopia, hemorrhage, or tumor.

Pathophysiology

Detachment interrupts the transmission of visual images from the retina to the optic nerve, causing progressive loss of vision to complete blindness.

Medical Management

Early surgery is the treatment of choice. Accumulated fluid is drained from the subretinal space. Inflammation is induced—by diathermy, photocoagulation, laser beam, or subfreezing temperatures—in order to stimulate adhesion formation.

Scleral buckling is also used to splint and hold the retina and choroid together.

Nursing Management
Assessment—subjective
Patient's complaints of
> Floating spots or flashing lights
> Progressive constriction of vision in one area
> Sensation of "curtain being drawn" across the eye (if tear is acute and extensive)

Nursing diagnoses
Anxiety related to loss of vision and uncertain outcome
Potential for injury related to eye patching
Altered visual sensory perception related to decreased vision or eye patching

Expected outcomes
Patient will experience manageable levels of anxiety and feel positive about outcomes of surgery.
Patient will not experience injury.
Patient's vision will improve.

Nursing interventions
Preoperative
Maintain patient on bed rest with eyes covered.
Position head with retinal tear in lowest portion of eyes.
Use side rails, place call bell within easy reach.
Encourage patient to discuss fears—provide correct information about surgery and outcomes.
Assist patient to avoid disorientation while eyes are patched:
> Visit frequently.
> Provide radio or TV for time orientation.

Postoperative
Position patient in bed as ordered by physician.
Restrict activities as ordered:
> Maintain bed rest 1 to 2 days.
> Avoid jerking movements of head, such as sneezing or hair combing.
Assist patient with activities of daily living as indicated by activity restriction.
Provide teaching about gradual resumption of activities and symptoms indicating possible redetachment.

Evaluation
Patient has been able to cope adequately with injury and outcome.

Patient safely completes activities of daily living during period of diminished vision.
Patient's vision improves.
Patient can discuss activity restrictions to be followed in the postdischarge period.

EAR INFECTION/INFLAMMATION

Ear infections may occur at any age and in any portion of the ear. They are common health problems. The possibility of serious complications following ear infection makes prompt identification and treatment important. Table 5-4 lists common infections of the ear. Figure 5-2 shows the external auditory canal, middle ear, and inner ear.

Pathophysiology
The pathophysiology of ear infections is related to the specific structures involved and basically results from local tissue inflammatory responses to bacteria or viruses. Pain is a common symptom. External and middle ear infections may cause drainage, itching, and redness. Some diminished hearing frequently accompanies these inflammations. Inner ear problems may affect balance by disturbing the vestibular system.

Medical Management
Standard medical interventions include systemic antibiotics and topical ear drops. Surgical intervention includes mastoidectomy, myringotomy, insertion of ventilation tubes, and tympanoplasty.

Nursing Management
Assessment—subjective
Patient complaints of:
> Pain or itching in ear
> Sense of fullness in ear
> Tinnitus (ringing in the ear) or roaring sound
> Vertigo
Assessment—objective
Decreased hearing
Fever
Redness, drainage, scaling

Nursing diagnoses
Diagnoses will depend on exact nature and severity of ear inflammation. Common diagnoses include the following:
> Alteration in comfort—pain and itching related to pressure and inflammation in the ear.
> Potential for injury related to vertigo and diminished hearing.
> Alteration in auditory sensory perception related to disruption of auditory conduction.

TABLE 5-4 Inflammations of the ear

Disorder	Description	Signs and Symptoms	Medical Therapy
External otitis	Inflammation of external ear; may be acute or chronic	Pain with movement of auricle, redness, scaling, itching, swelling, watery discharge, crusting of external ear	Application of astringents (Burow's solution), acidifiers (acetic acid), or antibiotics
Serous otitis media	Collection of sterile serum in middle ear; may be acute or chronic	Sense of fullness in ear, hearing loss, low-pitched tinnitus, earache	Removal of eustachian obstruction by aspiration or insertion of tubes for drainage
Acute purulent otitis media	Infection of middle ear, usually by pneumococci, streptococci, staphylococci, or *Haemophilus* influenza	Sense of fullness in ear, severe throbbing pain, hearing loss, tinnitus, fever	Antibiotics; if severe, bed rest, analgesics, nasal vasoconstrictors; myringotomy if necessary
Acute mastoiditis	Acute infection of middle ear with extension to adjacent mastoid process	Pain in ear and over mastoid, fever, headache, profuse discharge from ear, vertigo	Hospitalization with high doses of IV antibiotics, mastoidectomy
Chronic otitis media	Chronic inflammation of middle ear; sequela of acute otitis media	Deafness, occasional pain, dizziness, chronic discharge from ear	Local debridement, topical and systemic antibiotics; mastoidectomy and tympanoplasty may be necessary
Labyrinthitis	Inflammation of inner ear	Severe and sudden vertigo, nausea and vomiting, nystagmus, photophobia, headache, ataxic gait	No specific treatment; antibiotics; dimenhydrinate for vertigo; parenteral fluids if nausea and vomiting persist

From Long, B.C., and Phipps, W.J.: Essentials of medical-surgical nursing: a nursing process approach, St. Louis, 1985, The C.V. Mosby Co.

INSTILLATION OF EAR DROPS

1. Warm solution to body temperature—no more than 100° F (38° C). Vertigo can result from solutions that are too hot or too cold.
2. Have patient tilt head.
3. Straighten ear by pulling pinna up and back.
4. Instill drops to run along auditory canal wall.
5. Have patient hold position for 5 to 10 minutes.
6. Gently insert cotton into external auditory canal.

Expected outcomes
Patient will have decreased pain and discomfort.
Patient will compensate for vertigo and not experience injury.
Patient's hearing will improve.

Nursing interventions
Administer medications as ordered.
Teach patient correct technique for instilling ear drops (see box on p. 66).
Perform prescribed ear irrigations (see box on p. 66 and Figure 5-3).
If patient experiences vertigo, keep side rails up and supervise ambulation.

GUIDELINES FOR EAR IRRIGATION

NOTE: Avoid ear irrigation if
    Ear drum is punctured (increases inflammation).
    Attempting to remove foreign body (moisture may swell object).
1. Use tap water or normal saline; peroxide may be added to remove wax.
2. Warm solution to body temperature.
3. Straighten ear by pulling pinna up and back.
4. Use a steady stream of solution against roof of auditory canal.
5. Use gentle pressure; do not obstruct outflow with equipment.
6. Have patient lie on affected side after irrigation to promote drainage.

Teach patient about the nature of any planned surgery and the management of common symptoms such as nausea and vertigo.
Teach patient about preventive measures:
    Patient should avoid blowing nose or sneezing after surgery.
    After healing occurs patient should be taught to blow nose with both nostrils open and open mouth when sneezing.
    Patient should avoid frequent flying.

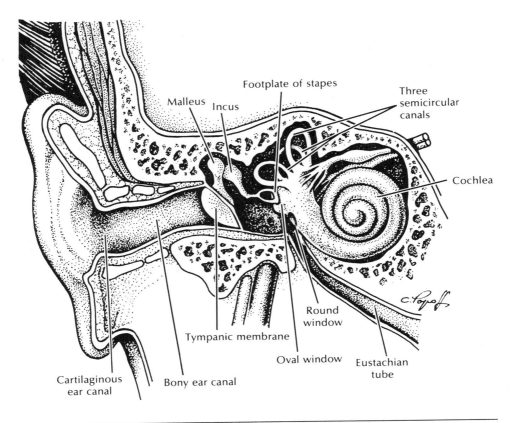

FIGURE 5-2 External auditory canal, middle ear, and inner ear. (From Malasanos, L., et al.: Health assessment, ed. 2, St. Louis, 1981, The C.V. Mosby Co.)

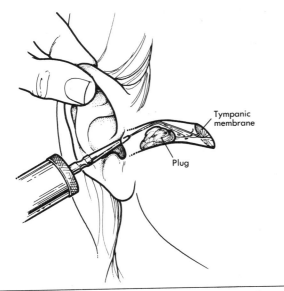

FIGURE 5-3 Irrigation of the external auditory canal.

Evaluation

Patient is free of pain and other annoying symptoms.

Patient has not fallen during periods of vertigo.

Patient's hearing has returned to preinfection levels; following surgery, patient's hearing has increased.

Patient can describe postdischarge routine and any measures appropriate for preventing reinfection.

OTOSCLEROSIS

Otosclerosis is a progressive condition in which the normal bone of the bony labyrinth in the ear is replaced by highly vascular spongy bone. It causes hearing loss by immobilizing the stapes. The cause is unknown; the disease occurs in young adulthood and seems to have a hereditary component.

Medical Management

Treatment of otosclerosis is surgical. Stapedectomy allows for removal of the stapes with prosthetic replacement.

Nursing Management

The nursing interventions after stapedectomy are similar to those for other types of ear surgery. Refer to the discussion of ear inflammations.

MENIERE'S DISEASE

Meniere's disease is a disorder of the inner ear that occurs most commonly in women between 50 and 60 years of age. Its cause is unknown. Usually several attacks occur yearly until the disease resolves spontaneously or progresses to complete deafness in the affected ear.

Pathophysiology
There is an increase of fluid in the cochlea, resulting from either increased production or decreased absorption, which increases the pressure within the labyrinth of the inner ear. This pressure produces attacks of severe vertigo, tinnitus, and progressive hearing loss. Usually only one ear is involved.

Medical Management
No medical treatment is entirely successful. Attempts are made to lower fluid pressure through oral fluid restriction, salt-free diet, and diuretics (thiazide or carbonic anhydrase inhibitors).

Antihistamines and antivertigo drugs such as dimenhydrinate (Dramamine) are used between attacks. IV administration of these drugs, plus atropine for its anticholinergic effects, is often needed during acute attacks. Surgical procedures may also be attempted to preserve hearing.

Nursing Management
Assessment—subjective
Patient complains of:
Episodes of vertigo (described as whirling sensation or room spinning, patient must lie down to keep from falling)
Nausea associated with vertigo
Tinnitus (buzzing sounds to painful loud ringing)
History of and patient's knowledge about disorder
Knowledge of circumstances that precipitate attack
Actions taken during attacks and degree of relief they provide

Assessment—objective
Unilateral or bilateral hearing loss
Vomiting, diaphoresis, or nystagmus during observed attack

Nursing diagnoses
Potential for injury related to severe vertigo
Alteration in auditory sensory perception related to progressive hearing loss
Self-care deficit related to inability to maintain an upright posture during attacks of vertigo
Knowledge deficit related to course and management of attacks

Expected outcomes
Patient will not experience injury during vertigo attacks.
Patient will experience sufficient disease control to maintain independence in the activities of daily living.

Patient's hearing loss will be minimized.
Patient will be knowledgeable concerning factors that precipitate or control attacks.

Nursing interventions
During attacks
Assist patient to meet hygiene needs as required.
Stand in front of patient to foster hearing and prevent head turning.
Encourage regular, slow position changes—try positioning patient on unaffected side.
Avoid use of bright or glaring lights.
Adjust diet to compensate for nausea or anorexia.
Keep side rails up.
Supervise position changes and all ambulation.
Administer medications as prescribed.
Preventing attacks
Teach use of low-salt diet and fluid limitations.
Patient should avoid reading when any vertigo or tinnitus is present.
Patient should avoid smoking.
Identify factors related to attacks, if possible.
Teach proper actions in case of attack:
If driving, patient should pull over and stop immediately.
If standing, patient should sit or lie down immediately.
Keep medications available at all times.

Evaluation
Patient successfully avoids injury during attacks.
Patient suffers minimal hearing loss and compensates appropriately for decreased perception.
Patient achieves sufficient disease control to maintain independence in the activities of daily living.
Patient can explain disease and its progress; discuss use of medications and side effects; describe diet and fluid restrictions to prevent attacks; and describe actions to take in case of an attack.

Bibliography

DeWeese, D.D., and Saunders, W.H.: Textbook of otolaryngology, ed. 6, St. Louis, 1982, The C.V. Mosby Co.
Gallagher, M.A.: Corneal transplantation, Am. J. Nurs. 81:1845, 1981.
How to test your patient's hearing acuity, Nurs. 80 10(7): 60-61, 1980.
Koch, K.H.: The deaf and hard of hearing: some hints, Nurs. Times 77(32):suppl 19-20, 1981.
Resler, M.M., and Tumulty, G.: Glaucoma update, Am. J. Nurs. 83:752-756, 1983.
Stern, E.J.: Helping the person with low vision, Am. J. Nurs. 80:1788-1790, 1980.
Wong, E.K., et al.: How ophthalmic drugs can fool you, RN 43:36-44, 1980.

NURSING CARE PLAN

PERSON WITH A RETINAL DETACHMENT

Nursing Diagnoses	Expected Patient Outcomes	Nursing Interventions

Alteration in visual sensory perception related to decreased vision of eye patching	Patients vision will be restored to predetachment level	1. Maintain prescribed activity restrictions.
		2. Position patient's head during initial period so that retinal tear is at lowest portion of eye.
		3. Assist patient with ADL within the activity limitations.
		4. If one eye has decreased vision and patient is restricted in movement:
		  a. Place bed such that patient is not facing wall and can see others approaching.
		  b. Place bedside table within patient's reach without need to turn head.
		5. If total vision is limited by eye patches or blurred vision:
		  a. Orient patient to temporal and physical surroundings.
		  b. Speak to patient when approaching and identify yourself.
		  c. Explain activities occurring in room.
		  d. Tell patient when you are leaving.

Potential for injury related to decreased vision	Patient will not experience injury during period of decreased vision	1. Keep side rails up if binocular patches are used postoperatively or vision is markedly reduced. 2. Keep call button within reach when patient is on bedrest. 3. Assist patient as necessary when ambulating after surgery if vision is still restricted, such as by eye patches.
Anxiety related to possible loss of vision	Patient will experience manageable levels of anxiety and verbalize concerns about pos-	1. Give patient opportunities to explore concerns about possible decreased vision. 2. Answer questions honestly. 3. Encourage realistic hope about maintaining vision as described by physician. 4. Explore patient's knowledge of disorder and planned therapy, and correct misunderstandings. 5. Explain rationale for activity restrictions (gravity may help detached portion of retina to fall back to normal position).
Knowledge deficit related to postoperative activity restrictions	Patient describes activity restrictions and medical follow-up	1. Teach patient to avoid jerking head (sneezing, coughing, vomiting). 2. Administer antiemetics or cough suppressants if necessary. 3. Teach patient about temporary restrictions to reading, sedentary work, and heavy activity (p. ●●●). 4. Teach patient to report signs of further retinal detachment.

NURSING CARE PLAN
MENIERE'S DISEASE

Nursing Diagnoses	Expected Patient Outcomes	Nursing Interventions
Anxiety related to effects of disorder	Patient will experience manageable levels of anxiety and verbalize concerns over prognosis.	1. Encourage patient to explore concerns about decreased hearing and dizziness attacks, and to take action related to the concerns. 2. Explore patient's knowledge of the disorder and correct misunderstandings. 3. Encourage realistic hope about expected hearing ability as described by physician. 4. Refer patient to necessary support services, such as social worker or audiologist.

Alteration in vestibular and auditory sensory perception related to fluid build-up in ear	Patient interacts with others accurately and experiences minimal hearing loss	1. If tinnitus is distressing, increase background noises such as music.
		2. If hearing is decreased:
		  a. Use measures to facilitate communication with hearing impaired.
		  b. Refer person to audiologist, if appropriate.

Potential for injury related to severe vertigo	Patient does not experience injury during attacks of vertigo	1. Keep side rails up when patient with dizziness is in bed. 2. Assist with ambulation as needed. 3. Encourage patient to sit or lie down and to remain immobile if signs of dizziness occur. 4. Encourage patient to move slowly and not turn head suddenly when dizziness is present. 5. Teach patient to stop car at side of road immediately at first signs of dizziness while driving.
Potential self-care deficit related to inability to maintain an upright posture	Patient will maintain independence in the activities of daily living	1. Provide desired foods and fluids if nausea is present. 2. Assist with hygiene as needed while encouraging independence; place hygiene supplies so that patient does not have to turn head. 3. Provide sufficient time for ADL so patient can move slowly.
Knowledge deficit related to the nature of the disorder and the management of attacks	Patient understands nature of disorder and factors that precipitate or control attacks	1. Teach patient about the disorder, therapy, and need for medical follow-up (see text). 2. Teach patient ways to protect self from injury and to prevent attacks of dizziness when possible. 3. Help patient to identify avoidable actions that precipitate dizziness attacks.

CHAPTER 6

Disorders of the Cardiovascular System

Cardiovascular diseases cause more deaths annually in the United States than all other diseases combined. This fact persists despite the steady decline in mortality that has occurred over the past several years. Over 40 million Americans have some form of heart or blood vessel disorder. This chapter will discuss coronary artery disease, congestive heart failure, inflammatory heart disease, valvular heart disease, and aneurysms. Figure 6-1 shows the circulation through the heart.

CORONARY ARTERY DISEASE

Coronary artery disease (CAD) is a general term used to describe conditions involving the coronary arteries and is the most significant of the cardiovascular disorders in terms of incidence and mortality. Extensive on-going research is aimed at identifying risk factors for the disease, especially those that are potentially modifiable, as well as at improving methods of treatment. The box on this page lists the major risk factors that have been associated with the development of CAD.

Pathophysiology

The exact cause of the atherosclerosis underlying most CAD is still unknown. The localized accumulation of lipids and fibrous tissue in the coronary arteries results in narrowing and possible occlusion. Vascular changes inhibit the ability of the arteries to dilate, thereby reducing blood flow to the myocardium. Symptoms are the result of imbalance between the supply and demand for oxygen by the myocardium. They tend to appear quite late. The two major manifestations are angina and myocardial infarction, with or without sudden death.

RISK FACTORS ASSOCIATED WITH CORONARY ARTERY DISEASE

NONMODIFIABLE RISK FACTORS
1. *Age.* Mortality with CAD rapidly increases with age.
2. *Sex.* Incidence of CAD in women is very low until after menopause.
3. *Race.* Non-white men and women experience higher mortality rates up to age 65.
4. *Family history.* A positive family history of CAD increases the risk.

MODIFIABLE RISK FACTORS
1. *Hyperlipoproteinemia.* Elevated cholesterol, triglyceride, and phospholipid levels are associated with development of CAD.
2. *Dietary patterns.* A diet chronically high in saturated fats, salt, refined sugar, and cholesterol is linked with CAD.
3. *Hypertension.* Elevated systolic or diastolic blood pressure often seems to accelerate atherosclerosis.
4. *Obesity.* Overweight individuals are more prone to develop associated risk factors.
5. *Cigarette smoking.* Relationship is unclear, but risk of death is 2 to 6 times greater in heavy smokers.
6. *Personality and life-style.* A sedentary life-style, chronic stress, and a hard-driving personality are often associated with CAD.

ANGINA

Angina is a chest pain resulting from temporary, reversible ischemia of the myocardium. Pain is usually retrosternal or substernal; it may radiate into neck, jaw, shoulder, or down left arm. It may be described as heaviness or tightness in chest. It is often precipitated by exercise, a heavy meal, exposure to cold, or strong emotion. Of short duration, it is usually relieved by rest or vasodilation.

Medical Management
Medical management includes:
    Control or elimination of modifiable risk factors

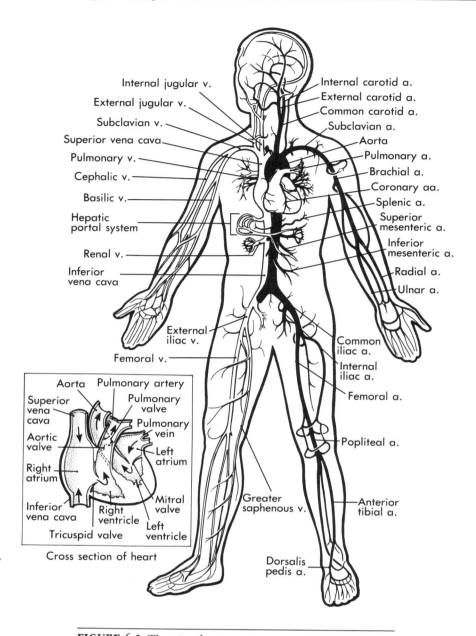

FIGURE 6-1 The circulatory system.

Elimination or spacing of precipitating factors
Administration of vasodilator medications (see Table 6-1)

Nursing Management
Assessment—subjective
History of the disease and its treatment
Pain pattern, severity
Precipitating factors
Medications in use, understanding of drugs
Diet and exercise patterns, occupation

Assessment—objective
Baseline vital signs
Weight

Nursing diagnoses
Diagnoses will depend on the severity of the disease but commonly include the following:
Activity intolerance related to occurrence of chest pain with exercise or exertion
Anxiety related to threat of pain and sudden death
Alteration in comfort—chest pain related to temporary myocardial ischemia
Knowledge deficit related to modification of risk factors, avoidance of precipitating factors, or diet and medications used to control anginal attacks.

Expected outcomes
Patient will appropriately space activities to continue usual life-style without attacks of pain.

TABLE 6-1 Drugs used in the management of angina

Drugs	Actions	Side Effects
Nitrites/Nitrates		
Nitroglycerin	Dilate coronary arteries and intercoronary collateral vessels	Postural hypotension
Isordil	Decrease peripheral resistance, systolic blood pressure, and	Burning sensation on tongue
Nitropaste	heart workload	Throbbing in head, flushing
		Headache
Beta-Adrenergic Blockers		
Inderal	Decrease myocardial oxygen demand by reducing heart rate,	Bradycardia (slowed heart beat)
Corgard	blood pressure, and myocardial contractility	Hypotension
Lopressor		Gastrointestinal complaints
Calcium Channel Blockers		
Nifedipine	Act at the cellular level to block movement of calcium ions,	Bradycardia
Diltiazem	thus reducing cardiac activity and workload of the heart	Hypotension
Verapamil	Decrease heart rate and act as potent vasodilators	
	Reduce coronary vasospasm	

Patient will feel less anxious through better control and management of the disease.

Patient will have fewer attacks of pain and will have pain relieved by vasodilator drugs.

Patient will assume knowledgeable control of life-style, appropriately modify diet patterns and exercise/activity routines, and will be able to discuss drugs used to control symptoms and their side effects.

Nursing interventions

Teach patient correct use of prescribed medications and their side effects (see Table 6-1 and box on this page).

Discuss with patient elimination of modifiable risk factors.

Plan diet for weight reduction.

Decrease patient's salt intake.

Modify patient's diet to decrease intake of cholesterol and saturated fats.

Eliminate cigarette smoking.

Maintain adequate control of hypertension if present.

Manage stress appropriately.

Explore modifications of patient's life-style to prevent pain attacks:

Patient should avoid physical and emotional overexertion.

Patient should avoid overeating, especially meals with red meat.

Patient should avoid prolonged exposure to climate extremes, dress appropriately and avoid extreme cold or hot, humid conditions.

Clarify with physician the resumption of regular planned exercise.

Discuss the use of nitroglycerin *prior* to planned exertion, such as exercise or sexual activity.

Emphasize need for ongoing medical management.

GUIDELINES FOR USING NITROGLYCERIN

SUBLINGUAL

Store tablets in tightly closed dark bottle; keep dry.

Sublingual administration causes burning sensation on the tongue.

Throbbing sensation in head and flushing sensation may be felt.

Make position changes slowly after taking nitroglycerin.

Use tablets prophylactically to avoid pain if known to occur with certain activities.

Take tablet at onset of pain and every 5 minutes if pain is unrelieved. Call physician if pain unrelieved after 3 to 4 tablets.

Always carry tablets.

Check expiration dates and be sure to obtain fresh supplies.

PASTES

Apply to any nonhairy area of skin.

Measure dose carefully with ruled papers.

Remove all old cream before applying new dose.

Evaluation

Patient is able to space daily activities to continue life-style without occurrence of pain.

Patient reports less anxiety as a result of decreased pain.

Vasodilator drugs keep patient free of pain.

Patient can describe effects of drugs, appropriate diet and activity, and signs and symptoms that indicate need to contact physician.

NOTE: Some patients with angina are candidates for coronary bypass surgery to shunt blood around the narrowed portions of the coronary arteries. Grafts from the saphenous vein or internal mammary artery are anastomosed from the ascending aorta to the coronary artery at a point distal to the obstruction. Care of the patient following heart surgery is discussed later in the chapter.

MYOCARDIAL INFARCTION

Myocardial infarction (MI) is caused by a sudden blockage of one of the branches of a coronary artery that interferes with the blood supply to a portion of the myocardium, producing ischemic death of tissue over a period of hours. It may cause sudden death or gradual scarring over of the necrotic area. The location and size of the infarct determine the consequences in terms of contractility and myocardial function.

Pathophysiology

Ischemia depresses cardiac function and triggers autonomic nervous system responses that worsen the imbalance between oxygen supply and demand. Ischemia that persists longer than 35 to 45 minutes produces permanent loss of contractile function in the area. Cardiogenic shock may develop as a result of inadequate cardiac output from decreased contractility and pumping capacity.

Medical Management

Diagnosis is based on the following symptoms and diagnostic study results:

Severe crushing chest pain unrelieved by rest or nitroglycerin

Signs of cardiogenic shock—rapid pulse, falling blood pressure, dyspnea, cyanosis, restlessness, intense anxiety (see box on this page)

ECG changes—may include pronounced Q waves, elevated ST segments, T wave abnormalities

Serum enzymes—CPK, LDH, SGOT enzymes are released into bloodstream from death of tissue

Interventions are aimed at reducing the workload of the heart, identifying and treating complications, and promoting physical and psychologic comfort and gradual cardiac rehabilitation.

Nursing Management

Assessment—subjective (acute phase)

Character of pain (there may be none in the elderly)

History of onset, treatment attempted, prior CAD history

Dyspnea

Assessment—objective (acute phase)

Vital signs (signs of shock), increased pulse, decreased blood pressure

Diaphoresis (perspiration), skin temperature

Skin color, cyanosis

Arrhythmias

Intense anxiety and apprehension

Presence of nausea/vomiting

CARDIOGENIC SHOCK

DEFINITION

Inadequate tissue perfusion of cardiac origin, most commonly caused by myocardial infarction

PATHOLOGIC SEQUENCE

1. Cardiac function is insufficient to perfuse body cells.
2. Vital organs do not receive nutrients and/or discharge cellular waste, producing metabolic acidosis.
3. Progressive damage occurs in vital organs from prolonged ischemia.

SIGNS AND SYMPTOMS

Hyperventilation—shallow respirations

Falling blood pressure—tachycardia, weak pulse

Decreasing urine output, oliguria

Cool clammy skin, pallor

Restlessness, decreasing level of consciousness

NURSING CARE

Identify early signs of evolving shock.

Accurately monitor vital signs frequently.

Provide support and reassurance to patient.

Assist with medical therapy:

Use vasopressors, cardiotonics, antiarrhythmics, sodium bicarbonate as ordered.

Provide supplemental oxygen.

Insert and monitor arterial lines and pulmonary artery catheters.

Nursing diagnoses

Diagnoses will depend on the severity of the MI and the stage of recovery. Common diagnoses include:

Acute phase

Extreme anxiety related to intense pain and fear of death

Alteration in comfort—pain related to severe myocardial ischemia

Alteration in cardiac tissue perfusion related to myocardial ischemia

Decreased cardiac output related to loss of myocardial contractility

Rehabilitation phase

Activity intolerance related to decreased myocardial function

Potential for ineffective individual and family coping related to life-style changes mandated by the MI

Knowledge deficit related to progressive cardiac rehabilitation and its treatment regimen

Disturbance in self-concept (self-esteem or role performance) related to life-style modifications resulting from MI

Expected outcomes

Acute phase

Patient will not experience disabling anxiety.

Patient's pain will be significantly reduced.

Vital functions will be supported and preserved.
Patient's metabolic demands will be reduced to the lowest possible level.

Rehabilitation phase

Patient will have sufficient energy to gradually increase self-care activities.
Patient and family will receive ongoing support and education about MI and be encouraged to openly discuss their feelings and fears.
Patient will learn about treatment regimen for MI—drug, diet, and exercise therapy.
Patient will successfully return to prior roles: familial, social, sexual, and occupational.

Nursing interventions

Acute phase

Administer drugs as prescribed:
  IV morphine for pain relief and vasodilation
  Valium to reduce anxiety and restlessness
  Prophylactic lidocaine to prevent arrhythmias
  IV heparin to prevent thromboembolism
Maintain patient on absolute bedrest—promote rest.
  Maintain calm environment, offer reassurance and support.
  Provide physical comfort measures to promote rest.
Attach monitoring devices and observe for arrhythmias.
Provide additional oxygen by nasal cannula.
Monitor vital signs—check intake and output balance carefully.
Caution patient to avoid straining and the Valsalva maneuver.
Take time for patient's family—offer support.
  Explain all equipment and procedures.

Rehabilitation phase

Maintain strict bedrest for 24 to 48 hours.
Add activities gradually based on metabolic demands and patient's response.
Add lying and sitting exercises as ordered.
Teach patient to take and monitor own pulse.
Terminate exercise if patient has chest pain or pulse rate greater than 100.
Teach patient and family about MI and its physical effects.
Patient can be discharged within 10 to 14 days if no complications arise.
Teach principles of diet modification:
  Plan weight control.
  Restrict salt.
  Reduce cholesterol and saturated fats.
Discuss patient's resumption of sexual activity after 4 to 6 weeks.
Help patient give up smoking.

PACEMAKERS

DEFINITION

A battery-powered pulse generator attached to a wire on catheter that delivers an electronic stimulus to the heart's atrial or ventricular conduction system. The device may be temporary (external) or permanent (implanted in subclavicular area).

TYPES

Fixed rate—pacemaker fixes stimuli at preset rate (rarely used as does not adapt to fluctuating body needs).
Demand—pacemaker produces stimulus only when patient's heart rate drops below a preset level.

ASSOCIATED NURSING CARE

External pacemaker
Monitor patient's heart rate—observe for pacing stimulus on monitor
Ensure catheter terminals are securely connected
Ensure that pacemaker is secured to patient so accidental dislodgement is prevented
Monitor patient for signs of infection at insertion site
Internal pacemaker
Teach patient to do the following:
  Monitor pulse daily
  Resume normal physical activity
  Use only electrical equipment in good working order
  Carry pacemaker ID card

Evaluation

Acute phase

Patient reports decrease of pain and anxiety.
Patient does not have undetected complications.
Patient's cardiac workload is reduced to minimal levels.

Rehabilitation phase

Patient engages in progressive cardiac rehabilitation program and gradually resumes former activities.
Patient and family participate in cardiac education program.
Patient can describe dietary restrictions, medications to be taken, and exercise plan to follow at home.
Patient can describe symptoms indicative of need for immediate physician's attention.
Patient successfully resumes occupational, familial, and sexual roles.

NOTE: Pacemakers, electronic devices employed to control the heart rate, are occasionally needed by patients whose cardiac damage is such that they are unable to sustain a stable cardiac rhythm. The box above outlines basic data about pacemakers and associated nursing care.

CONGESTIVE HEART FAILURE

In congestive heart failure (CHF) the heart is no longer able to pump an adequate supply of blood to meet the demands of the body. The failure may be acute or chronic. The chronic form generally produces milder symptoms. Congestive heart failure is caused by:

1. Conditions resulting in direct heart damage, such as MI
2. Conditions that produce ventricular overload:
   a. Preload: amount of blood in ventricle at end of diastole is increased as in fluid overload or valvular and septal defects
   b. Afterload: force that the ventricle must exert to eject blood into the circulatory system is increased as with valvular stenosis, or pulmonary or systemic hypertension

Pathophysiology

The active symptoms of congestive heart failure appear as the heart's compensatory mechanisms are first set in motion and then exhausted. Symptoms include the following:

Tachycardia: heart rate increases to increase cardiac output

Ventricular dilation: myocardial fibers stretch to provide more forceful contractions

Myocardial hypertrophy: increased muscle mass causes more efficient contraction

As cardiac output becomes inadequate for renal perfusion, the kidneys compensate by retaining sodium and water to increase output. This creates fluid overload and edema.

Congestive heart failure often is classified as being either right-sided or left-sided. The mechanisms of these two disorders are outlined in the box on this page. Excessive fluid retention by the body results in venous stasis, an increase in venous pressure, and congestion in either the pulmonary system or systemic venous system.

Medical Management

Primary goals of treatment are aimed at restoring the balance between the supply of and demand for blood by body tissue and removing excess fluid. Major approaches include the following:

Providing supplemental oxygen, usually by nasal cannula

Reducing body's need for oxygen

Restricting sodium and fluid intake

Administering medications:

Digitalis to improve strength and force of contractions

Diuretics to reduce circulatory volume (thiazides)

Nursing Management

Assessment—subjective

History and development of symptoms, history of heart disease

Shortness of breath, degree of orthopnea

CONGESTIVE HEART FAILURE

LEFT-SIDED FAILURE:

Left ventricle cannot pump all the blood coming from the left atria; left atria cannot accept all the blood coming from the pulmonary bed.

Blood backs up into pulmonary bed.

Increased hydrostatic pressure causes fluid to accumulate in the lungs.

Blood flow is decreased to brain, kidneys, and systemic cells.

Symptoms

Severe dyspnea, orthopnea, rales, cyanosis

Irritability, restlessness, confusion

Severe weakness, fatigue

Oliguria

RIGHT-SIDED FAILURE:

Right ventricle cannot pump all the blood coming from the right atria; right atria cannot accept all the blood coming from the systemic circulation.

Blood backs up into systemic circulation.

Increased hydrostatic pressure causes peripheral and dependent pitting edema.

Venous congestion in kidneys, liver, and gastrointestinal tract.

Symptoms

Peripheral and dependent edema—pitting type

Distended neck veins

Anorexia, nausea, bloating

Recent abrupt weight gain

Ankle swelling

Increasing fatigue, loss of appetite

Assessment—objective

Visible dyspnea

Edema: site, degree

Abdominal distention

Neck vein distention

Baseline vital signs

Baseline weight

Presence of adventitious breath sounds

Level of consciousness

Nursing diagnoses

Diagnoses will vary based on the severity of the disorder but common diagnoses include:

Activity intolerance related to decreased muscle oxygenation

Anxiety related to dyspnea and feelings of air hunger

Ineffective breathing pattern related to pulmonary congestion

Decreased cardiac output related to excess fluid level

Fluid volume excess related to decreased cardiac output

Potential impairment of skin integrity related to tissue edema

TABLE 6-2 Diuretics used in the treatment of heart failure

Type	Example	Onset/Peak/Duration	Side Effects
Thiazide	Chlorothiazide (Diuril)	2 hr/4 hr/6-12 hr	Gastrointestinal upsets (can be minimized by taking medication with meals); hypokalemia; hyperglycemia
	Hydrochlorothiazide (Esidrix, Hydrodiuril)	2 hr/4 hr/6-12 hr	
Loop	Furosemide (Lasix)	1 hr/1-2 hr/6-8 hr	Similar to thiazide diuretics; also ototoxicity and blood dyscrasias
	Ethacrynic acid (Edecrin)	30 min/2 hr/6 hr	
Potassium sparing	Spironolactone (Aldactone)	Gradual/3 days/2-3 days after therapy discontinued	Gastrointestinal irritation; hyperkalemia
	Triamterene (Dyrenium)	Rapid/7-9 hr/12-16 hr	

From Phipps, W.J., Long, B.C., and Woods, N.F.: Medical-surgical nursing: concepts and clinical practice, ed. 2, St. Louis, 1983, The C.V. Mosby Co.

Knowledge deficit related to the control of and management of congestive heart failure

Sleep pattern disturbance related to night time orthopnea

Expected outcomes

Patient will gradually resume self-care activities without excessive fatigue.

Patient will breathe freely and experience decreased anxiety.

Patient's oxygen and carbon dioxide exchange in the lungs will improve.

Patient's cardiac output will improve.

Patient will gradually excrete excess fluid.

Patient will maintain an intact skin.

Patient will be knowledgeable about the treatment regimen and prevention of CHF.

Patient will experience uninterrupted restful sleep.

Nursing interventions

Ensure rest by providing support and anticipating needs.

Place patient in semi-Fowler's or high Fowler's position.

Provide oxygen as ordered.

Position patient with pillow on overbed table to facilitate breathing during acute phase.

Administer prescribed medications and teach patient about desired effects and side effects (see Table 6-2 and box on p. 78).

Explain all care routines fully.

Monitor vital signs frequently.

Monitor daily weight, assess status of edema.

Maintain accurate intake and output records.

Teach patient principles of restricted sodium diet.

Prevent constipation and straining through use of stool softeners.

Monitor skin and prevent skin breakdown:

Wash and dry skin frequently and gently.

Use lotion and massage.

Use anti-pressure devices on bed.

Change patient's position frequently.

Pay special attention to sacrum; avoid abrasion and shearing force.

Increase patient's self-care activities slowly as condition improves.

Teach patient and family the signs and symptoms of incipient failure and the importance of planning and spacing activities to avoid fatigue and stress.

Evaluation

Patient's energy level increases; patient moves toward independent self-care.

Patient is able to breathe freely, experiences no dyspnea.

Improved oxygen and carbon dioxide exchange increases patient's energy level, kidney function, and appetite.

Patient's cardiac output improves; lungs are clear.

Patient is without edema, and maintains a stable weight.

Patient's skin is intact.

Patient is able to sleep at night without episodes of dyspnea.

Patient and family can accurately describe the activity restrictions, diet modifications, and medication schedule to follow for successful home maintenance.

NOTE: Pulmonary edema is a medical emergency that may be associated with left-sided congestive heart failure. It

NURSING ACTIONS RELATED TO ADMINISTRATION OF DIGITALIS

ADMINISTERING DIGITALIS:
Take apical pulse before administering digitalis preparations; withhold medication and notify physician if pulse is below 60 or above 120.

If giving digoxin intramuscularly, inject it deeply and massage area well since drug is a tissue irritant.

Monitor serum potassium blood levels (hypokalemia is the most common cause of digitalis toxicity).

Give potassium supplements (if prescribed).

MONITORING PATIENT FOR DIGITALIS TOXICITY:
Cardiovascular effects
  Bradycardia
  Tachycardia
  Bigeminy (double beats)
  Ectopic beats
  Pulse deficit (difference between apical and radial pulse)

Gastrointestinal effects
  Anorexia
  Nausea and vomiting
  Abdominal pain
  Diarrhea

Neurologic effects
  Headache
  Double, blurred, or colored vision
  Drowsiness, confusion
  Restlessness, irritability
  Muscle weakness

Adapted from Phipps, W.J., Long, B.C., and Woods, N.F.: Medical-surgical nursing: concepts and clinical practice, ed. 2, St. Louis, 1983, The C.V. Mosby Co.

results from the rapid effusion of serous fluid from the pulmonary vasculature into the interstitial tissue and alveoli. Gas exchange fails and the patient begins to drown in pulmonary secretions. The box on this page describes the major symptoms and management.

INFLAMMATORY HEART DISEASE

Bacterial, viral, and fungal disorders, as well as inflammatory reactions, may produce inflammatory heart disease. Any layer of the heart muscle may be involved. The process may be acute and life threatening or mild and relatively asymptomatic. It may cause no residual damage or trigger serious problems in later years. A description of the major forms of inflammatory heart disease is presented in Table 6-3. Infective endocarditis is described in the text as a model.

INFECTIVE ENDOCARDITIS (ACUTE ENDOCARDITIS, SUBACUTE BACTERIAL ENDOCARDITIS)

Infective endocarditis is an infection of the endocardium usually involving the heart valves. Acute endocarditis has a rapid onset and a high mortality even with treat-

MANAGEMENT OF PULMONARY EDEMA

SYMPTOMS:
Profound dyspnea and pallor

Cough that produces large quantities of blood-tinged frothy sputum

Audible wheezing

Tachycardia

MANAGEMENT:
Administer medications as ordered:
  Morphine IV to decrease anxiety and reduce venous return,
  Aminophylline IV to dilate the bronchial tree,
  Digitalis to strengthen cardiac contractions,
  Diuretics to reduce fluid load.

Place patient in high Fowler's position.

Give 40% to 70% oxygen by face mask.

Monitor serum potassium as large amounts will be excreted with treatment.

Administer rotating tourniquets, if prescribed, to trap blood in the extremities, reducing cardiac overload:
  Place tourniquets high up toward axilla or groin.
  Tourniquets should be tight enough to occlude veins but pulses must remain palpable.
  Tourniquets should be on three extremities at a time; rotate in a clockwise manner every 15 minutes. Each extremity is occluded for 45 minutes each hour.
  When treatment ends, remove one tourniquet at a time at 15 minute intervals.

ment. Subacute endocarditis develops more slowly and responds well to treatment. The disease may also be classified according to causative organism. Viridans (alpha) streptococci, staphylococci, and enterococci are the major infective agents.

Pathophysiology
Patients who experience intrusive procedures, mainline drugs, or have cardiac anomalies and faulty valves that increase blood turbulence are at high risk for endocarditis. The infecting organisms are carried in the bloodstream and deposited on heart valves or other portions of endocardium. The organisms bombard the valves and become imbedded. Vegetative growths then develop which scar and perforate leaflets. The vegetative growths also may break off as emboli.

Medical Management
Medical management includes intravenous antibiotic therapy specific to cultured organism (usually a penicillin). Therapy is continued even after symptom cessation. Heart action is reduced and supported as needed.

Nursing Management
  Assessment—subjective
  History of heart or valvular disease

TABLE 6-3 Pericarditis, myocarditis, and rheumatic heart disease

Disorder	Etiology	Signs and Symptoms	Medical Management
Pericarditis	Inflammation of the sac that contains the heart as a result of trauma, neoplasm, systemic disease or infection; fluid accumulates in the pericardial space (acute); fibrous thickening of pericardial layers	Severe chest pain, aggravated by deep breathing. Pain is precordial, radiates to left shoulder, relieved by sitting up and leaning forward. Pericardial friction rub Fever; increased white blood cells Signs of CHF (chronic) Cardiac tamponade (acute): excess fluid impairs diastolic filling and cardiac output	Treatment of underlying condition Pain relief Pericardiocentesis for effusion or tamponade Pericardectomy for severe cases
Myocarditis	Inflammation of heart muscle—may occur alone or with systemic illnesses, especially infectious ones	May be nonspecific, such as fever, fatigue, dyspnea Signs of CHF	Identification and treatment of underlying condition Supportive CHF therapy General comfort measures
Rheumatic heart disease	Inflammatory disease involving all three heart layers; residual damage through scarring and deformity of heart valves; seen in conjunction with beta-hemolytic streptococcal infections; autoimmune response causes antibody formation	Joint pain, recurrent heart murmur, friction rub Follows upper respiratory infection by 1 to 4 weeks May advance to signs of arrhythmias, CHF	Parenteral antibiotics Anti-inflammatory drugs Comfort measures Symptom management

Recent history of intrusive procedure, such as dental work, minor surgery, Foley catheters, or cystoscopy
History of IV drug abuse
Malaise, fatigue, joint pain

Assessment—objective
Presence of fever (low grade or high grade)
Dyspnea
Edema
New murmur or change in quality of existing murmur
Anemia and petechiae

Nursing diagnoses
Diagnoses will depend on the severity of the disease. Common diagnoses include the following:
Activity intolerance related to systemic illness and decreased tissue oxygenation
Knowledge deficit related to treatment regimen and prevention of future episodes
Decreased cardiac output related to failing valvular function

Expected outcomes
Patient's energy level will gradually increase until patient can resume normal activity pattern.
Patient will be knowledgeable about the disease: its origins, treatment regimen, and prevention of future attacks.
Patient's cardiac function will return to normal with effective antibiotic therapy.

Nursing interventions
Administer prescribed antibiotics.
Teach patient role of antibiotics in controlling the disease.
Monitor vital signs frequently.
Assess temperature patterns.
Provide for adequate rest, but strict bed rest is not necessary.
Be alert for complications, such as signs of CHF or emboli.
Provide comfort measures for fever and joint aches.
Encourage well-balanced diet.
Assist patient to find adequate diversionary activities.
Teach patient about need for prophylactic antibiotics in the future, especially before dental work.
Teach patient importance of scrupulous oral hygiene and regular dental care.

Evaluation
Patient resumes normal activities and experiences no unusual fatigue.
Patient can discuss origins of disease, purposes and goals of treatment regimen, and measures to follow to prevent reoccurrence.
Patient's cardiac function returns to pre-illness levels or patient is scheduled for surgical replacement of damaged heart valves.
NOTE: The major features of pericarditis, myocarditis, and rheumatic heart disease are summarized in Table 6-3.

VALVULAR HEART DISEASE

Valvular disorders commonly occur as sequelae to the inflammatory diseases previously discussed. They may also be congenital. Rheumatic heart disease is the most common precipitating disorder. Diseased heart valves may either become stenosed or insufficient. Stenosed valves obstruct the normal flow of blood through the heart. Insufficient valves cause regurgitation or backflow of blood into the chamber from which it was expelled.

Pathophysiology

Initially the heart is able to compensate for the diseased valves through myocardial hypertrophy. Effective medical treatment may extend the compensatory period by years. If the condition worsens congestive heart failure will develop. Table 6-4 describes the specific forms of valvular dysfunction.

Medical management

Conservative treatment is aimed at controlling the symptoms of heart failure and improving cardiac output (see

TABLE 6-4 Valvular heart disorders

Disorder	Etiology	Signs and Symptoms	Medical Management
Mitral insufficiency	Papillary muscle dysfunction allows valve to flap in direction of atria during systole. Caused by: Rheumatic heart disease Congenital factors Bacterial endocarditis	Fatigue and weakness Right-sided heart failure Frequently accompanied by atrial fibrillation Blowing, high-pitched systolic murmur Third heart sound	Restricted activity Low-sodium diet Diuretics Cardiac glycosides Surgical valve repair or replacement
Mitral stenosis	Fusing of thickened fibrotic valve which progressively narrows and immobilizes the valve. Caused by: Rheumatic heart disease Congenital factors	Fatigue Dyspnea Pulmonary hypertension Right-sided failure Atrial fibrillation with pooled blood in atria, causing thrombus Low-pitched, rumbling presystolic murmur Snapping, loud first heart sound	Low-sodium diet Diuretics Cardioversion or drug treatment for fibrillation Surgical valve repair or replacement
Aortic insufficiency	Deforming of the valve leaflets causes them to close improperly, allowing blood to backflow. Caused by: Rheumatic heart disease Congenital factors	Symptoms are rare until left ventricular failure is imminent Palpitations, exertional dyspnea Angina Soft blowing aortic diastolic murmur Widened pulse pressure	Cardiac glycosides Low-sodium diet Diuretics Nitroglycerin Surgical valve replacement is usually necessary
Aortic stenosis	Aortic valve becomes stenosed obstructing left ventricular outflow during systole. Caused by: Congenital valvular problem (most common cause) Rheumatic heart disease Atherosclerosis in elderly	Exertional dyspnea Angina Exertional syncope (loss of consciousness) Harsh, rough midsystolic murmur Systolic thrill over aortic area	Rest Cardiac glycosides Diuretics Low-sodium diet Nitroglycerin Surgical valve replacement
Tricuspid insufficiency	Rare disorder since the normal valve leaflets are very small and play less of a role in valve closure. Impaired valve allows backflow of blood into right atrium. Caused by: Rheumatic heart disease (rare) Congenital factors	Symptoms of right-sided heart failure Hepatomegaly, jugular vein distention	Cardiac glycosides Low-sodium diet Diuretics Surgical valve repair or replacement
Tricuspid stenosis	Rare disorder in which shortening and fusion of the commissures cause orifice to narrow and block blood returning to the heart. Caused by: Rheumatic heart disease	Symptoms of right-sided heart failure Hepatomegaly, jugular vein distention	Cardiac glycosides Low-sodium diet Diuretics Surgical valve repair or replacement

Table 6-4). If condition worsens, surgical repair or replacement of the valve is performed.

Nursing Management
Assessment—subjective (preoperative)
History and course of disease
Current medical treatment
  Diet and activity
  Medications
Knowledge and attitude about proposed surgery
Patient's complaints of
  Fatigue
  Dyspnea
  Pain
  Palpitations or syncope (fainting with drop in blood
    pressure)

Assessment—objective
Activity and energy level
Respiratory rate and quality—breath sounds

CARDIAC CATHETERIZATION

RIGHT-SIDED:
Purpose
Confirm presence of congenital or acquired valvular disease.

Procedure
1. Cutdown is made in large vein, such as the basilic.
2. Catheter is threaded through vena cava, right atrium, and ventricle, pulmonary artery, and capillaries.
3. Blood samples are taken and pressures recorded.

LEFT-SIDED:
Purpose
Evaluate valve competency and assess left ventricular function, selective coronary angiography.

Procedure
1. Cutdown is made in large artery, such as femoral or brachial.
2. Catheter is threaded through the aorta, aortic arch, and into left ventricle or coronary arteries.
3. Blood samples are taken and pressures recorded or contrast medium is inserted to outline the coronary circulation.

GENERAL CONSIDERATIONS:
Procedure is performed under local anesthetic.
Procedure lasts from 1 to 3 hours, patient must lie still.
Right-sided catheterization produces little discomfort.
Left-sided catheterization may produce:
  Warm flushing sensation when contrast medium injected
  Nausea
  Fluttering sensation (ectopic beats) from catheter irritation
  Chest pain when contrast media is injected

Baseline vital signs
Presence of abnormal heart sounds
Presence of edema
Prominent neck veins
Peripheral oxygenation—nail beds, skin tone, temperature
NOTE: Diagnostic workup usually involves cardiac catheterization. The boxes on this page outline the two major procedures and give basic nursing care associated with this procedure.

Nursing diagnoses
Diagnoses will be variable based on the severity of the disorder, but commonly include:
Activity intolerance related to insufficient cardiac output
Ineffective breathing pattern related to fluid accumulation in lung spaces
Decreased cardiac output related to failing valves and cardiac pumping mechanism
Anxiety related to seriousness of open heart surgery
Knowledge deficit related to post–heart surgery routines and procedures
Fluid volume excess related to physiologic response to inadequate cardiac perfusion

NURSING CARE ASSOCIATED WITH CARDIAC CATHETERIZATION

PRE-TEST CARE:
Reinforce teaching provided by the physician as needed. Encourage patient to ask questions.
Shave and scrub specified insertion site, such as groin or antecubital space.
Give nothing by mouth prior to test—IV is generally started.

POST-TEST CARE:
Monitor patient by prescribed routine, which usually includes the following:
  Vital signs (BP taken on unoperative arm)
  Peripheral pulses on operative side
  Color and sensation on operative side
  Site for evidence of bleeding or hematoma (sandbag, pressure dressing, or ice bag may be used)
  Intake and output
Femoral approach necessitates bed rest for 12 to 24 hours; head of bed should be elevated no more than 30 degrees, and leg should be kept straight.
Brachial approach necessitates keeping arm straight for several hours; patient may be out of bed when vital signs are stable.
ALERT: Procedure may cause vessel spasm or thrombus, arrhythmia, hypotensive reaction to contrast material, and significant diuresis from contrast material.
Checks are usually performed every 15 minutes for 1 hour, every 30 minutes for 3 hours, and then hourly.

Expected outcomes

Patient will gradually return to normal activity schedule after surgery.

Patient will experience optimum oxygen and carbon dioxide exchange in lungs.

Patient will steadily improve cardiac output after surgery.

Patient will experience only manageable levels of anxiety over anticipated surgical procedure.

Patient will be knowledgeable about proposed surgery and the postoperative treatment regimen to be followed.

Patient will have normal fluid volume as cardiac function improves.

Nursing interventions
Preoperative

Explain and discuss planned surgical procedure.

Describe and, if possible, take patient to visit intensive care unit.

Discuss expected tubes and equipment and their purposes:

Venous and arterial lines

Monitors

Chest tubes

Intubation tube/ventilator

Urinary catheter

Teach patient bed exercises and breathing exercises to be performed after the operation.

Assist in stabilizing medical condition

Administer medications as prescribed.

Monitor cardiopulmonary status.

Establish baseline perfusion, pulses.

Foster balance of rest and activity.

Monitor intake and output carefully.

Postoperative

Maintain turn, coughing, and deep breathing schedule.

Provide cough pillow for adequate splinting.

Encourage patient to engage in progressive ambulation.

Monitor lung sounds, blood gases.

Maintain patency of water seal drainage.

Assess for fluid overload and CHF.

Check daily weights, and for signs of peripheral edema, and dyspnea.

Provide prescribed analgesics.

Provide comfort measures—allow rest periods.

Provide TED stockings; encourage leg exercises.

Monitor for incisional or intrapericardial bleeding.

Monitor for and correct arrhythmias.

Monitor urine output and fluid balance carefully.

Teach patient and family about activity and diet restrictions and medications.

Evaluation

Patient returns to normal occupational and recreational patterns, and has increased activity tolerance.

Patient has effective respiratory pattern; lungs are clear to auscultation.

Patient is without systemic signs of cardiac failure.

Patient is knowledgeable about post-discharge diet and activity patterns; can state purpose and side effects of all medications.

Patient maintains a normal fluid balance.

Patient can state signs that indicate need for immediate medical follow-up.

Patient's incisions heal without complications.

ANEURYSMS

An aneurysm is a localized or diffuse enlargement of an artery at some point along its course. Aneurysms occur when the vessel wall becomes weakened by trauma, congenital disease infection, and atherosclerosis. They can occur virtually anywhere, but the most common site is along the course of the aorta.

Pathophysiology

Once an aneurysm develops and the middle arterial layer is damaged, there is a tendency toward progressive dilatation, degeneration, and risk of rupture.

The types of aneurysms are saccular, fusiform, and dissecting. A saccular aneurysm is a pouch-like dilation on one side of the artery. A fusiform aneurysm involves the entire circumference of the arterial wall. A dissecting aneurysm splits and dissects the arterial wall, causing it to widen.

Medical Management

After angiographic studies, surgery is usually performed to resect the aneurysm and replace the diseased section with a Teflon or Dacron graft. Surgical approaches vary based on the site and extent of the aneurysm.

Nursing Management
Assessment—subjective

History of disease and symptoms (often discovered on routine examination and asymptomatic)

Knowledge and fears about planned surgery

General health status

Assessment—objective

Baseline vital signs

Peripheral circulation

Baseline intake and output

Nursing diagnoses

Diagnoses may vary based on location and severity of the disorder. Common diagnoses include the following:

Anxiety related to seriousness of surgery and uncertainty of outcome.

Alteration in comfort related to pressure of the aneurysm.

Knowledge deficit related to proposed surgical procedure and the postoperative care.

Potential alteration in urinary elimination related to inadequate postsurgical renal perfusion.

Expected outcomes

Patient will have only manageable levels of anxiety concerning the impending surgery.

Patient will not be in pain.

Patient will be knowledgeable about proposed surgery and the associated postoperative care.

Patient will maintain a normal urine output.

Nursing interventions

Preoperative

Teach patient about surgery and postoperative care routines.

Take patient on tour of intensive care unit if permitted.

Assess and mark peripheral pulses and baseline vital signs.

Postoperative

Monitor vital signs, central venous pressure (CVP), peripheral pulses frequently.

Observe color and temperature of extremities.

Monitor urine output hourly (at least 30 ml/hour).

Position flat in bed, avoid hip flexion.

Turn side to side, encourage flexion and extension of feet.

Provide TED stockings; check Homans' sign.

Use abdominal binder and pillow splinting for coughing and deep breathing.

Provide adequate pain medication.

Monitor nasogastric tube if ileus present.

Encourage patient to ambulate as permitted to prevent thrombophlebitis.

Evaluation

Patient has minimal discomfort and is able to do coughing and deep breathing effectively.

Patient maintains a normal urinary output.

Patient understands postoperative care regimen and postdischarge activity restrictions.

Patient has adequate peripheral blood flow, palpable peripheral pulses, and negative Homans' sign.

BIBLIOGRAPHY

Andreoli, K.G., *et al.*: Comprehensive cardiac care: a text for nurses, physicians, and other health practitioners, ed. 5, St. Louis, 1983, The C.V. Mosby Co.

Baum, P.L.: Abdominal aortic aneurysm? The patient takes AAA care, Nurs. 82 12(12):34-41, 1982.

Bitran, D., *et al.*: Intra-aortic balloon counterpulsation in acute myocardial infarction, Heart Lung 10:1021-1027, 1981.

Brzenski, T.S.: Pacemakers: pulse of life, AORN J. 32:967-976, 1980.

Cohen, S.: New concepts in understanding congestive heart failure. Pt. I, How the clinical features arise, Am. J. Nurs. 81:119-142, 1981.

Cohen, S.: New concepts in understanding congestive heart failure. Pt. II, How the therapeutic approaches work, Am. J. Nurs. 81:357-380, 1981.

Connors, J.P., and Avioli, L.V.: An update on cardiac surgery, Heart Lung 10:323-328, 1981.

Crumlisch, C.M.: Cardiogenic shock: catch it early! Nurs. 81 **11**(8):34-41, 1981.

Jasinkowski, N.: Aortic bypass: trimming the postop risks, RN **46**:41-45, 1983.

Klein, D.M.: Angina: physiology, signs and symptoms, Nurs. 84 **14**:44-46, 1984.

Lakier, J.B.: Myocardial infarction management: the first 24 hours, Hosp. Med. **19**:66D-66Q, 1983.

Scordo, K.A.: Taming the cardiac monitor. Part 1, Nurs. 82, **12**(8):58-64, 1982.

Scordo, K.A.: Taming the cardiac monitor, Pt. 2, Nurs. 82 **12**(9):60-69, 1982.

Stanford, J.F., *et al.*: Antiarrhythmic drug therapy, Am. J. Nurs. **80**:1288-1295, 1980.

VanMeter, M.: Balloon flotation catheters today: what they tell you, why they're vital, RN **46**:36-41, 1983.

Waggoner, P.C.: Postoperative care of the patient undergoing cardiac valve replacement: a nursing perspective, Crit. Care Quart. **4**:57-65, Dec. 1981.

Wenger, N.K., Hurst, J.W., and McIntyre, M.C.: Cardiology for nurses, New York, 1980, McGraw-Hill Book Co.

NURSING CARE PLAN

MYOCARDIAL INFARCTION (MI)—ACUTE PHASE

Nursing Diagnoses	Expected Patient Outcomes	Nursing Interventions
Anxiety related to intense pain and fear of death.	Patient will not experience disabling anxiety	1. Assure patient that the most dangerous stage of MI has passed. 2. Give family opportunities to discuss their concerns and keep them informed of patient's progress to deter transmission of their anxiety to patient. 3. Provide a calm unhurried environment. 4. Be sure patient understands the function of the continuous ECG is to monitor, not to keep the heart beating. 5. Give prescribed tranquilizers or sedatives as needed.
Alteration in comfort—acute pain related to myocardial ischemia	Patient's pain will be significantly reduced or relieved	1. Monitor degree of pain and effectiveness of interventions. 2. Give prescribed analgesics as needed (initially by IV). 3. Encourage relaxation exercises.

Alteration in cardiac tissue perfusion related to coronary artery obstruction	Patient's vital functions will be preserved
	ECG monitor shows normal sinus rhythm
		1. Monitor vital signs for signs of shock and irregular pulse.
		2. Monitor ECG continuously for arrhythmias
		  a. Record strips every 4 hours
		  b. Notify physician if PVBs occur
		  c. Give prescribed lidocaine
		3. Monitor breath sounds for respiratory congestion.
		4. Give prescribed oxygen by nasal catheter during initial period.
		5. Place patient in semi-Fowler's position.
		6. Encourage fluids but avoid overhydration.
		7. Give anticoagulant, if prescribed.

Alteration in cardiac output related to loss of myocardial contractility	Patient's metabolic demands will be reduced to minimal	1. Monitor vital signs for signs of shock. 2. Use measures to decrease anxiety. 3. Provide absolute rest. 4. Assist with all activities of daily living. 5. Teach patient to avoid Valsalva maneuvers.

NURSING CARE PLAN

MYOCARDIAL INFARCTION (MI)—REHABILITATIVE PHASE

Nursing Diagnoses	Expected Patient Outcomes	Nursing Interventions

Activity intolerance related to decreased myocardial function	Patient will have sufficient energy to gradually resume self-care activities	1. Space activities with rest.
		2. After 48 hours encourage a gradual increase in self-care activities.
		3. Decrease mealtime fatigue:
		  a. Offer small, frequent meals.
		  b. Avoid very hot or very cold foods.
		  c. Allow sufficient time for meals.
		4. Begin rehabilitation teaching early, so patient has sense of expected recovery.
		5. Encourage and supervise an increased activity schedule:
		  a. Start with lying and sitting exercises.
		  b. Increase length of ambulation gradually.
		  c. Encourage exercises for 20 minutes twice a day.
		6. Teach patient to monitor pulse during exercises and to stop exercise if pulse does not increase or if it increases >20 over resting pulse.
		7. Reinforce plans for home activity program.

Potential for sexual dysfunction related to fears of recurrent MI	Patient will gradually resume preillness sexuality	1. Give patient opportunities to explore concerns about own sexuality and resumption of sexual activity. 2. Correct misunderstandings about effect of coitus after infarction. 3. Encourge patient and partner to identify coital positions that are less stressful to patient. 4. Suggest that coitus be delayed until 3 hours after a heavy meal or excessive alcohol intake. 5. Teach patient symptoms occurring during coitus that need to be reported to physician.

Knowledge deficit related to the regimen of progressive cardiac rehabilitation	Patient will be knowledgeable about treatment regimen and can describe drug, diet, and exercise restrictions	1. Teach the patient:
		  a. Nature of MI and rationale for prescribed therapies.
		  b. Measures to prevent further MIs.
		  c. Effect of stressors and methods to relieve stress.
		  d. Benefits of a regular planned activity program.
		  e. Principles of sodium- and cholesterol-restricted diet.
		  f. Action and side effects of all prescribed medications.

Potential for ineffective family coping related to lifestyle changes required by the MI	Patient and family will receive ongoing support and education and be encouraged to discuss their feelings and fears	1. Provide patient and family with teaching and reteaching as needed. 2. Clarify misconceptions and misunderstandings. 3. Discuss return to employment and leisure patterns. 4. Refer for counseling follow-up if appropriate.

NURSING CARE PLAN

CONGESTIVE HEART FAILURE

Nursing Diagnoses	Expected Patient Outcomes	Nursing Interventions
Alteration in cardiac output—decreased—related to excess fluid load	Patient will experience an improvement in cardiac output	1. Monitor respirations q4h for increased effort and rate, and pulse for tachycardia or for rate <60. 2. Monitor heart sounds q4h for presence of S_3 or gallop rhythm. 3. Give prescribed digitalis preparations or vasodilators. Monitor patient's response. 4. Teach patient to avoid Valsalva maneuver.
Ineffective breathing pattern related to pulmonary congestion	The exchange of O_2 and CO_2 in the lungs will improve Patient will not need supplemental oxygen	1. Monitor for adventitious breath sounds q4h. 2. Assess neck vein distention q4h (presence, degree). 3. Provide oxygen by nasal cannula or face mask at 2 to 6 L/min as prescribed during early period. 4. Place patient in well-supported high Fowler's or semi-Fowler's position; elevate feet if sitting in chair.
Anxiety related to severe dyspnea	Patient will breathe freely and experience decreased anxiety	1. Give patient opportunities to explore feelings about effect of illness on life-style. 2. Assist patient to identify personal strengths. 3. Give medications to reduce anxiety, if prescribed. 4. Teach measures to control heart failure and reduce stress.
Potential impairment of skin integrity related to tissue edema	Patient's skin remains intact	1. Keep patient's legs elevated when sitting in chair. 2. Encourage frequent position changes when lying in bed. 3. Keep skin soft and supple with special attention to sacrum and heels. 4. Use additional measures, as necessary, to protect skin from pressure. Avoid abrasion or shearing force.

Knowledge deficit related to the management of congestive heart failure	Patient understands nature and management of CHF and how to prevent recurrence	1. Teach patient:
		  a. Nature of CHF and rationale for therapy.
		  b. Self-monitoring for recurring signs of CHF.
		  c. How to be active yet avoid fatigue.
		  d. Management of prescribed sodium-restricted diet.
		  e. Need for follow-up care.
		  f. Importance of weighing daily.

Activity intolerance related to decreased muscle oxygenation	Patient will gradually resume self-care activities without excessive fatigue	1. Plan rest periods. 2. Encourage gradually increasing activity within prescribed restrictions; monitor for intolerance. 3. Assist with ADL as necessary; encourage self-care as tolerated. 4. Provide small frequent feedings. Prevent constipation.
Fluid volume excess related to decreased cardiac output	Patient will gradually excrete excess fluid	1. Assess extremities for edema (site, degree of pitting) and coolness of skin q4h. 2. Weigh daily. 3. Give prescribed diuretics. 4. Give sodium-restricted diet as prescribed.

CHAPTER 7

Disorders of the Peripheral Vascular System

Peripheral vascular disease refers to a number of disease entities affecting either the arteries or the veins outside the heart. Patients exhibit signs and symptoms of these disorders because of some interference in normal blood supply to the tissues, either obstructive or as a result of anatomic abnormalities. Figure 7-1 shows the anatomical structure of the cardiovascular system.

ARTERIAL DISEASE

The symptoms of arterial disease are the result of disturbances in the delivery of blood and oxygen to the tissues. The severity of the symptoms reflects the degree of circulatory deprivation. Many of the specific disorders are related to the development of atherosclerosis and arteriosclerosis in the peripheral tissues. Table 7-1 describes some of the more common arterial disorders. Arteriosclerosis obliterans is discussed as a model.

ARTERIOSCLEROSIS OBLITERANS
Pathophysiology
Arteriosclerosis is a late stage of atherosclerosis involving both the medial and intimal layers of the artery. The intima develops atheromas (lipid deposits) and the media loses elasticity, producing gradual obstruction of the artery. Symptoms are the result of tissue ischemia and may progress to ulceration, necrosis, and gangrene.

Medical Management
Medical management includes comfort measures, carefully planned exercise programs, vasodilating medications, and preventive measures.

Surgery to improve blood supply may be indicated in severe cases. Procedures include bypass grafts, endarterectomy, sympathectomy, or amputation in the event of complications.

Nursing Management
Assessment—subjective
History of disease and its treatment
History of pain and intermittent claudication
  Type and severity, location
  Relationship to exercise and rest
Healing of simple cuts and abrasions
Usual diet, life-style, occupation, and exercise habits
Smoking history

Assessment—objective
Presence, strength, and equality of peripheral pulses
Skin
  Temperature, color, hair growth
  Texture changes, appearance of nails
Diminished sensation, paresthesias

Nursing diagnoses
Diagnoses will vary slightly depending on the severity of the disease. Common diagnoses include the following:
  Activity intolerance related to the onset of ischemic pain with exercise
  Alteration in comfort—pain related to ischemic changes and spasms in extremities
  Potential for injury related to decreased sensory awareness in extremities
  Knowledge deficit related to preventive and comfort measures appropriate with peripheral vascular disease
  Potential impairment of skin integrity related to lack of nutrients to peripheral tissue.
  Alteration in peripheral tissue perfusion related to arterial obstruction

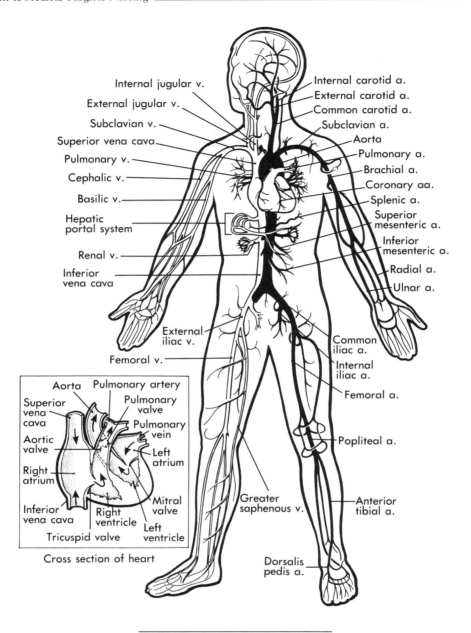

FIGURE 7-1 Cardiovascular system.

Expected outcomes

Patient will increase tolerance for exercise with treatment.

Patient will balance rest and activity and be able to perform activities of daily living without pain.

Patient will not have tissue injury from heat, cold, or pressure.

Patient will be knowledgeable about the treatment regimen.

Patient will maintain intact skin over legs, feet, and hands.

Patient will have increased peripheral tissue perfusion.

Nursing interventions

Assist patient to develop an exercise plan that carefully balances rest and activity.

Moderate exercise improves arterial circulation.

ALERT: Too much exercise puts excess metabolic demand on the circulation. Walking is ideal exercise.

Teach patient to:

Avoid remaining in one position or standing for too long.

Arrange frequent rest periods while traveling.

Avoid crossing legs while sitting.

Ensure that chairs do not impair circulation.

TABLE 7-1 Peripheral arterial disorders

Disorder	Etiology	Signs and Symptoms	Medical Management
Arteriosclerosis obliterans	Late stage of atherosclerosis Atheroma in intimal layers Loss of elasticity in medial layer	Tingling and numbness in toes Coolness in extremities Achy feeling in muscles with exercise Later, intermittent claudication (cramping pain) with walking or exercise Weak or absent pulses Shiny atrophic skin changes Loss of hair growth	Vasodilators Rest and exercise program Surgical intervention for advanced disease Stopping smoking
Thromboangiitis obliterans (Buerger's disease)	Obstructive inflammatory process in small arteries and veins Associated with smoking Appears in males and slightly more often in Jewish persons	Pain: intermittent claudication, pain at rest, or general aching Numbness and tingling Superficial thrombophlebitis	Stopping smoking (may be enough to reverse symptoms) Sympathectomy if unresponsive to conservative measures Preventive measures
Raynaud's phenomenon	Episodes of arterial spasm—most often in the hands May appear alone or secondary to another disease process. Occurs primarily in women.	Cold, numbness, and tingling of one or more fingers Bilateral process, affects both hands Fingers appear white or mottled Cold aggravates spasms	Avoiding cold Stopping smoking Vasodilators Sympathectomy if unresponsive to conservative measures

Avoid constricting clothing and exposure to cold.
Avoid use of direct heat to extremities.
Maintain proper foot care.
Avoid trauma and pressure to extremities.
Refrain from massaging legs.
Describe to patient importance of giving up smoking.
Administer vasodilator, anticoagulant medications as prescribed.
Assist patient to reduce weight and dietary cholesterol and fat.

Evaluation

Patient is able to maintain a normal activity pattern without experiencing claudication.
Patient effectively spaces activities throughout the day to remain free of pain.
Patient maintains skin integrity in the extremities and does not experience injury.
Patient is knowledgeable about the disease process and measures to increase comfort and perfusion.
Patient maintains desired body weight.
Patient adjusts diet to decrease cholesterol and fat intake.
Patient successfully quits smoking.

AMPUTATION

Although amputations may be necessitated by trauma or tumor, most are the result of progressive peripheral vascular disease. The presence of diabetes increases the likelihood of the need for amputation.

Surgeons attempt to remove all diseased tissue while leaving a stump that permits effective use of a prosthesis. BK (below knee) amputation is preferred because it preserves knee function and requires less energy and balance for walking. However, AK (above knee) amputation may be necessary because of the extent of the disease process.

Postoperative attention must be paid to preventing flexion contractures, reducing edema, and shaping the stump so that effective prosthesis fitting and gait training can proceed. The box on p. 90 outlines the basic features of preoperative and postoperative care for a patient facing amputation.

VENOUS DISEASE

THROMBOPHLEBITIS

Thrombophlebitis is a venous disorder characterized by vein inflammation and clot formation. It is associated with venous stasis, endothelial damage, and hypercoagulability of the blood. It is a serious potential complication of any illness that requires immobilization.

Pathophysiology

Exact etiology of the disorder is still not fully understood. The combination of thrombosis and inflammation produces swelling, warmth, and tenderness along the vein. Superficial veins may feel hard and thready. Serious pain is present with any dorsiflexion of the foot.

NURSING CARE OF THE PATIENT EXPERIENCING AMPUTATION

PREOPERATIVE CARE:

Discuss surgical procedure with patient and family.
Discuss post-op routines and exercises.
Teach patient about the occurrence of phantom limb sensations.
Encourage patient to verbalize feelings of anger or grief about impending procedure.
Assess physical strength and abilities to initiate rehabilitation.

POSTOPERATIVE CARE:

Immediate
Monitor vital signs and assess frequently for signs of hemorrhage.
Keep stump elevated on pillows for first 24 hours.
Monitor Hemovac drainage regularly.

Ongoing
Remove pillows from under stump.
Place patient prone for 20 minute periods at least twice daily.
Teach patient exercises and supervise practice:
  Hyperextension exercises
  Straight leg lifts
  Swing through or range of motion exercise over side of bed
  Gluteal sets, quadriceps sets, and bed push-ups to increase triceps strength
  Balance exercises at bedside
Teach stump care:
  Clean stump and sock carefully each day.
  Inspect daily for signs of pressure breakdown.
  Use firm smooth figure-eight ace wrapping to reduce swelling and shape stump—teach patient how to wrap.
Teach proper technique for crutch walking.
Help patient adjust to change in body image.

Medical Management

Thrombophlebitis is treated by rest and the use of anticoagulants. Warm, moist heat may be used in treatment although some physicians feel that heat increases the risk of emboli.

Nursing Management

Assessment—subjective
History of precipitating activity
  Immobility, especially prolonged sitting
  Minor trauma
Pattern and severity of pain

Assessment—objective
Unilateral swelling
Redness and heat in affected leg
Positive Homans' sign

Nursing diagnoses
Associated diagnoses commonly include:
  Alteration in comfort—pain related to inflammation and ischemia
  Knowledge deficit related to prevention and treatment of venous disease.
  Impaired physical mobility related to bed rest treatment of thrombophlebitis.
  Potential for injury or bleeding related to anticoagulant therapy.

Expected outcomes
Patient's pain will decrease.
Patient will be knowledgeable about the development, treatment, and prevention of thrombophlebitis.
Patient will not develop complications from bed rest.
Patient will not experience bleeding while receiving anticoagulant therapy.

Nursing interventions
Maintain patient on bed rest or activity restriction as prescribed.
Apply warm, moist heat or cold packs as ordered.
Keep affected limb elevated.
Administer anticoagulants as ordered and check for signs of bleeding. Avoid rectal temperature and IM route for injections.
  Hematest urine, guaiac test all stools.
  Examine skin for petechiae.
  Teach patient to use soft toothbrushes and avoid use of straight razors.
Administer streptokinase if prescribed (resolves thrombus).
Observe for signs of pulmonary embolism, such as sudden sharp chest pain or dyspnea.
Measure calf or thigh circumference daily.
Assess adequacy of peripheral circulation.
Apply TED stockings, teach patient proper use for home care.
  Put on before getting out of bed in morning.
Teach patient general principles of leg and foot care appropriate to general circulation impairment.

Evaluation
Patient is able to resume normal activities without discomfort.
Patient can discuss treatment plan and outline preventive measures to prevent recurrence.
Patient maintains intact skin, full range of motion and muscle strength, clear lungs, and adequate bowel and bladder function.
Patient manages anticoagulation therapy without incidence of spontaneous bleeding.

VARICOSE VEINS

Varicose veins are abnormally dilated veins with incompetent valves. They occur most often in the lower extremities and lower trunk, usually in the great and small saphenous veins. Congenitally defective valves, prolonged standing, and systemic conditions that interfere with venous return all contribute to the development of varicose veins.

Pathophysiology
Weakened vein walls do not adequately withstand normal pressure and dilate with blood pooling. Dilation increases the valve stretching and worsens the condition.

Medical Management
Mild problems with varicosities may be treated by teaching patients to elevate their legs at regular intervals throughout the day, to avoid constriction and stasis, and to wear support stockings.

Surgical treatment involves ligation and removal of varicosed vein.

Nursing Management
Assessment—subjective (preoperative)
History of the problem and patient management
Obstetrical history if patient is female
Patient's occupation
Patient's complaints of:
Pain
Fatigue
Swelling or cramping

Assessment—objective
Visible evidence of varicosities
Presence of edema
Posture

Nursing diagnoses
Common diagnoses include:
Alteration in comfort—discomfort related to cramping in legs
Activity intolerance related to edema and feelings of fatigue in legs
Alteration in peripheral tissue perfusion related to incompetent venous valves in lower extremities

Expected outcomes
Patient's discomfort will decrease.
Patient will be able to complete usual occupational and leisure activities without developing fatigue or leg edema.
Patient will have improved perfusion to lower extremities.

Patient will be knowledgeable about measures to prevent reoccurrence of varicosities.

Nursing interventions—preoperative
Teach patient about surgical procedure and regimen for post-operative positioning and activity.

Nursing interventions—postoperative
Elevate foot of bed for first 24 hours.
Provide adequate analgesia.
Initiate early ambulation and encourage frequent walking.
Assist patient with walking and transferring if needed.
Monitor incisions for bleeding.
Teach patient how to prevent recurrence of varicosities. Patient should:
Establish and maintain desired weight.
Avoid prolonged sitting, standing, or crossing legs.
Avoid constricting clothing.
Practice frequent foot dorsiflexion and ankle exercise.
Wear elastic stockings; put them on before arising.

Evaluation
Patient is free of cramping, pain, swelling, and fatigue.
Patient resumes desired activity pattern without reoccurrence of symptoms.
Patient is able to discuss measures to help prevent recurrence of varicosities.

HYPERTENSION

Hypertension is defined as a consistent elevation of blood pressure above 140/90 (150/90 for older adults). This disorder affects some 20 million persons, occurring slightly more often in males. The incidence of hypertension increases with age and is twice as prevalent among the black population. Many people with hypertension receive inadequate care or none at all.

Hypertension is commonly classified into two groups: primary and secondary. The cause of primary or essential hypertension is basically unknown. Secondary hypertension results from a known cause such as glomerulonephritis, Cushing's disease, or renal stenosis.

Pathophysiology
Blood pressure is determined by the following:
Volume of blood flow and strength, rate, and rhythm of heart
Diameter of blood vessels and the viscosity of the blood

Increased peripheral resistance from narrowing of the arterioles is the single most common characteristic of hypertension. This peripheral resistance is influenced by renal regulation of the renin angiotensin network, and stimulation of sympathetic system and release of catecholamines.

With prolonged hypertension, the elastic tissue of arterioles is replaced by fibrous collagen tissue. As resistance increases, so does ventricular workload, leading to possible congestive heart failure. Inadequate blood supply to the coronary arteries can lead to angina and myocardial infarction. Permanent damage may occur in the kidney and cerebral vessels.

Medical Management
Management of hypertension is based on antihypertensive medications (see Table 7-2) supplemented by use of a low-fat, low-sodium diet, control of weight, and lifestyle modifications to reduce stress.

A major thrust of care is prevention and early detection of hypertension in the general population. National programs have been developed for education, screening, and to improve compliance.

Nursing Management
  Assessment—subjective
ALERT: Early hypertension is usually asymptomatic.
  Headaches (occipital and present in the morning)
  Flushing of face
  History of nose bleeds
  Occupation and life-style
  Usual dietary patterns
  Smoking history

Assessment—objective
Vital signs
Obesity
Increased cholesterol and lipid levels

Nursing diagnoses
Diagnoses may be variable but commonly include:
  Knowledge deficit related to treatment of hypertension, side effects of medications, principles of diet control, and seriousness of complications.
  Noncompliance with medication and diet regimen prescribed for hypertension.

TABLE 7-2 Drugs commonly used to treat hypertension

Type	Action	Side Effects
First-Level Intervention		
Thiazide diuretics Chlorothiazide (Diuril) Hydrochlorothiazide (HydroDiuril) Furosemide (Lasix) Ethacrynic Acid (Edecrin)	Block sodium reabsorption in tubules; water is excreted with sodium	Decreased potassium, increased glucose, uric acid Hypovolemia, dehydration Anorexia, nausea
Potassium sparing diuretics: Spironolactone (Aldactone)	Antagonize effect of aldosterone; sodium is excreted in exchange for potassium	Hyperkalemia
Second-Level Intervention		
Rauwolfia compounds Reserpine (Serpasil)	Deplete catecholamines in sympathetic postganglionic fibers	Drowsiness, lethargy, depression, nasal congestion, nausea, and impotence.
Central nervous system drugs Methyldopa (Aldomet)	Reduce sympathetic activity by replacing norepinephrine with false, weaker neurotransmitter	Orthostatic hypotension, drowsiness, impotence, edema, weight gain
Propranolol (Inderal) Metoprolol (Lopressor) Nadolol (Corgard)	Act as beta-adrenergic blockers at peripheral autonomic sites	Gastrointestinal upset, rash, fever
Third-Level Intervention		
Central nervous system drugs: Hydralazine (Apresoline) Prazosin (Minipres) Nitroprusside (Nipride)	Relaxes arteriolar smooth muscle for vasodilation	Hypotension, headache, weakness, dizziness, tachycardia
Guanethidine (Ismelin)	Blocks norepinephrine release from nerve endings	Orthostatic hypotension, diarrhea, impotence
Clonidine (Catapres)	Stimulates adrenergic receptors in brain, causes inhibition of sympathetic vasoconstriction	Orthostatic hypotension, dry mouth, sedation, headache, fatigue

Expected outcomes

Patient will be knowledgeable about nature of hypertension and its physiologic effects.

Patient will be able to state action and side effects of prescribed medications and measures to control their side effects.

Patient will modify diet to meet prescribed restrictions.

Patient will express desire to maintain treatment regimen and control effects of the disease.

Nursing interventions

Assist patient to reduce and maintain desired weight.

Teach patient principles of modified fat and sodium diets.

Assist patient to explore and reduce factors contributing to personal and occupational stress. Patient should:

Balance rest, recreation, and activity.

Plan regular exercise patterns.

Use relaxation techniques.

Help patient reduce or stop smoking.

Teach patient about prescribed medications.

Teach patient how to manage side effects of medications. Patient should:

Take diuretics early in the day.

Maintain adequate intake of potassium.

Recognize symptoms of hypovolemia.

Prevent or control orthostatic hypotension by avoiding hot baths and making position changes slowly.

Be alert for symptoms of depression or impotence.

Explore adjustment of drugs or doses with physician.

Monitor lying, sitting, and standing blood pressures.

Teach patient to accurately monitor own blood pressure.

Support patient's adjustment to long-term management of the disease.

Evaluation

Patient can discuss effects and complications of hypertension.

Patient can discuss action and expected side effects of prescribed medications.

Patient employs measures to counteract expected side effects of medications.

Patient lowers fat and sodium intake in diet and maintains desired weight.

Patient employs relaxation techniques and modifies life-style to reduce stress; engages in regular exercise.

Patient exhibits willing compliance with diet and drug regimens.

BIBLIOGRAPHY

Craven, R.F., and Curry, T.D.: When the diagnosis is Raynaud's, Am. J. Nurs. **81:**1007-1009, 1981.

Fahey, V.A.: An in-depth look at deep vein thrombosis, Nurs. 84 **14:**33-41, 1984.

Falotico, J.B.: Pulmonary embolism, Crit. Care Update **8:**5-15, 1981.

Frank-Stromberg, M., and Stromberg, P.: Test your knowledge of managing the patient with hypertension, Nurs. 81 **11:**56-59, 1981.

Hill, M.N., and Foster, S.B.: High blood pressure, Nurs. 82 **12:**72-75, 1982.

Juergens, J.L., Spittell, J.A., and Fairbairn, J.F.: Peripheral vascular diseases, ed. 5, Philadelphia, 1980, W.B. Saunders Co.

Lowther, N.B., and Carter, V.D.: How to increase compliance in hypertensives, Am. J. Nurs. **81:**963, 1981.

Maschak-Carey, B.J., and Moore, K.: Anticoagulation therapy, Crit. Care Update **8:**5-16, 1981.

Porter, J.M., Baur, G.M., and Taylor, L.M.: Lower extremity amputations for ischemia, Arch. Surg. **116:**89-98, 1981.

Quinless, F.: Peripheral vascular disease, physiology, signs and symptoms, Nurs. 84 **14:**52-53, 1984.

CHAPTER 8

Disorders of the Blood and Blood-forming Organs

Diseases associated with the blood and blood-forming organs involve the development and functioning of red blood cells, white blood cells and platelets, as well as the mechanism of coagulation. They vary widely in pathology, overt symptoms and response to treatment. The nursing care associated with major problems of each type will be discussed in this chapter.

DISORDERS OF THE RED BLOOD CELLS

Red blood cells (RBCs) are produced in the bone marrow and circulate in the blood for about 120 days, transporting oxygen to the tissues. Anemia is a broad category of disorders involving a deficiency in RBCs or quantity of hemoglobin. Anemias may also be classified in terms of cell characteristics. Table 8-1 defines the common terms used to classify red blood cell abnormalities with common causes of each type. Anemia may result from blood loss, impaired production, increased destruction, or nutritional deficiencies. Table 8-2 categorizes the most common types of anemia by these causes.

The general body responses to anemia are quite similar regardless of cause. Some specific symptoms are unique to specific disease processes, however: as is medical management. Table 8-2 details specific information about signs, symptoms, and treatment of the common forms of anemia.

Pathophysiology
Regardless of the cause, anemia interferes with the RBC function of transporting oxygen to the tissues. This leads to tissue hypoxia. The body responds with a variety of compensatory mechanisms to keep the individual quite asymptomatic until the severity of the anemia worsens. The heart and lungs bear the brunt of the compensatory

efforts and frequently exhibit the strongest symptoms up to and including cardiac failure and shock.

Medical Management
General medical treatment is aimed at decreasing demands on the body and replacing RBCs while treating the deficiency. Treatment may include giving iron and vitamins to support production, preventing or halting conditions causing hemolysis, or replacing volume and cells through blood transfusion. Treatments for specific anemias are outlined in Table 8-2.

Nursing Management
Assessment—subjective
History and progression of symptoms
Menstrual history, if female
Prior medication or treatment
Usual dietary pattern
Associated health problems
Occupational exposure to drugs and chemicals

TABLE 8-1 Common anemias and red blood cell morphology

Anemia	Cause
Normocytic (normal cell size) Normochromic (normal hemoglobin content)	Acute blood loss, most hemolytic processes
Microcytic (small cell size) Normochromic (normal hemoglobin content)	Tumor, infection, chronic illness
Microcytic (small cell size) Hypochromic (decreased hemoglobin content)	Iron deficiency
Macrocytic (abnormally large cell size) Normochromic (normal hemoglobin content)	Folic acid deficiency, vitamin B_{12} deficiency

Patient's complaints of:
Fatigue and malaise
Cold intolerance
Complaints of paresthesias
Joint/bone pain

Assessment—objective
Vital signs—orthostatic blood pressure and pulse
Evidence of dyspnea
Skin color, temperature, presence of cyanosis/jaundice
Oral mucous membranes
Laboratory results

Nursing diagnoses
Diagnoses will depend on the specific type of anemia and degree of severity. Common diagnoses include:
Activity intolerance related to chronic tissue hypoxia
Impaired gas exchange related to either decreased

numbers of RBCs or impaired oxygen capacity of RBCs
Potential for injury related to systemic weakness and dizziness
Alteration in nutrition, less than body requirements related to inadequate ingestion or absorption

Expected outcomes
Patient will gradually be able to resume normal occupational and leisure activity pattern without incidence of fatigue.
Patient will have improved gas exchange and an increased number of red blood cells.
Patient will not fall during ambulation or position changes.
Patient will be able to identify foods rich in iron and vitamins and adapt diet to increase intake of needed nutrients.

TABLE 8-2 The anemias

Disorder	Etiology	Signs and Symptoms	Medical Management
I. Blood loss A. Acute	Hemorrhage (trauma, gastrointestinal [GI] bleeding)	Physiological signs of shock: Restlessness or irritability Cool, moist skin; pallor Increased pulse; decreased blood pressure	Stop source of bleeding; restore losses with IV fluid, whole blood or packed cell transfusions Support vital functions with oxygen, vasopressors
B. Chronic	Slow GI loss (malignancy) Vaginal bleeding (menstrual disorders) Hemorrhoids	Patient may remain asymptomatic with RBC and hemoglobin at 50% of normal level, then have chronic fatigue, weakness, elevated pulse, exertional dyspnea	Stop source of blood loss Promote proper nutrition; give supplemental iron
II. Impaired production A. Aplastic anemia	Bone marrow depression from drugs, chemicals, virus, radiation, unidentified causes Special attention to: Chloramphenicol Anticonvulsants Sulfonamides Butazolidine	Symptoms as with chronic blood loss; problem often affects white cells and platelets as well; infection; petechiae, spontaneous GI, genitourinary (GU), or CNS bleeding	Remove causative agent if possible Provide supportive care until bone marrow regeneration possible: transfusions of RBCs, platelets; laminar air flow to protect from infection; steroids to stimulate erythropoiesis
III. Increased destruction of red blood cells (hemolysis) A. Congenital 1. Sickle cell anemia (hemoglobinopathy)	Hereditary abnormality in hemoglobin protein which occurs primarily in black population; intermolecular rearrangement causes hemoglobin S to be formed, which tends to sickle in shape during lowered oxygen tension	General symptoms of anemia plus: generalized, localized or migratory bone or joint pain, leg ulcers, cardiomegaly, murmurs, CHF, jaundice Crisis may be precipitated by any condition increasing body's need for oxygen: acute onset, severe pain, vomiting, fever	Treat symptoms with analgesics, oxygen, IV hydration Provide supportive care during exacerbations Provide genetic counseling Prevention imbalance in oxygen needs

Continued.

TABLE 8-2 The anemias—cont'd

Disorder	Etiology	Signs and Symptoms	Medical Management
2. Thalassemia	Inherited disorder of decreased synthesis of hemoglobin and malformation of red blood cells which increases their hemolysis	Thalassemia minor—mild anemia with associated symptoms Thalassemia major—severe anemia, enlarged spleen, jaundice	No therapy indicated for mild form Transfusions for severe form to maintain patient in relatively symptom-free state
3. Enzyme deficiency (G-6-PD)	Inherited deficiency of enzyme in pathways that metabolize glucose, leading to premature RBC destruction	General symptoms of anemia are produced through acute hemolysis occurring when cells exposed to oxidant drugs such as ASA or sulfonamides	Diagnose condition and remove the drug stimulus
B. Acquired hemolytic	Most often drug-induced or autoimmune. Antibodies are produced that cause premature destruction of the RBCs	General symptoms of anemia reflecting severity of the disorder	Attempt to suppress the antigen antibody reactions through administration of corticosteroids
IV. Nutritional deficiency A. Iron deficiency	Deficiency of iron leads to synthesis of red blood cells with a decreased amount of hemoglobin; eventually leads to decreased number of cells	Few overt clinical signs in early stages, then gradual development of general symptoms, plus: Brittle concave nails Shiny smooth tongue Cracks in corner of mouth	Determine cause Provide adequate balanced diet Administer ferrous sulfate orally or parenterally if GI absorption is insufficient
B. Megaloblastic anemia 1. Vitamin B_{12} deficiency (pernicious)	Insufficient amount of B_{12} absorbed from intestine through combining with intrinsic factor; B_{12} is essential for synthesis of RBCs	General signs of anemia plus: Peripheral neuropathy Ataxia Smooth inflamed tongue	Administer vitamin B_{12} parenterally
2. Folic acid deficiency	Often occurs with chronic alcoholism, or malabsorption syndromes; folic acid essential for synthesis of RBCs	General signs of anemia plus symptoms of underlying disease	Administer oral folic acid and a well-balanced diet Treat underlying disorder

Nursing interventions

Balance rest and activity.
  Assist patient with activities of daily living as needed.
  Keep outside stimulation at a controlled level.
Supervise weak patient to prevent injury.
  Avoid abrupt changes of position.
  Check orthostatic blood pressure.
  Avoid use of hot baths.
Administer supplemental oxygen as needed.
  Provide extra pillows, keep head of bed elevated.
  Monitor for exertional dyspnea.
Turn and change position every 2 hours.
  Offer skin care and massage.
  Provide blankets if patient feels cold.
Teach patient about balanced diet and iron-rich foods.
Administer and teach patient about prescribed medications.
Administer blood transfusions if prescribed.

Administer transfusions slowly.
Observe and monitor patient for signs of transfusion reaction.
NOTE: The box on p. 97 discusses nursing care during RBC transfusion.

Evaluation

Patient performs self-care, resumes normal activities without fatigue, weakness, or onset of dyspnea.
Patient experiences improved tissue perfusion as evidenced by decrease in symptoms and laboratory values in normal range.
Patient discusses elements essential to balanced diet and selects and eats iron-rich foods.
Patient can discuss purpose and side effects of medications.
Patient does not experience injury or complications of treatment regimen.

DISORDERS OF THE PLATELETS

Platelets are formed in the bone marrow and serve as the first barrier to blood loss through vessel injury. Eighty percent of the body's platelets are generally in circulation and their normal life span is only 10 days. Platelet production is suppressed by most of the same drugs and chemicals that suppress RBC production. Aspirin is the primary drug with active anti-platelet activity in common use.

THROMBOCYTOPENIA

By definition, thrombocytopenia exists when a lower than normal number (150,000 to 400,000/cu. mm) of circulating platelets exists. Idiopathic thrombocytopenia purpura is a primary disorder of young adults in which an autoantibody is produced against a platelet antigen. Malignant disease, drugs, chemicals, and radiation may produce thrombocytopenia as a secondary effect.

Pathophysiology
The decreased number of circulating platelets interferes with hemostasis, producing excessive and spontaneous bleeding, often reflected in purpuric lesions and visible bruising on the skin.

Medical Management
Attempts are made to isolate and remove the cause of platelet depression if possible. A splenectomy may be indicated to remove the organ primarily involved in the destruction and removal of circulating platelets. Steroids may be administered to decrease antibody production and reduce phagocytosis of circulating platelets.

Nursing Management
Assessment—subjective
History and pattern of symptoms
Medications used, especially over the counter
Occupational exposure to drugs and chemicals
Patient's reports of:
Bleeding from gums, nose
Excessive menstrual flow
Blood in stool or urine

Assessment—objective
Presence of visible bruises, petechiae
Positive urine hematest
Positive stool guaiac test
Evidence of gingivitis
Laboratory reports of depressed platelets

Nursing diagnoses
Potential for injury related to easy bruising and interrupted or delayed clotting

NURSING CARE DURING BLOOD TRANSFUSIONS

BEFORE TRANSFUSION:
Take baseline set of vital signs.
Keep blood refrigerated in the blood bank until ready for use.
Use two nurses to check blood bag data and ensure positive identification.
Verify data with patient ID band before starting blood.
Prime tubing with normal saline solution—IV should have 18-gauge needle.
ALERT: Never hang blood products with glucose solutions as they induce red blood cell hemolysis and clumping.
Tell patient to immediately report signs of reactions (see below).

DURING TRANSFUSION:
Stay with patient during first 15 minutes of transfusion to observe for reaction.
Run blood slowly during first 15 minutes.
Compare serial vital signs.
Administer remainder of unit in less than 4 hours.
If whole blood is used, watch for signs of fluid overload.
Monitor vital signs at regular intervals throughout transfusion.
Monitor for signs of delayed transfusion reactions (see below).

SIGNS OF ACUTE HEMOLYTIC REACTION (USUALLY OCCUR IMMEDIATELY):
Burning sensation along the vein
Flushed face, abrupt fever and chills
Chest pain, labored breathing
Headache, backache, flank pain
Nursing Interventions
Stop transfusion immediately—run saline.
Call physician immediately.
Treat shock as prescribed if present.
Collect urine samples.
Send urine specimens, unused blood, and identifying tags to lab for analysis.

SIGNS OF ALLERGIC REACTION (USUALLY OCCUR WITHIN 30 MINUTES):
Hives and itching
Facial edema
Dyspnea, wheezing, anaphylaxis
Nursing Interventions
Stop transfusion immediately—run saline.
Notify physician.
Administer antihistamine as prescribed.
Transfusion may be continued under close observation if reaction is mild.

SIGNS OF PYROGENIC REACTIONS (USUALLY OCCUR WITHIN 1 TO 1½ HOURS)
Chills and fever
Headache and tachycardia
Palpitations or abdominal pain
Nursing Interventions
Stop transfusion immediately—run saline.
Notify physician.
Treat symptomatically as prescribed.
Monitor patient status closely.

Knowledge deficit related to measures to employ to prevent bleeding

Expected outcomes
Patient will be knowledgeable about safety precautions to follow to avoid bleeding and bruising.
Patient will not experience preventable bleeding.

Nursing interventions
Monitor patient for new bruising or extension of existing bruises.
Institute and teach patient about bleeding precautions:
Test urine and stool for blood.
Avoid taking rectal temperature.
Do not give intramuscular injections.
Apply at least 5 minutes of pressure to all venipuncture sites.
Avoid use of straight razors.
Patient should use soft toothbrush or Water Pik for oral hygiene.
Patient should avoid trauma—no contact sports.
Patient should avoid use of any product containing aspirin.
Teach patient to contact physician with any sign of worsening of bruising or overt bleeding.
Teach patient about all medications prescribed.
Administer platelet transfusions if prescribed.
Teach patient importance of informing dentist of condition before any dental work.
ALERT: Serious bleeding from injury is likely when platelet count is below 60,000/ml, spontaneous hemorrhage is a life-threatening possibility below 20,000/ml.

Evaluation
Patient can describe signs indicative of increased bleeding.
Patient can describe safety measures to employ while platelet level is low.
Patient does not experience preventable bleeding.

DISORDERS OF COAGULATION

Coagulation of blood results from the interaction of a number of clotting factors in a series of events called the coagulation cascade. Coagulation disorders may result from the depletion or absence of one or more of these clotting factors and may be either congenital or acquired. The bleeding problem may be mild or severe.

HEMOPHILIA

Both hemophilia A (factor VIII) and hemophilia B (factor IX) are hereditary sex-linked recessive disorders that are almost exclusively limited to males.

Pathophysiology
Patients with hemophilia present with life-long histories of bleeding tendencies. Complications are the direct result of the bleeding tendency:
Joint deformities from repeated spontaneous bleeds
Life-threatening bleeding into soft tissue areas such as intracranial or retroperitoneal areas

Medical Management
Treatment consists of replacement of deficient clotting factors if bleeding episodes do not respond to local treatment. Transfusions of cryoprecipitate or concentrates of other deficient factors are given.

Nursing Management
Assessment—subjective
History and pattern of disease and treatment
Treatment regimen: side effects, costs, impact
Pain: type, location, severity
Life-style adaptations required by disease
General knowledge base concerning transmission

Assessment—objective
Presence of active visible bleeding site

Nursing diagnoses
Diagnoses will depend on the severity and control of the disease but may include:
Alteration in comfort—pain related to bleeding into joints and tissues
Knowledge deficit related to self-control and mastery of the disease
Ineffective individual or family coping related to chronic nature of disease and the ongoing cost of treatment
Potential for injury related to spontaneous bleeding developing from minor injury

Expected outcomes
Patient will have disease controlled, providing freedom from pain.
Patient will understand disease symptoms and treatment regimen.
Patient and family will receive available community assistance for dealing with the financial and psychic hardship associated with the disease.
Patient will maintain effective control and not experience spontaneous bleeding.

Nursing interventions
Teach patient about clotting factor replacement therapy used to control disease.
Teach patient and family the technique of home administration of clotting factors if feasible.
Teach patient appropriate preventive measures. Patient should:

Avoid trauma and minor injury.
Carry Medic Alert information at all times.
Know first-stage first aid for minor bleeding.
Provide patient and family with information about local
agencies that can provide support or financial as-
sistance.
Provide patient and family with accurate genetic coun-
seling.

Evaluation
Patient maintains knowledgeable control of hemo-
philia and is free of pain.
Patient can discuss disease, treatment regimen, and
appropriate life-style modifications.
Patient and family maintain optimistic outlook and are
assisted in coping with financial costs of treatment.
Patient adjusts activities to avoid injury.

DISSEMINATED INTRAVASCULAR COAGULATION (DIC)

Disseminated intravascular coagulation (DIC) is a re-
cently recognized pathophysiologic response of the body
to disease or injury. A primary disease causes initiation
of the clotting process which occurs throughout the vascular system. Fibrinolytic processes are stimulated and
clotting factors become depleted, leading to severe hemorrhage. The box below outlines common primary diseases that may trigger DIC and basic principles of management of this complex clinical complication.

MANAGEMENT OF DISSEMINATED INTRAVASCULAR COAGULATION

ASSOCIATED DISEASE STATES:
Introduction of foreign substance:
Endotoxin
Venoms
Placental matter from abruptio placentae
Conditions associated with thrombus formation:
Hypotension
Shock
Massive tissue damage:
Trauma
Neoplasm

MEDICAL MANAGEMENT:
Control or eliminate underlying disease
Administer blood or blood products to replace depleted
factors:
Platelets
Packed cells
Cryoprecipitate
Manage acute renal failure through dialysis

NURSING INTERVENTIONS:
Administer medical plan
Observe and test for evidence of new bleeding
Provide symptomatic comfort and support for critically ill
patient

DISORDERS OF THE WHITE BLOOD CELLS

The primary function of the white blood cells is to
provide for humoral and cellular response to infection.
Any compromise in the integrity of the white blood
cell system leaves the individual extremely susceptible
to infection.

Neutrophils are primarily responsible for phagocytosis
and destruction of bacteria and other infectious organisms. Lymphocytes are the principal cells of immunity
and the production of antibodies.

Chemotherapy drugs, exposure to other drugs and
chemicals, and radiation may all suppress white cell function but the most common disorder involves malignant
disease.

LEUKEMIA
The leukemias are malignant disorders involving the
bone marrow and lymph nodes and are characterized by
uncontrolled proliferation of WBCs and their precursors.
Table 8-3 lists the common leukemias and their characteristics.

Pathophysiology
Large numbers of WBCs accumulate first at the site of
origin and then spread to hematopoietic organs, causing
enlargement. The proliferation of one type of cell interferes with production of other blood components. Im-
mature cells decrease immunocompetence and increase
susceptibility to infection. Peripheral WBC count may
show an increase or decrease in numbers.

Medical Management
Medical management is specific to the particular type of
leukemia (see Table 8-3), but utilizes aggressive chemotherapy as its base. Dramatic increases in survival
have been achieved for some forms of the disease, particularly ALL. Combination drug therapy, coupled with
maintenance therapy while disease is in remission, is a
normal protocol. Therapy is intense and rigorous, often
demanding extensive hospitalization and intensive nursing care to sustain the patient.

Nursing Management
Assessment—subjective
History and duration of symptoms
History of prior treatment, if any
Patient's complaint of fatigue and weakness
History of frequent infection
Possible weight loss or anorexia
Family's response to symptoms and diagnosis
Medications in use

Assessment—objective
Fever
Presence of anemia, thrombocytopenia

TABLE 8-3 Leukemias

Leukemia	Type	Peak Age	Prognosis	Symptoms	Medical Management
Acute lymphocytic leukemia (ALL)	Acute	2–4 yrs.	Good response to treatment; over 50% of patients under 15 achieve 5 year survival	Fever, respiratory infections, anemia, bleeding mucous membranes, lymphadenopathy, fatigue, and weakness	Combined chemotherapy Radiotherapy Drugs: Vincristine Prednisone 6-mercaptopurine Methotrexate
Acute myelogenous leukemia (AML)	Acute	12–20 yrs., after 55	High mortality from infection and hemorrhage, poor prognosis	Same symptoms as ALL, but less lymphadenopathy	Chemotherapy: Cytosine arabinoside Thioguanine Adriamycin Daunorubicin
Chronic lymphocytic leukemia (CLL)	Chronic	50–70 yrs.	Most patients do quite well; survive 10 or more years with disease	Weakness, fatigue, massive lymphadenopathy, pruritic vesicular skin lesions, anemia, thrombocytopenia	Chemotherapy: Alkylating agents— Chlorambucil and glucocorticoids
Chronic myelogenous leukemia (CML)	Chronic	30–50 yrs.	Death usually occurs in less than 5 years from infection and hemorrhage	Weakness, fatigue, anorexia, weight loss, splenomegaly, anemia, thrombocytopenia, fever	Chemotherapy with same agents used with AML, also vincristine, busulfan

Bruising, petechiae
Lymphadenopathy
Bleeding or ulceration on mucous membranes
General systems assessment

Nursing diagnoses
Diagnoses will depend on the disease type and severity. Common diagnoses include:
Activity intolerance related to severe fatigue and weakness
Ineffective individual or family coping related to the treatment regimen and prognosis of the disease
Alteration in comfort related to side effects of the chemotherapy regimen
Potential for injury and infection related to the disease symptoms and side effects of the treatment regimen
Alteration in nutrition, less than body requirements, related to anorexia and gastrointestinal side effects of chemotherapy
Potential alteration in oral mucous membranes related to side effects of chemotherapy
Knowledge deficit related to the management of the side effects of chemotherapy

Expected outcomes
Patient will maintain sufficient energy to remain independent in the activities of daily living.

Patient and family will receive support and honestly share their feelings and fears about the disease.
Patient will remain comfortable during chemotherapy regimen.
Patient will be protected from bleeding and infection during chemotherapy.
Patient will maintain an adequate nutrient intake to meet minimal body requirements.
Patient's mucous membranes will remain intact to allow for oral nutrition.
Patient will be knowledgeable about treatment regimen, expected side effects, and their management.

Nursing interventions
Administer combined chemotherapy, if covered by hospital policy.
Ensure patency of vascular access (see Chapter 2 for specific interventions for IV administration of chemotherapy).
Institute bleeding precautions.
See discussion under thrombocytopenia.
Monitor for signs of bleeding.
Administer blood and blood products as ordered.
Assist patient to space activity to conserve energy.
Assist patient with activities of daily living as needed.
Protect patient against nosocomial infection.
Promote scrupulous hygiene, particularly oral.
Insist on rigorous handwashing by staff.

Prep skin prior to skin puncture.

Monitor for early signs of infection.

Establish protective isolation if indicated: laminar air flow rooms may be needed to preserve life in severely leukopenic patients.

Employ nursing measures to counter anorexia and nausea (see Chapter 2 for specific nutrition interventions for chemotherapy).

Teach patient and family about treatment regimen including:

Purposes of combination drug therapy

Expected side effects of drugs

Management of side effects

Purpose of isolation

Measures to prevent infection or bleeding

Symptoms indicating complications

Provide emotional support to patient and family.

Ensure adequate time for questions; encourage expression of fears and concerns.

Include family in all aspects of care.

Explore community agencies that can provide patient and family with support and specific assistance.

Evaluation

Patient rests at frequent intervals but is able to maintain independence in activities of daily living.

Patient and family openly discuss disease, treatment and prognosis, and actively deal with fears and frustrations.

Patient has minimal discomfort during treatment.

Patient maintains adequate blood levels and does not experience spontaneous bleeding or acquired infection.

Patient maintains a stable body weight and adjusts diet to ensure intake of minimal nutritional requirements while receiving chemotherapy.

Patient does not develop extensive mouth ulceration and is able to comfortably ingest food and fluid orally.

Patient can describe purpose and side effects of treatment regimens, plans with nurse to adjust diet, hygiene, and activity to minimize the side effects of treatment.

DISORDERS ASSOCIATED WITH THE LYMPH SYSTEM

The chief functions of the lymph nodes and lymph system are to assist in phagocytosis of cellular debris and to provide an immune response to antigens received from the structures drained by the lymph node. Lymph nodes enlarge in the presence of a wide variety of infectious processes. Infectious mononucleosis is the best known primary disorder. Most of the other disorders of the lymph system are malignant in nature.

LYMPHOMA

The category of lymphoma includes a variety of malignant disorders in which the lymph tissue is infiltrated with malignant cells and the affected nodes enlarge. The disease then spreads to lymph tissue of other nodes such as the liver or spleen. Lymphomas usually follow a pattern of exacerbation and remission.

Pathophysiology

Lymphomas are generally classified as:

1. *Hodgkin's disease:* potentially curable disease characterized by presence of Reed-Sternberg cells in affected nodes. Treatment plans and prognosis are closely tied to accurate disease staging.
2. *Non-Hodgkin's lymphoma:* broad spectrum of diseases with different histologic features and prognoses. Treatment again is closely tied to accurate histologic identification and disease staging.

Table 8-4 compares the major aspects and treatment of Hodgkin's disease and non-Hodgkin's lymphoma.

Medical Management

Treatment for all lymphomas is carefully tied to accurate identification of cell types and degree of disease spread. Successful treatment protocols have been well defined for Hodgkin's disease in particular. Repetitive courses of combined chemotherapy are the basis of remission induction and maintenance. Treatment may be augmented by radiation, particularly for the early stages. Surgery is used to facilitate the staging and diagnosis.

Nursing Management
Assessment—subjective

History, duration, and severity of symptoms

Prior treatment and response if appropriate

Patient's complaints of:

Fever

Weakness

Anorexia

Night sweats

General pruritus (itching)

Assessment—objective

Nontender enlarged lymph nodes

Weight loss

Fever

Enlarged liver and spleen

Positive lymph node biopsy or lymphangiogram

TABLE 8-4 Disorders of the lymph system

Disorder	Etiology	Signs and Symptoms	Medical Management
Hodgkin's disease	Unknown, viruses implicated	Lymph node enlargement (firm, nontender, painless), fever, weight loss, night sweats, pruritus (itching), fatigue and weakness, presence of Reed-Sternberg cells	Radiation therapy for early stages; radiation and chemotherapy for middle stages; combination chemotherapy for late stages MOPP regimen most commonly used: nitrogen mustard, vincristine, procarbazine and prednisone
Non-Hodgkin's lymphoma	Unknown, viruses implicated Affects 50 to 70 year olds	Nontender "bulky" lymphadenopathy, moderate hepatomegaly and splenomegaly; patient may experience unexplained weight loss, fever, night sweats	Radiotherapy for initial treatment for localized disease Combination chemotherapy is the mainstay of treatment for diffuse disease; a variety of drug combinations are employed

Nursing diagnoses

Diagnoses will vary based on the severity and stage of the disease. Common diagnoses include:

Activity intolerance related to systemic fatigue and fever

Alteration in comfort related to pruritus, fever, and sweating

Knowledge deficit related to treatment regimen and side effects of chemotherapy

Alteration in nutrition, less than body requirements related to side effects of chemotherapy

Expected outcomes

Patient will maintain sufficient energy to be independent in self-care.

Patient will employ effective measures to reduce the discomfort of disease symptoms.

Patient will be knowledgeable of the treatment regimen and the management of the side effects of drugs.

Patient will maintain an adequate nutritional intake and stabilize body weight.

Nursing interventions

Assist patient to deal with the side effects of chemotherapy and radiation (see Chapter 2 for specific interventions).

Help patient to arrange activities to conserve energy.

Provide comfort measures appropriate to symptoms.
    Keep bedding and linen fresh and dry.
    Offer baths and skin care.
    Administer antipyretic and antipruritic medication as prescribed.

Plan with patient to adjust diet to insure adequate nutritional intake and fluids.

Teach patient about treatment regimen and measures to control side effects.

Explain importance of detailed diagnostic workup.

Provide teaching about the effects of broad field radiation and chemotherapy on reproductive capacities.

Males are frequently sterile and should consider sperm banking.

Females usually regain fertility in time; may have ovaries relocated outside radiation treatment zone.

Provide on-going support to patient and family.

Evaluation

Patient has sufficient energy to maintain self-care independence.

Patient experiences lessened discomfort from symptoms and treatment side effects.

Patient is knowledgeable about disease, treatment regimen, and the treatment of side effects.

Patient maintains stable weight and eats a diet that contains the minimal nutritional requirements.

BIBLIOGRAPHY

Brinkmeyer, S.D.: Fluid resuscitation; an overview, J. Am. Osteopath. Assoc. 82:326-330, 1983.

Buickus, B.A.: Blood therapy: administering blood components, Am. J. Nurs. 79:937-941, 1979.

Campbell, V.B., Preston, R., and Smith, K.Y.: The leukemias: definition, treatment and nursing care, Nurs. Clin. North Am. 18(3):523-542, 1983.

Cullins, L.C.: Blood therapy: preventing and treating transfusion reactions, Am. J. Nurs. 79:935-936, 1979.

Gibbons, P.T.: Transfusion therapy in sickle cell disease, Nurs. Clin. North Am. 18(1):201-205, 1983.

Hutchison, M.M.: Aplastic anemia: care of the bone-marrow failure patient, Nurs. Clin. North Am. 18(3):543-552, 1983.

Knobf, M., et al.: Cancer chemotherapy treatment and care, Boston, 1981, G.K. Hall & Co.

Lopez, J.A., and Hausz, M.: Therapeutic apheresis, Am. J. Nurs. 82:1572-1578, 1982.

Perry, A.G., and Potter, P.A.: Shock: comprehensive nursing management, St. Louis, 1983, The C.V. Mosby Co.

NURSING CARE PLAN

SICKLE CELL CRISIS

Nursing Diagnoses	Expected Patient Outcomes	Nursing Interventions
Alteration in comfort; pain related to sickling process in joints and organs	Patient's pain is held at manageable level	1. Give prescribed analgesics as needed and evaluate effectiveness of medication. 2. Identify measures patient has found helpful and include these measures in the care. 3. Support joints gently when assisting patient to do ROM exercises. 4. Use moist heat or massage, if helpful. 5. Change linens as needed if fever is present. 6. Use other pain-relieving measures; person with frequent crises may benefit from learning special techniques such as biofeedback or self-hypnosis. 7. Assist patient in avoiding habituation and dependence on narcotics if possible.
Impaired gas exchange related to trapping of RBCs in capillaries	Patient maintains a sufficient oxygen level to meet body needs	1. Provide prescribed oxygen as needed. 2. Reduce body's metabolic needs. 3. Provide prescribed medications for fever/infection (antibiotics, antipyretics). 4. Administer prescribed transfusion (packed red cells).
Alteration in tissue perfusion related to blockage in small arterioles and capillaries	Patient does not develop thrombosis, skin ulcerations, or retinal infarction	1. Give prescribed intravenous fluids; because large amounts may be given, monitor patient for fluid overload. 2. Encourage oral fluids, if permitted. 3. Monitor for signs of thrombosis (pain in chest or abdomen, headache, decreased vision, oliguria or low urinary specific gravity). 4. Assess legs, especially medial malleoli, for signs of skin breakdown; use measures to prevent skin dryness or injury from trauma.
Disturbance in self-concept, self-esteem, and role performance related to disease exacerbations	Patient fulfills expectations of social roles and speaks positively of self	1. Provide opportunities for patient to discuss feelings about inability to fulfill expected roles. 2. Assist patient to identify personal strengths. 3. Assist patient to explore alternative ways to meet role expectations. 4. Suggest joining a support group or obtaining counseling to minimize dependency behaviors.
Activity intolerance related to pain and decreased tissue oxygenation	Patient will have sufficient energy to remain independent in the activities of daily living	1. Space daily activities and encourage frequent rest periods. 2. Assist with activities of daily living as needed. 3. Assist with gentle ROM exercise each shift.
Knowledge deficit related to disease origins and treatment and genetic implications	Patient/family understand the nature of the disorder and its treatment and receive appropriate genetic testing and counseling	1. Assess patient's knowledge of sickle cell anemia and correct misunderstandings. 2. Teach patient the basis of sickle cell disease and genetic effects. 3. Provide resources for family planning and genetic counseling. 4. Teach patient to avoid situations that cause crises. 5. Teach patient to drink 4 to 6 quarts fluid daily. 6. Discuss genetic counseling and contraceptive methods if patient is concerned about transmitting disease.

NURSING CARE PLAN

AIDS

Nursing Diagnoses	Expected Patient Outcomes	Nursing Interventions
Potential for ineffective individual coping related to the persistent stress of the AIDS diagnosis and prognosis	Patient utilizes effective coping strategies to deal with diagnosis and prognosis	1. Give patient opportunities to discuss feelings about having AIDS. 2. Give friends and family opportunities to discuss their feelings and concerns related to AIDS. 3. Provide appropriate factual information. 4. Assist patient to identify usual coping mechanisms. 5. Assist patient to explore alternative coping strategies. 6. Reinforce all positive coping behaviors. 7. Teach relaxation techniques if appropriate.
Anticipatory grieving related to uncertainty of disease course and prognosis	Patient, family, and friends make realistic plans for the future and appropriately resolve grief feelings	1. Assist patient and friends or family to explore and share their concerns about the future probabilities. 2. Support grief responses. 3. Help the involved persons identify personal strengths. 4. Help patient identify specific support persons and facilitate interactions with these persons. 5. Maintain realistic hopes. 6. When patient and others are ready, help them discuss plans for the immediate future.
Potential for social isolation related to stigma of the disease	Patient maintains contacts with family and friends and is not ostracized	1. Help patient identify feelings about interacting with or being rejected by others. 2. Help other persons to identify their concerns about acquiring AIDS; provide data about modes of transmission (blood products and needles, sexual relationships, and mother-to-fetus, but *not* casual contact). 3. Help patient explore ways of maintaining contacts with others at desired level. 4. Facilitate interaction of patient with others when possible.
Potential for infection related to incompetent immune system and frequent hospitalization	Patient is free of opportunistic infections	1. Encourage patient to follow scrupulous personal hygiene. Emphasize importance of good skin care and oral care. 2. Patient should avoid contact with persons with infections. 3. Patient should avoid activities that may result in minor skin trauma. 4. Teach ways to prevent spread of AIDS to others. 5. Teach patient to report early signs of infection. 6. Monitor hospitalized patient daily for signs of new infection, particularly respiratory, gastrointestinal, or skin. Employ protective isolation if appropriate. 7. Use blood/body fluids precautions when patient is hospitalized.
Alteration in nutrition: less than body requirements related to anorexia and effects of chronic illness	Patient maintains a stable weight	1. Monitor weight and nutritional intake. 2. Provide a high protein, high calorie diet. 3. Plan frequency of meals to promote increased intake; several small meals may be better tolerated. 4. Provide between-meal snacks. Offer supplements as appropriate 5. Use measures to encourage eating. 6. Provide oral hygiene before meals. 7. Provide TPN care, if needed. 8. Ensure adequate fluids and bulk to prevent constipation.

NURSING CARE PLAN

AIDS—cont'd

Nursing Diagnoses	Expected Patient Outcomes	Nursing Interventions

Alteration in comfort related to local effects of the disease	Patient experiences effective symptom management and is comfortable	1. When fever is present:
		  a. Bathe patient frequently in tepid water.
		  b. Keep bed linens clean and dry.
		  c. Administer antipyretics as ordered.
		  d. Provide extra fluid and monitor I & O.
		  e. Keep lips and mouth lubricated to prevent cracking.
		  f. Assist with ADLs to conserve energy.
		2. When mouth lesions are present:
		  a. Inspect mouth each shift.
		  b. Keep lips lubricated and mouth moist.
		  c. Encourage patient to rinse mouth q2-4hrs. with solutions of saline and peroxide. Avoid commercial mouthwashes.
		  d. Modify diet to eliminate spicy foods. Offer viscous xylocaine before meals if appropriate.
		3. When diarrhea is present:
		  a. Monitor frequency and characteristics of stool.
		  b. Administer antidiarrheal medication.
		  c. Ensure adequate fluid to replace losses.
		  d. Cleanse anal area carefully after each defecation. Encourage use of sitz baths and anal ointments.
		  e. Modify diet to decrease stool.
		  f. Encourage rest to decrease peristalsis.

Knowledge deficit related to condition, treatment modalities and modes of transmission	Patient understands the disease and the proposed treatment plan. Patient is knowledgeable about measures to prevent transmission.	1. Teach patient:
		  a. Nature of the disease process.
		  b. Treatment plan including action and side effects of all medications.
		  c. How to maintain adequate levels of nutrition, exercise, and rest.
		  d. How to avoid infection.
		  e. To avoid smoking, drugs, and excessive alcohol.
		  f. To inform necessary persons, such as dentists, of AIDS diagnosis.
		  g. How to prevent transmission by practicing "healthy" sex, by not sharing personal articles, and by not donating blood.
		  h. Resources available in community to provide financial, physical, or psychosocial assistance.

CHAPTER 9

Disorders of the Respiratory System

Disorders of the respiratory system are numerous and varied. They range from transient infectious processes to chronic degenerative and malignant problems. This chapter will separate respiratory disorders into two major categories: disorders of the upper airway and disorders of the lower airway. Figure 9-1 shows the anatomical structure of the respiratory system.

DISORDERS OF THE UPPER AIRWAY

Disorders of the upper airway include problems of the nose and sinuses, pharynx and tonsils, and larynx. Common health problems of the upper airway are infection, structural defects, and cosmetic appearance.

CARE OF THE PATIENT WITH NASAL SURGERY

PREOPERATIVE CARE:
Teach patient about procedure and type of anesthesia (general or local) to be used.
Teach patient about necessity for mouth breathing after surgery.
Teach patient about anticipated swelling and discoloration.

POSTOPERATIVE CARE:
Monitor vital signs regularly.
Monitor for signs of bleeding:
  Observe for excessive swallowing.
  Assess bleeding through nasal drip pad.
Change drip pad under nose as needed.
Place patient in upright position—apply ice over nose.
Encourage fluid intake.
Provide oral mouth care frequently.
Provide adequate analgesia and relief for nausea if indicated.
Maintain or provide adequate room humidity.
Inform patient that first stools may be tarry from swallowing blood.

NOSE AND SINUSES

Disorders of the nose and sinuses include a variety of allergic, infectious, and obstructive problems. Uncomplicated cases of rhinitis, allergic rhinitis, and sinusitis are frequently treated with over-the-counter antihistamine medications and antibiotics. Nasal obstructions from structural abnormalities, tumors, or trauma are usually surgically treated. The box on p. 106 outlines basic principles of care for a patient experiencing nasal surgery.

PHARYNX AND TONSILS

The most common disorders affecting the pharynx or tonsils in adults are acute infections that may be relieved by symptomatic care or antibiotics if indicated. Surgical interventions through tonsillectomy and adenoidectomy are usually more serious procedures in the adult patient than in the child. The box on p. 106 outlines basic principles for a patient with a tonsillectomy.

CARE OF THE PATIENT WITH TONSILLECTOMY

PREOPERATIVE CARE:
Teach patient about the surgical procedure.
Teach patient about diet and analgesia after surgery.

POSTOPERATIVE CARE:
Position patient on side until fully awake.
Use Fowler's position once patient is awake.
Provide adequate analgesia.
Apply ice collar if prescribed.
Observe for bleeding:
  Teach patient not to cough or clear throat.
  Observe patient for frequent swallowing.
  Prevent vomiting if possible; observe for blood.
Offer fluids and soft bland diet when patient is stable:
  Avoid use of straw as it creates throat suction.
  Suggest patient use large swallows since they hurt less.
  Cold items are better tolerated.
  Avoid irritating foods for one week.
Keep fluid intake high.
Patient should avoid rigorous activity and exercise during first 3 to 5 days.

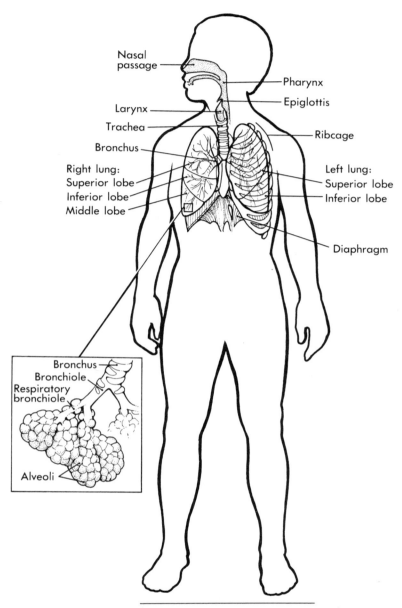

FIGURE 9-1 Respiratory system.

LARYNX

Disorders involving the larynx range from relatively benign laryngitis to cancer of the larynx. Cancer of the larynx is a relatively common disorder that occurs most frequently in men over 60 years of age. It may be confined to the vocal cords or extend rapidly to the deep lymph nodes of the neck. Its development appears to be related to heavy smoking, alcohol abuse, chronic laryngitis, and vocal abuse.

Pathophysiology

Tumor growth prevents the free vibration of the vocal cords. This produces the classic early sign of hoarseness of a progressive nature. More advanced disease may produce signs of dysphagia, a feeling of a "lump in the throat," or pain.

Medical Management

The treatment of choice is surgical. A partial or total laryngectomy is performed, depending on the extent of the disease. Radical neck dissection often accompanies total laryngectomy because of the danger of neck metastases. Surgery removes the cervical lymph nodes, but may also sacrifice the sternocleidomastoid muscle, internal jugular vein, and accessory nerve.

Nursing Management

Assessment—subjective (preoperative)

History and severity of symptoms

Patient's history of smoking or alcohol use

Patient's knowledge of surgical procedure and outcomes

Patient's response to potential loss of vocal function

Assessment of past coping mechanisms

Assessment—objective

General health status, especially respiratory system

Degree of hoarseness

Difficulty with swallowing

Nursing diagnoses

Common postoperative nursing diagnoses include:

Ineffective airway clearance related to edema around surgical area and increased volume of secretions

Impaired verbal communication related to loss of vocal mechanism

Potential for ineffective coping related to loss of verbal communication and its impact on social and family roles

Knowledge deficit related to artificial airway management and mechanisms of speech rehabilitation

Disturbance in self-concept (body image and role performance) related to loss of verbal communication

Expected outcomes

Patient will maintain a clear airway through appropriate use of positioning and suctioning.

Patient will effectively communicate needs to nursing staff.

Patient will begin to resolve grief over vocal loss and receive appropriate support from family and staff.

Patient will learn how to manage artificial airway and will be knowledgeable about rehabilitation options.

Patient will begin to incorporate body changes into a revised but positive body image and continue presurgical social and family roles.

Nursing interventions

Preoperative

Prepare patient for surgery and postoperative care. Explain:

Presence and appearance of stoma

Hemovac or other wound drainage if planned

Technique of suctioning and equipment

Devices to deliver humidity

Purpose and management of nasogastric tube

Encourage patient and family to ask questions and discuss fears and concerns about surgery and rehabilitation.

Discuss with patient communication device to be used after the operation, such as magic slate, chalkboard, or pad and pencil.

Present options of speech rehabilitation:

Assess patient for readiness for visit from a rehabilitated patient.

Establish location of nearest Lost Chord or New Voice Club.

Put family in touch with services of the American Cancer Society.

Postoperative

Suction tracheostomy as needed to clear airway (see box below for suctioning procedure).

Keep head of bed elevated.

Auscultate lungs.

TRACHEOSTOMY CARE AND SUCTIONING

TRACHEOSTOMY SUCTIONING:

Explain procedure to patient.

Auscultate lungs prior to procedure.

Prepare sterile equipment for use, using strict sterile technique.

Use sterile gloves and catheter.

Use sterile container and water.

Have patient take five to six deep breaths of 100% oxygen prior to procedure.

Use Ambu bag and administer breaths if patient is unable to cooperate.

Lubricate catheter with sterile water prior to insertion.

Insert catheter *without suction* about 6 to 8 inches or deep enough to produce an effective cough.

Apply intermittent suction and withdraw catheter slowly, rotating while withdrawing.

Rinse catheter in sterile water between insertions.

Hyperoxygenate again between insertions.

Repeat procedure if needed—limit suctioning to 10 to 15 seconds.

Auscultate lungs at conclusion to ensure effectiveness.

Clean inner cannula every four hours or as necessary.

TRACHEOSTOMY CARE:

After suctioning, unlock and remove inner cannula if present.

Immerse in H_2O_2 and cleanse with brush.

Rinse in sterile water or saline, shake dry, reinsert and lock in place.

Cleanse around stoma with H_2O_2 and saline on applicators or 4 × 4 inch gauze pads.

Apply Betadine solution or ointment if part of hospital protocol.

Change trach dressing as needed.

Change ties as needed.

Insert ties through slits to secure to outer cannula.

Tie tapes with double knot at side of neck.

ALERT: Tracheostomy tube should be manually secured in place whenever tapes are not in place.

Tapes should be snug but allow passage of fingertips when tied.

ALERT: Suctioning may be needed every 5 minutes during the first few hours.

Maintain humidity to stoma.

Have call bell within easy reach—answer immediately.

Ensure that agreed-upon communication device is at bedside.

Avoid using patient's writing arm for IV tubes.

Monitor wound drainage including Hemovac.

Provide skin care around stoma as needed.

Provide frequent mouth care.

Provide nasogastric tube feedings (usually for about 10 days); ensure adequate hydration.

   Begin feedings by mouth cautiously; keep head of bed elevated.

Teach patient to support head when changing positions.

Rehabilitation

Teach patient self-care of tube if permanent stoma has not been created (suctioning is rarely needed after discharge).

Involve speech therapist in beginning rehabilitation.

Encourage supportive visits from family and friends.

Encourage contacts with volunteer groups.

Assist patient to plan life-style modifications that will be necessary after discharge. Patient should:

   Prevent water and foreign objects from entering stoma.

   Adjust hygiene routines:

      Take precautions when bathing or showering.

      Take precautions when shaving—avoid use of talc.

   Make clothing adjustments such as scarf or collar of porous material to cover stoma.

   Make recreational adjustments—swimming and water sports are contraindicated.

Teach patient signs of complications:

   Increased or purulent secretions

   Fever and cough

Support patient in all appropriate expressions of coping.

Evaluation

Patient's airway is clear; does not require mechanical suctioning.

Patient is able to effectively communicate needs and has been referred to speech therapist/center for rehabilitation.

Patient is exhibiting positive coping behaviors and expresses desire to resume usual activities.

Patient cares independently for stoma and discusses measures to protect stoma and ensure adequate humidity.

Patient cares for self and maintains active involvement with family and friends. Patient communicates determination to resume former roles and responsibilities.

DISORDERS OF THE LOWER AIRWAY

There are many disorders of the lower airway, but the most significant are those that are chronic. They cause significant impact on life-style and are a frequent cause of permanent disability. The discussion of lower airway disorders will follow the restrictive and obstructive disorders classification.

Restrictive disorders are those causing a restriction in lung volume and reduction in lung compliance. They include diseases that restrict lung movement and inhibit proper inspiration.

Obstructive disorders are those that exhibit an increase in airway resistance resulting in prolonged exhalation.

RESTRICTIVE LUNG DISORDERS

The major subcategories of restrictive lung disorders are infections, malignancies, and adult respiratory distress syndrome.

PNEUMONIA

Pneumonia may be caused by a variety of bacterial and viral organisms. It occurs most commonly in winter and early spring, affects individuals of all ages, and accounts for over 10% of all hospital admissions. It usually results from aspiration of infected material although its specific communicability is dependent on the infecting organism (see Table 9-1).

Pathophysiology

The infecting organism causes inflammatory exudate to fill the alveolar air spaces, producing lung consolidation. Gas exchange cannot occur in affected alveoli. Hypoxemia may occur depending on amount of lung tissue affected. Typical symptoms are listed in Table 9-1.

Medical Management

Once sputum smears and cultures have been obtained, antibiotic therapy is instituted for the causative organism. Supportive care is offered for fever, fatigue, and decreased respiratory function. Response to appropriate therapy usually occurs within 24 to 48 hours.

Supplemental oxygen may be needed for patients who are markedly hypoxemic. Supportive measures are offered to assist the patient to open and clear the airway.

Strict isolation is necessary for staphylococcal pneumonia. Staff protection is ensured by good handwashing for most other types.

TABLE 9-1 Pneumonia

Type of Pneumonia	Etiology	Signs and Symptoms	Medical Therapy
Typical (classical) pneumonia	Common cause *Streptococcus pneumoniae;* uncomplicated	Sudden onset with shaking chill Fever (39° to 40° C), pleuritic chest pain, productive cough, restricted chest movement Sputum—green and purulent and may be blood tinged; "rusty" Respirations—rapid and shallow with "grunting" at end of each breath Nasal flaring, intercostal rib retraction, use of accessory muscles, and cyanosis may be present	*Drugs of choice* Penicillin G procaine, IM Aqueous crystalline penicillin G, IV Penicillin V *Other effective drugs* Erythromycin, clindamycin, cephalosporins, other penicillins, trimethoprim with sulfamethoxazole
	Streptococcus pneumoniae; complicated (empyema, metastatic infection) *Haemophilus influenzae*	Inspiratory rales and dullness to percussion; pleural effusion and empyema may develop	Penicillin G Ampicillin *Other effective drugs* Chloramphenicol, cefamandole, trimethoprim with sulfamethaxozole
	Staphylococcus aureus		Nafcillin *Other effective drugs* Methicillin, oxacillin, cefazolin, cephalothin, vancomycin, clindamycin
	Staphylococcus aureus (methicillin resistant), *Klebsiella pneumoniae*		Vancomycin, IV Cefazolin, IV, plus gentamicin or tobramycin
Atypical pneumonia	Common cause *Mycoplasma pneumoniae*	Onset gradual over 3–4 days Malaise, headache, sore throat, dry cough May have chest wall soreness from coughing	*Drug of choice* Erythromycin *Other effective drugs* Tetracycline
	Uncommon cause *Legionella pneumophila*	Above plus abdominal pain and diarrhea Temperature 40° C or greater Shaking chills, respiratory distress Renal failure, hyponatremia, hypophosphatemia, elevated creatine phosphokinase	*Drug of choice* Erythromycin *Other effective drugs* Rifampin, gentamicin

From Long, B.C., and Phipps, W.J.: Essentials of medical-surgical nursing: a nursing process approach, St. Louis, 1985, The C.V. Mosby Co.

Nursing Management

Assessment—subjective

History and duration of symptoms

History of recent upper respiratory infection

Location and degree of pain

Patient's complaints of:

Fatigue

Anorexia

Dyspnea

Fever and chills

Assessment—objective

Baseline vital signs, elevated temperature

Auscultate lungs—presence of decreased breath sounds, inspiratory rales, cyanosis

Productive cough: greenish, purulent, rusty sputum

Splinting chest during inspiration

Tachypnea; use of accessory muscles, nasal flaring

Presence of expiratory grunt

Nursing diagnoses

Diagnoses may vary slightly depending on the severity of the disease, but commonly include:

Activity intolerance related to hypoxemia and general systemic illness

Ineffective airway clearance related to increased mucous production, inflammation, and alveolar consolidation

Alteration in comfort—pain related to pleural irritation

TABLE 9-1 Pneumonia—cont'd

Type of Pneumonia	Etiology	Signs and Symptoms	Medical Therapy
Aspiration pneumonia	Common factor in all forms of aspiration pneumonia is aspiration of material into airways	Mixed anaerobic aspiration pneumonia: the clinical course is mild and gradual in the early stages. There are cough and low-grade fever over several days or weeks, slowly progressing to expectoration of large amounts of foul-smelling sputum. When aspiration pneumonia is acquired in the hospital it may be insidious in onset, and the only early symptoms may be an unexplained fever and mild tachypnea. If the involved organisms are staphylococcal or gram-negative pathogens, the patient's condition can take a rapid downhill course accompanied by bacteremia and septic shock.	Symptomatic bacterial infection present—antibiotics specific to that organism will be used.
Hematogenous pneumonia	Occurs when pathogenic organisms are spread to the lungs via the bloodstream. *Staphylococcus aureus* and *Escherichia coli* are the most commonly involved agents. Most often the patient has an endovascular focus of infection (infected intravascular catheter, endocarditis, or intravenous drug abuse) *Escherichia coli* pneumonia is seen in patients with deep-seated *Escherichia coli* infections, such as intraabdominal abscess, pyonephrosis, or empyema of the gallbladder.	Pulmonary symptoms minimal compared with the symptoms of septicemia Nonproductive cough and pleuritic chest pain similar to that seen in pulmonary embolism are most common complaints	*Drugs of choice* Nafcillin, IV, ampicillin, IV, plus gentamicin or tobramycin Clindamycin, IV, plus gentamicin or tobramycin

Ineffective breathing pattern related to restricted chest movement and splinting

Potential fluid volume deficit related to fever and anorexia

Expected outcomes

Patient will experience a gradual return to normal energy level.

Excess mucus production and lung inflammation will resolve with antibiotic therapy; lungs will become progressively clearer to auscultation.

Patient will have less chest pain.

Patient will fully inflate both lungs on inspiration and will not restrict chest movements.

Patient will receive sufficient fluids orally and intravenously to compensate for losses and will maintain normal fluid balance.

Nursing interventions

Position patient in semi-Fowler's position to facilitate breathing.

Monitor vital signs frequently, especially temperature and respirations.

Assess adequacy of ventilatory effort.

Observe for cyanosis, use of accessory muscles.

Auscultate lungs.

Collect adequate sputum specimens.

Administer medications as prescribed:

Antibiotics

Analgesics

Antipyretics, expectorants, antitussives

Provide comfort measures: linen, bathing, mouth care for elevated temperature.

Administer parenteral fluids as ordered.

Offer fluids orally as tolerated.

Record intake and output accurately.

Encourage adequate rest.

Assist patient with activities of daily living as needed.

Prevent spread of disease through scrupulous hand-washing.

Teach patient about coughing and tissue disposal.

Use respiratory isolation for staphylococcal pneumonia.

Ensure adequate room humidity.

Administer oxygen if prescribed.

Encourage patient to cough and deep breathe effectively.

Splint chest while coughing.

Utilize chest physical therapy if patient cannot clear airway by coughing.

Encourage patient to restrict activity level until disease resolves to prevent relapse.

Complete full course of antibiotic therapy.

Evaluation

Patient resumes normal activities without reoccurrence of fatigue or dyspnea.

Patient's vital signs are normal, cough is resolving, and lungs are clear to auscultation.

Patient's chest pain has resolved.

Patient's ventilatory movements return to normal—no chest splinting is used.

Patient meets body needs for fluid through ingestion of normal oral diet.

TUBERCULOSIS

Tuberculosis, although controllable, is still a significant health problem in the United States. Statistics have shown a slight increase in urban regions, and it is a significant health problem among immigrant populations. The over-65 population is at particular risk.

Pathophysiology

Tuberculosis (TB) is caused by the *Mycobacterium tuberculosis* bacillus, a gram-positive and acid-fast bacillus. The disease is spread by the inhalation of tubercle-laden droplets. An individual's reaction to the bacillus depends on individual susceptibility, size of the dose, and virulence of the organism. The response sequence includes:

1. Alveoli are inflamed.
2. Inflammatory response and cellular reaction produces small firm white nodule (primary tubercle).
3. Tubercle is walled off by fibrotic tissue and becomes either necrotic or calcified. Liquified material is coughed up, leaving a cavity in parenchyma.

NOTE: Most individuals infected by organism do not develop active disease but demonstrate only positive skin testing and x-ray evidence of calcified nodes or cavities. Active disease may later occur during a period of intense or prolonged physical or emotional stress.

If the initial immune response is not adequate, clinical disease will then occur. A hypersensitivity response may trigger classic symptoms of fatigue, malaise, weight loss, anorexia, low grade fever, and night sweats. In certain cases the onset is similar to the course of an acute pneumonia. The local inflammation causes productive cough although the sputum is rarely bloody unless the disease is in an advanced stage.

Medical Management

The diagnosis is carefully established through a combination of skin testing, x-ray examinations, and culture of the sputum.

NOTE: tubercle bacillus grows slowly and culture reports are not available for 3 to 6 weeks.

Basic treatment involves the antituberculosis drugs (see Table 9-2). Second-line drugs are employed if the bacillus proves resistant to first-line drugs. Drugs are ad-

TABLE 9-2 Drugs used to treat tuberculosis

Drug	Dosage	Side Effects
First-Line Drugs:		
Isoniazid (INH)	5–10 mg/kg/day	Peripheral neuritis, hepatic toxicity, hypersensitivity (skin rash, fever, arthralgia)
Ethambutol (EMB)	15–25 mg/kg/day	Optic neuritis, peripheral neuritis, skin rash, GI upset
Rifampin	10–20 mg/kg/day	Hepatitis, fever, GI upset, peripheral neuropathy
Streptomycin	15–20 mg/kg/day	Auditory toxicity, nephrotoxicity
Second-Line Drugs:		
Para-aminosalicylic acid (PAS)	150 mg/kg/day	GI upset, hypersensitivity, hepatotoxicity
Ethionamide	750–1000 mg/day	GI upset, hepatotoxicity
Kanamycin	0.5–1 g/day	Auditory toxicity, nephrotoxicity
Capreomycin	1 g/day	Auditory toxicity, nephrotoxicity
Pyrazinamide (PZA)	15–30 mg/kg/day	Hyperuricemia, hepatotoxicity
Cycloserine	750 mg/day	Psychosis, personality change, skin rash

ministered for 9 to 24 months depending on the virulence of the organism.

Basic treatment also aims at preventing the spread of the disease. Adequate drug therapy and freely circulating room air are the basic elements. A patient who cannot observe basic hygiene precautions for coughing and sputum disposal may be asked to wear a high filtration mask. Standard masks for personnel have not proven effective. Strict isolation even at home is not necessary.

Nursing Management

Assessment—subjective
History and progression of symptoms
Family composition—members at risk
Patient's complaints of
    Fatigue
    Malaise
    Anorexia
    Afternoon or night sweats
Patient's perceptions of or attitudes toward the diagnosis of tuberculosis

Assessment—objective
Vital signs, presence of fever
Productive cough, character of sputum
Decreasing weight

Nursing diagnoses
Diagnoses may be variable with acuity and stage of the disease but commonly include:
Activity intolerance related to fatigue generated by inflammatory response
Ineffective airway clearance related to excess mucus production
Alteration in comfort related to sweats and gastrointestinal side effects of medications
Potential for ineffective individual or family coping related to long-term therapy or social stigma associated with tuberculosis
Knowledge deficit related to tuberculosis, its contagious aspects, and its treatment
Alteration in nutrition, less than body requirements, related to the anorexia and nausea associated with both the acute stage of tuberculosis and side effects of medications

Expected outcomes
Patient will experience increased energy and be able to resume normal activities of daily living.
Patient will experience decreased sputum production and maintain a clear airway.
Patient will experience fewer side effects of the disease and treatment and feel increased comfort.
Patient and family will make positive adaptation to the diagnosis and implications of treatment regimen.

Patient will be knowledgeable about the tuberculosis disease process, need for long-term therapy, and measures to prevent its spread.
Patient's appetite will increase; patient will plan and eat a well-balanced diet and maintain a stable body weight.

Nursing interventions
Administer medications as prescribed (see Table 9-2).
    Teach patient about expected side effects, especially gastrointestinal disturbances.
    Teach patient importance of taking all medications for as long as prescribed (may be 9 to 24 months).
    Stress importance of routine follow-up to monitor for toxic effects of medications.
Establish degree of respiratory isolation indicated.
    Teach patient rationale for restrictions.
    Teach patient importance of covering mouth when coughing or sneezing.
    Teach patient proper technique for disposal of contaminated tissues.
Follow strict handwashing precautions.
Employ appropriate nursing measures to increase patient's comfort level.
Encourage patient to allow for adequate rest until energy level improves.
    Space and limit activities.
    Assist patient with activities of daily living as required.
    Offer baths and linen changes as needed.
    Explore ways to modify food patterns to meet nutritional needs within the constraints of persistent anorexia.
Encourage patient and family to verbalize feelings and concerns about diagnosis of tuberculosis.
Teach family importance of ongoing screening for family members exposed to tuberculosis.
Teach patient facts about possibility of future recurrence and importance of being alert to symptoms.

Evaluation
Patient's energy level returns to normal; patient resumes normal occupational, social, and leisure roles.
Patient's mucus production decreases—lungs are clear to auscultation.
Patient does not suffer from the discomfort of disease symptoms or side effects of medications.
Patient and family accept tuberculosis diagnosis and make a positive commitment to compliance with treatment regimen.
Patient is knowledgeable about tuberculosis, its transmission, and the therapy regimen.
Patient's appetite returns, patient eats a balanced diet and maintains a stable body weight.

LUNG CANCER

Lung cancer is the primary cause of cancer death in men and is showing a dramatic increase in women. The increased death rate is directly related to the increased number of women with a prolonged history of cigarette smoking. Mortality is primarily dependent on the cell type and size of the tumor on diagnosis. The disease tends to occur in individuals 50 years or older.

Pathophysiology

Most lung tumors arise from the bronchi. Presenting symptoms will vary depending on tumor location.

Peripheral lesions are frequently asymptomatic and are diagnosed on routine chest x-ray examination. They may penetrate the pleural space and produce pleural effusion. Infiltration of adjacent ribs and vertebrae may produce severe pain.

Central lesions are in larger bronchioles and cause inflammation and obstruction. Symptoms include cough, dyspnea, chills, and fever. Lung cancer tends to metastasize to both adjacent and distant structures.

Medical Management

The major challenge of medical management for lung cancer is detecting the disease early enough to intervene successfully. Immediate surgery with local resection, lobectomy, or pneumonectomy is employed. Radiotherapy and chemotherapy are employed as treatment adjuncts and as palliative measures for inoperable lesions. Table 9-3 describes basic surgical procedures.

TABLE 9-3 Types of lung surgery

Procedure	Description
Pneumonectomy	Entire lung is removed. Phrenic nerve is crushed to allow diaphragm to rise and partially fill space. Drainage tubes are not used.
Lobectomy	One lobe of a lung is removed. Remaining tissue must be capable of overexpanding to fill up the space. Two chest tubes are used for postoperative drainage.
Segmental Resection	One or more lung segments are removed. Procedure attempts to preserve maximum amount of functional lung tissue. Two chest tubes are used for postoperative drainage. Air leaks may delay reexpansion.
Wedge Resection	Well-circumscribed diseased portion is removed without regard for segmental planes. Two chest tubes are used for postoperative drainage.

Nursing Management

Assessment—subjective (preoperative)

Patient's complaint of:
Cough and dyspnea, pain associated with breathing
Hemoptysis
Fever and chills
Fatigue and weight loss
Smoking history: amount, duration, type

Assessment—objective

Visible shortness of breath
Unilateral wheezing
Positive chest x-ray and bronchoscopy findings

PRINCIPLES AND BASIC MANAGEMENT OF WATER SEAL CHEST DRAINAGE

WATER SEAL DRAINAGE:

Purpose: to remove fluid and air from the intrapleural space to allow for lung reexpansion

Equipment: 1-, 2-, or 3-bottle chest drainage setups or self-contained disposable units such as Pleurevac (see Figure 9-2.)

1 bottle water seal—provides for gravity drainage of the chest; air and fluid are forced out on inspiration
2 bottle water seal—allows for the addition of suction to aid in chest reexpansion
3 bottle water seal—has separate bottles for water seal, drainage collection, and suction
Pleurevac—provides for 3-bottle setup in one unit, but may be used as 1- or 2-bottle unit also

NURSING INTERVENTIONS:

Mark level in drainage bottle regularly—check every hour while drainage is heavy.
Check all connections to ensure that they are taped securely.
Fasten tubing to bed to prevent dependent loops.
Check frequently to be sure water is oscillating in water seal.
Water level rises during inspiration and falls on expiration.
If water is not moving, check system for obstruction, such as patient lying on tubes.
Water will cease oscillating when lung is reexpanded.
Milk or strip chest tubes if ordered:
This procedure is controversial since it significantly increases negative pressure in the chest.
Keep clamps at bedside to clamp chest tube if bottle is accidentally broken.
ALERT: Clamping is never done except in emergency or with direct order. It can cause tension pneumothorax. If emergency occurs, reconnect tubes with new sterile setup as quickly as possible.
Never lift chest tube bottles above level of the chest.
Ensure that side rails and bed will not come down on top of bottle.
Encourage patient to cough and deep breathe.
Ambulation may be encouraged with water seal drainage.
Monitor patient's status regularly—answer all questions about equipment and precautions.

Nursing diagnoses

Diagnoses will vary based on the acuity and stage of the disease. Common diagnoses include:

Ineffective airway clearance related to increased mucus production

Alteration in comfort—pain related to bone infiltration or postoperative incision pain

Potential for ineffective individual or family coping related to the diagnosis and prognosis of lung cancer

Alteration in nutrition, less than body requirements, related to metabolic disturbances of cancer

Expected outcomes

Patient will maintain a clear airway and optimum oxygen and carbon dioxide exchange.

Patient's pain will decrease.

Patient and family will be supported as they work through their feelings about both diagnosis and prognosis.

Patient will continue to eat a diet that meets the body's minimal nutritional requirements.

Nursing interventions

Preoperative

Teach patient about diagnostic tests and proposed surgical procedure.

Teach patient about equipment to be used in care.

Prepare patient for ICU equipment if appropriate.

Teach patient proper coughing technique and the use of position changes and oxygen in the postoperative period.

Postoperative

Monitor for patency of water seal drainage system (see the box on p. 114 for basic principles).

Monitor for signs of excessive bleeding.
Record vital signs frequently.

Initiate coughing and deep breathing every 1 to 2 hours—manually splinting the chest wall.

Provide adequate pain relief. ALERT: Patient cannot adequately cough and deep breathe without sufficient pain relief.

Keep fluid intake high to liquify secretions.

Ensure adequate room humidity.

Initiate range of motion exercises for arms and shoulders.

Encourage ambulation early in postoperative period.

Position patient on good side with operative side uppermost to promote reexpansion of lung tissue.

Pneumonectomy patients are positioned on the operative side since no functional lung tissue remains to reexpand.

Evaluation

Patient's lungs are clear to auscultation; remaining lung tissue provides for adequate oxygen and carbon dioxide exchange.

Patient's pain is controlled enough to allow for ambulation and effective coughing.

Patient and family openly discuss diagnosis and prognosis and make decisions about additional treatment.

Patient eats a nutritious diet and maintains a stable weight.

Patient recovers from surgery without complications.

CHEST TRAUMA

Injuries to the chest range from fractured ribs to major trauma of chest, heart, lungs, and blood vessels. Most patients receive initial treatment in the emergency room

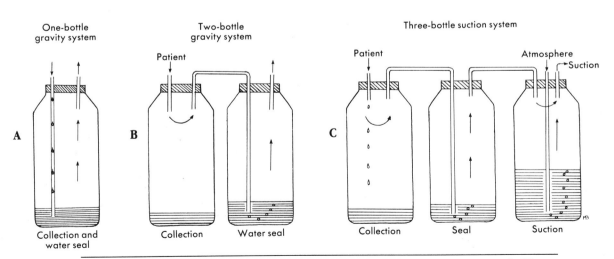

FIGURE 9-2 A, One-bottle drainage system. **B,** Two-bottle drainage system. **C,** Three-bottle drainage system. (Illustrations from Hirsch, J., and Hannock, L.: Mosby's manual of clinical nursing procedures, St. Louis, 1981, The C.V. Mosby Co.)

CHEST TRAUMA

BLUNT INJURIES:

Trauma involving the chest cage without penetration of chest itself.

1. *Fractured ribs.* Damage normally involves fourth to eighth ribs, caused by blows or crushing injury.

    Unless rib fragments penetrate the pleura, treatment is conservative with tight strapping of the affected side.

2. *Flail chest.* When ribs are fractured in more than one place, the chest wall on the affected side becomes unstable. There is insufficient bony support to maintain bellows functions of lungs, and paradoxic breathing results.

    Treatment is by internal stabilization. A tracheostomy is performed and patient is placed on a volume controlled ventilator to stabilize and control respiration until bone union occurs.

PENETRATING INJURIES:

Trauma involving the chest cage and underlying structures

1. *Pneumothorax.* Air enters the pleural space between the lung and chest wall. Atmospheric pressure builds up in pleural space, and lung on affected side collapses.

    Treatment involves reinflation of the lung with chest tube drainage

    Tension pneumothorax. Positive pressure buildup on the affected side may cause mediastinal shift, compressing the opposite lung and interfering with cardiac action.

2. *Hemothorax.* Blood leaks into pleural space and collapses the affected lung; this often occurs with pneumothorax.

    Treatment involves drainage and reexpansion with chest tubes.

3. *Cardiac tamponade.* Blood accumulates in the pericardial sac, gradually compressing the heart and interfering with function.

    Treatment involves emergency pericardiocentesis to remove pressure, followed by appropriate surgical repair.

and then follow-up surgical repair. Nursing management basically parallels that of the patient with lung cancer treated with thoracic surgery and water seal drainage. The box above describes the common forms of chest trauma.

OBSTRUCTIVE LUNG DISEASES

CHRONIC OBSTRUCTIVE PULMONARY DISEASE

Chronic obstructive pulmonary disease (COPD) refers to diseases that obstruct air flow and commonly includes the major disorders of asthma, chronic bronchitis, and pulmonary emphysema. All stages and severity of problems are included from reversible abnormalities to irreversible and progressive insufficiencies. The generic term COPD is commonly used although each disorder has its own characteristics.

Incidence statistics continue to escalate. An aging population and the prevalence of cigarette smoking are considered major contributors. COPD is a major cause of both death and disability in the adult population in the United States.

CHRONIC BRONCHITIS

Chronic bronchitis is defined by its symptoms: hypersecretion of mucus, and recurrent or chronic productive cough for at least 3 months per year for at least 2 years. Physiologically there are hypertrophy and hypersecretion of the bronchial mucous glands. It is caused by inhalation of chemical or physical irritants, or by bacterial and viral infections.

Pathophysiology

The inability to clear the airway of excess mucus causes susceptibility to infection. Repeated infection leads to fibrotic tissue changes. The airways show scarring, stenosis, and obstruction. Changes occur first in the smaller airways.

EMPHYSEMA

Emphysema is a disorder characterized by increased lung compliance, decreased diffusing capacity, and increased airway resistance. The cause is unknown but imbalances in proteolytic enzymes and inhibitors have been widely researched. Cigarette smoking is a frequent contributor to emphysema.

Pathophysiology

The diagnosis of emphysema is made from pulmonary function tests showing a decrease in airflow. Pathologically there are destructive changes in the alveolar walls and enlargement of air spaces distal to the terminal bronchioles.

Medical Management

Chronic bronchitis and emphysema are discussed together because they frequently coexist in the same individual and many of the treatment measures are similar. Major goals include decreasing the severity of active symptoms and reducing the progression of the disease. Therapy revolves around general supportive measures; physical rehabilitation; respiratory therapy including aerosols, oxygen, intermittent positive pressure breathing (IPPB), postural drainage, and chest physical therapy; and medications, particularly the bronchodilators, expectorants, and antibiotics.

Nursing Management
Assessment—subjective
History and severity of disease symptoms
Medications and treatments in use
Smoking history
History of upper respiratory infections
Knowledge of disease process
Patient's and family's response to progressive disability
Patient's complaints of:
    Shortness of breath
    Sleep disturbances
    Chronic cough
    Fatigue
General health status

Assessment—objective
Anorexia, weight loss
Presence of dyspnea with speech or exercise
Use of accessory muscles in respiration
Diminished chest excursion
Tachypnea
Amount and appearance of sputum
Presence of cyanosis
Presence of barrel chest
Bronchovesicular breath sounds
Prolonged expiration
Signs of right-sided CHF, edema
Results of pulmonary function and blood gas tests

Nursing diagnoses
Diagnoses depend on the stage and severity of the disease. Common diagnoses include:
    Activity intolerance related to shortness of breath and peripheral tissue hypoxia
    Ineffective airway clearance related to excessive mucus production and decreased expiratory force
    Impaired gas exchange related to destructive changes in the alveolar membrane
    Knowledge deficit related to measures to increase general health status and lessen symptoms
    Alteration in nutrition, potential for more than or less than body requirements, related to decreased activity or severe dyspnea
    Sleep pattern disturbance related to severe dyspnea in the recumbent position

Expected outcomes
Patient will maintain sufficient energy to remain independent in the activities of daily living.
Patient will be able to clear the airway with appropriate use of medications and therapy.
Patient will employ available preventive measures to facilitate adequate gas exchange.
Patient will be knowledgeable about disease process,

OXYGEN THERAPY

METHODS OF ADMINISTRATION:
1. Nasal catheter
    Continuous O_2 delivery even if patient mouth breathes
    Irritating to nasal tissue and poorly tolerated by patients
2. Nasal prongs
    Safe, simple, and well tolerated method of O_2 delivery—best for low doses
    Difficult to position properly, easily dislodged, poor delivery if patient mouth breathes
3. Face mask
    Efficient for rapid short-term delivery
    Poorly tolerated as tight seal is required about mouth
4. Venturi mask
    Allows for accurate delivery of high O_2 concentrations
    Poorly tolerated
5. Rebreathing mask
    Accurate O_2 delivery
    High humidity not possible
    Lightweight but poorly tolerated

GENERAL CONSIDERATIONS:
Oxygen therapy is drying and irritating to mucous membranes.
High-dose oxygen must be adequately humidified and nebulized.
Humidification and delivery equipment must be changed frequently to prevent or contain bacterial growth.
No smoking regulations must be posted and enforced.
Flow rates should be monitored frequently, especially for COPD patients.

---

    prescribed medications, and measures to delay disease progression.
    Patient will maintain an adequate nutritional intake and a stable weight, or reduce weight to optimum level.
    Patient will adjust position appropriately to obtain restful sleep.

Nursing interventions
General health
Teach patient about disease progression and home management.
Assist patient and family members to give up smoking.
Discuss modification of life-style and home environment to reduce exposure to pollutants.
Teach patient measures to avoid infection.
    Minimize contacts with crowds and young children.
    Consult with physician about flu immunization.
Avoid extremes of hot and cold.
    Ensure adequate humidity in winter.
Teach patient importance of balanced nutritious diet and maintaining normal weight.
    Use small, frequent feedings if anorexic.
    Ensure protein adequacy.
Ensure adequate fluid intake.

Medications

Administer medications as prescribed:

Bronchodilators (theophylline, terbutaline, aminophylline)

Expectorants, antibiotics, digitalis preparations

Teach patient about prescribed medications and side effects.

Respiratory therapy

Administer and teach patient proper use of aerosol therapy.

Teach use of humidifiers and nebulizers.

Teach proper use of hand-held inhalators.

Administer oxygen if prescribed (see box on p. 117).

ALERT: Only low flow oxygen is used (1 to 2 L) because chronic carbon dioxide retention causes decreased pO_2 to be the primary respiratory drive and this decreased pO_2 level cannot be removed.

Exercise

Teach patient progressive relaxation exercises.

Assist patient to adjust breathing pattern. Patient should:

Use pursed lips breathing.

Use abdominal breathing.

Exhale with exertion.

Lean forward during exhalation.

Assist patient with muscle reconditioning as tolerated.

Teach patient and family how to do postural drainage and chest physiotherapy (see Figure 9-3 and box on p. 119).

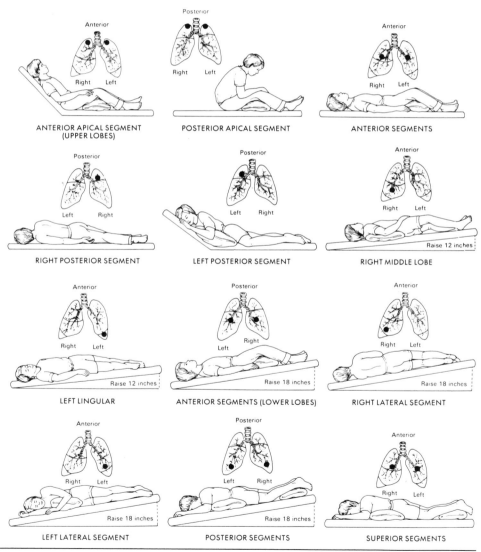

FIGURE 9-3 Correct positions for postural drainage. (From Hirsch, J., and Hannock, L.: Mosby's manual of clinical nursing procedures, St. Louis, 1981, The C.V. Mosby Co.)

Evaluation

Patient maintains independence in self-care and participates in usual daily activities.

Patient is able to clear airway daily.

Patient avoids situations that interfere with alveolar gas exchange, and improves alveolar exchange through appropriate exercises.

Patient is knowledgeable about disease and can discuss prescribed medications and correctly demonstrate prescribed treatments.

Patient can discuss safe use of oxygen therapy in the home.

Patient maintains a stable weight and adequate nutrient intake.

Patient sustains a pattern of restful sleep.

ASTHMA

Asthma is discussed separately because the airway obstruction involved is sudden and intermittent. There are two main types: immunologic and nonimmunologic. Immunologic asthma usually occurs in childhood and is associated with another allergic disease. Nonimmunologic asthma usually occurs in adulthood and is associated with recurrent respiratory tract infections rather than an allergy.

In either type of asthma, attacks are easily provoked by a variety of factors: changes in temperature and humidity, fumes and smoke, exertion, and emotional stress.

Pathophysiology

The airway is basically asymptomatic between attacks and exhibits no structural damage. Antigen-antibody reactions trigger the asthma attack through the release of chemical mediators. They cause three major responses:

1. Bronchospasm from constriction of smooth muscle in the large and small airways.
2. Mucosal edema and airway narrowing from increased capillary edema.
3. Increased mucous gland secretion and mucous production.

Medical Management

The treatment plan attempts to provide symptomatic relief from attacks, control specific causative factors, and promote optimum health. Oxygen therapy is used as needed during acute attacks. Bronchodilator drug programs include theophylline preparations and sympathomimetics. Other medical efforts are aimed at identifying and controlling precipitating factors in the environment.

Nursing Management
Assessment—subjective
History of disease and its treatment
History of onset of attack
Factors that precipitate attack
  Allergy history
Medications in use and patient's knowledge of them and their correct usage
Patient's complaints of:
  Shortness of breath
  Anxiety
  Feeling of suffocation

CHEST PHYSIOTHERAPY—CLAPPING AND VIBRATION

PURPOSE:
To combine the force of gravity with natural ciliary activity of the small bronchial airways to move secretions upward toward the main bronchi and the trachea.
Usually combined with postural drainage (see Figure 9-2 for positions).

PROCEDURE:
Help patient assume appropriate position for lung segment to be drained.
Clap over area with cupped hands for approximately 1 minute to loosen secretions and stimulate coughing.
At conclusion of clapping, instruct patient to breathe deeply; apply vibrating pressure during the expiratory phase.
Repeat as needed and include all appropriate positions.

GENERAL INFORMATION:
Modify desired positions as needed to increase patient tolerance.
Clapping is not done over bare skin—provide cloth barrier.
Time treatments for maximal benefit:
  Soon after arising
  At bedtime
  More often as prescribed and tolerated
  Complete procedure at least 1 hour before meals
Provide rest and mouth care following procedures.
Auscultate lungs before and after treatment to assess effectiveness.

Assessment—objective

Presence of wheezing, prolonged expiration, rhonchi
Productive or nonproductive cough
Presence of dyspnea, tachycardia, and tachypnea
Apparent respiratory distress
  Use of accessory muscles to breathe
  Forward positioning to breathe
Transient cyanosis, diaphoresis

Nursing diagnoses

Diagnoses commonly include:
Anxiety related to inability to effectively move air in lungs
Ineffective airway clearance related to excess mucous production in lungs
Impaired gas exchange related to bronchospasm and excess mucus in the airway
Knowledge deficit related to disease mechanism and optimum treatment

Expected outcomes

Patient's anxiety will decrease as a result of improved disease control.
Patient will successfully employ treatment measures to keep a clear airway.
Patient will experience improved gas exchange in the lungs.
Patient will be knowledgeable concerning disease and proposed treatment plan.

Nursing interventions

Acute attack

Establish calm environment, reassure patient.
Position patient in high Fowler's position—stay with patient.
Monitor vital signs and respiratory status regularly.
  Auscultate lungs.
  Observe for cyanosis.
Administer humidified oxygen as ordered.
Administer bronchodilators as ordered.
Monitor IV rates carefully.
Monitor patient for medication's side effects: tachycardia, palpitations, sweating.
Encourage fluids by mouth.
Encourage patient to cough up secretions.
Promote comfort measures for diaphoretic patient.

Chronic management

Teach patient to avoid potential allergens and precipitating factors if possible, such as smoking, exertion, cold air, dust.
Teach patient to seek prompt treatment of upper respiratory infections.

Teach patient breathing exercises and use of chest physiotherapy if appropriate.
Teach patient to maintain optimum nutrition, adequate rest, and sufficient fluids.
Teach patient about medications and their safe use. Teach patient to use inhaled bronchodilators before planned exercise.
Teach patient relaxation and stress management techniques.

Evaluation

Patient is in knowledgeable control of disease process, experiences infrequent attacks, seeks appropriate care promptly.
Patient is able to cough effectively and maintain a clear airway to auscultation.
Patient has adequate gas exchange in lungs, does not experience hypoxemia or hypercapnia.
Patient is knowledgeable about disease process and can discuss the purpose and side effects of prescribed medications and treatments.

RESPIRATORY INSUFFICIENCY AND FAILURE

Respiratory *insufficiency* occurs when the exchange of oxygen and carbon dioxide is inadequate to meet body needs during normal activities. *Failure* occurs when the exchange of oxygen and carbon dioxide is inadequate to meet body needs at rest.

These conditions may occur as a result of any of the disorders discussed in the chapter as well as a variety of other acute or chronic, surgical, neurologic, and neuromuscular disorders. Diagnosis is made from blood gas results, pulmonary function testing, and the patient's clinical status.

Criteria:

$PO_2 < 50$ mm Hg on room air
$PCO_2 > 50$ mm Hg
  vital capacity < 15 ml/kg
  respiratory rate > 30/min or <8/min
  In patients with COPD, a falling pH becomes the critical factor since the other parameters are present chronically.

Pathophysiology

Regardless of the cause, without adequate ventilation and gas exchange, the arterial pO_2 falls and body cells become hypoxic. Accumulating CO_2 alters the pH and the patient becomes acidotic. Clinical manifestations are related to either the elevated CO_2 or decreasing oxygen levels.

Medical Management

Therapy begins with identifying the underlying disease state and removing or decreasing the cause if possible. Specific interventions are aimed at improving oxygenation and ventilation. Supplemental oxygen is given at the lowest effective rate. The airway is kept clear through position, suction, and physiotherapy. Mechanical ventilation is used if needed.

Nursing Management

Assessment—subjective

History of condition and respiratory problems
Patient's complaints of:
Severe fatigue
Shortness of breath
Headache

Assessment—objective

Quality of ventilatory effort:
Respiratory rate and rhythm
Breath sounds
Use of accessory muscles
Signs of cyanosis in mucous membranes, lips, ear lobes
Position used for breathing
Diaphoresis; cool, clammy skin
Drowsiness, restlessness, mood fluctuation
Visible dyspnea—inability to complete sentences because of shortness of breath

Nursing diagnoses

Common diagnoses include:
Activity intolerance related to the fatigue of tissue hypoxia
Ineffective airway clearance related to excess mucus or fluids or neuromuscular weakness
Impaired gas exchange related to obstructive or restrictive lung disorders
Alteration in general tissue perfusion related to hypoxemia and hypercapnia

Expected outcomes

Patient's energy level will increase with improved oxygenation of tissues.
Patient will maintain a clear open airway through effective intervention.
Patient will experience improved oxygen and carbon dioxide exchange and diffusion in the lung.
Patient will have improved perfusion to body organs and tissues.

Nursing interventions

Monitor patient carefully for subtle changes in oxygenation status.
Administer humidified oxygen as prescribed.
Monitor COPD patient for carbon dioxide narcosis.
Help patient tolerate mask delivery systems if needed.
Monitor vital signs and lung sounds.
Keep airway open.
Suction as necessary.
Position patient comfortably in upright position.
Administer ultrasonic mist if prescribed.
Perform postural drainage and chest physiotherapy.
Administer intermittent positive pressure breathing (IPPB) if prescribed.
Manage artificial airway and ventilator if in use.
Keep patient calm and at rest to decrease oxygen needs.
Maintain neutral environmental temperature.
Reassure patient and control anxiety.
Explain all procedures and treatments.
Maintain adequate hydration.
Monitor IV fluids.
Keep accurate intake and output records.
Facilitate communication for intubated or trached patient.
Keep call bell close—answer promptly.
Provide pad and pencil or magic slate.

Evaluation

Patient progressively resumes responsibility for self-care.
Patient's airway is clear to auscultation.
Patient's respirations are unlabored; blood gases are within normal limits.
Patient exhibits no signs of cyanosis and is mentally alert and aware.

ADULT RESPIRATORY DISTRESS SYNDROME

Adult respiratory distress syndrome (ARDS) is an often fatal syndrome associated with shock, trauma, overdose of drugs, inhaled substances, and pulmonary infections. It is characterized by severe dyspnea, hypoxemia, and diffuse bilateral pulmonary infiltrations. Figure 9-4 describes the pathophysiologic process of ARDS.

Patients with ARDS are critically ill. They are treated with mechanical ventilatory support and frequently require the addition of positive end expiratory pressure (PEEP) to support ventilation. Other interventions are similar to those used for the patient in respiratory failure.

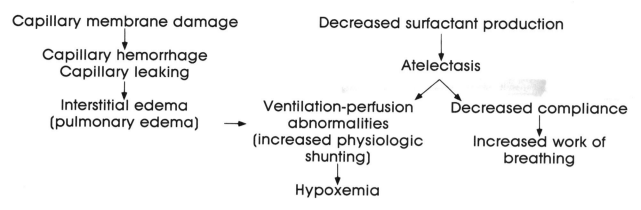

Symptoms appear after a post-injury latent period of 18 to 24 hours
Tachypnea
Labored breathing, air hunger
Cyanosis
Hypoxemia from blood gas studies
Bilateral interstitial and alveolar infiltrations

FIGURE 9-4 Pathophysiology of adult respiratory distress syndrome.

BIBLIOGRAPHY

Albanese, A., and Toplitz, A.: A hassle-free guide to suctioning a tracheostomy, RN 45:24-30, 1982.

American Lung Association: Chronic obstructive pulmonary disease, New York, 1981, The Association.

Argawal, M.K., et al.: Fibrosarcoma of nose and paranasal sinuses, J. Surg. Oncol. 15:53-57, 1980.

Blues, K.: A framework for nurses providing care to laryngectomy patient, Ca. Nurs. 1:441-446, 1978.

Bricker, P.L.: Chest tubes. The crucial points you mustn't forget, RN 43:21-26, 1980.

Cardin, S.: Acid-base balance in the patient with respiratory disease, Nurs. Clin. North Am. 15:593-601, 1980.

D'Agostino, J.S.: Teaching tips for living with C.O.P.D. at home, Nurs. 84 14:57, 1984.

Elpern, E.H.: Asthma update: Pathophysiology and treatment, Heart Lung 9:665-670, 1980.

Fuchs, P.L.: A.R.D.S.: physiology, signs, and symptoms, Nurs. 83 13:52-53, 1983.

Hunter, P.M.: Bedside monitoring of respiratory function, Nurs. Clin. North Am. 16:211-224, 1981.

Kerth, C.C.: Wound management following head and neck surgery, Nurs. Clin. North Am. 14:761-778, 1979.

Landis, K., and Smith, S.: The mechanically ventilated patient: a comprehensive nursing care plan, Crit. Care Q. 6:43, 1983.

Larsen, G.L.: Rehabilitation for the patient with head and neck cancer, Am. J. Nurs. 82:119-120, 1982.

McCormick, G.P., et al.: Artificial speech devices, Am. J. Nurs. 82:121-122, 1982.

Rokosky, J.S.: Assessment of the individual with altered respiratory function, Nurs. Clin. North Am. 16:195-209, 1981.

Straus, M.J.: Lung cancer: clinical diagnosis and treatment, ed. 2, New York, 1982, Grune & Stratton, Inc.

NURSING CARE PLAN

CHRONIC OBSTRUCTIVE PULMONARY DISEASE

Nursing Diagnoses	Expected Patient Outcomes	Nursing Interventions
Ineffective airway clearance related to increased mucous production and decreased expiratory force	Patient is able to clear the airway effectively	1. Assess breath sounds. 2. Give prescribed bronchodilators by aerosol; dilute in water. 3. Teach patient correct use of aerosol and to use only prescribed number of inhalations (excess use may result in overdosage with side effects). 4. Provide fluid intake of 2000 to 2500 ml/day to thin secretions (unless contraindicated, such as with cor pulmonale). 5. Avoid giving patient fluids that are very hot or cold (may cause bronchospasm or increased secretions). 6. Give postural drainage and clapping as prescribed. 7. Keep room air humid (30% to 50%) and free of inhalant irritants (such as smoke). 8. Avoid abrupt changes in temperature and use air conditioning as appropriate.
Impaired gas exchange related to destructive changes in the alveolar membrane	Patient will follow regimen to increase alveolar gas exchange	1. Assess respiratory status. 2. Provide prescribed low flow oxygen. 3. Provide breathing retraining: pursed lip breathing, leaning forward position for exhalation, abdominal breathing techniques, inhalation-exhalation exercises, and exhalation with exertion. 4. Teach relaxation techniques as appropriate (relaxation exercises, meditation).
Activity intolerance related to dyspnea and peripheral tissue hypoxia	Patient will have sufficient energy to maintain independence in the activities of daily living	1. Provide additional time to carry out the activities of daily living. 2. Provide for rest periods. 3. Teach patient to use controlled breathing techniques and to time exertion with exhalation. 4. Encourage the patient to follow a progressive muscle conditioning and exercise program. 5. Teach patient to avoid bed rest and immobility.
Alteration in nutrition, less than body requirements related to severe dypsnea and the effort of breathing	Patient ingests required nutrients and maintains a stable body weight	1. Monitor nutrient intake daily and weigh weekly. 2. Provide meals at intervals that promote increased intake; several small meals may be better tolerated. 3. Give high protein supplementary feedings. 4. Avoid heavy meals and foods that patient perceives as gas-producing. 5. Avoid very hot or cold foods. 6. Provide mouth care prior to eating if secretions are excessive. 7. Provide comfortable, pleasant environment and time for eating to decrease fatigue and encourage increased intake. 8. Encourage patient to use supplemental O_2 during meals if ordered.
Potential for ineffective individual coping related to the limitations of chronic disease	Patient will make a positive adjustment to disease restrictions	1. Give patient opportunities to express concerns about limitations imposed by COPD. 2. Provide rationale for necessary activities and information about positive effects. 3. Discuss with family/friends the need for patient to maintain role relationships and to feel worthwhile. 4. Assist patient to identify personal strengths. 5. Provide information about community resources, such as group meetings with other persons with COPD.

Continued.

NURSING CARE PLAN

CHRONIC OBSTRUCTIVE PULMONARY DISEASE—cont'd

Nursing Diagnoses	Expected Patient Outcomes	Nursing Interventions
Knowledge deficit related to measures to increase general health status and disease management	Patient is knowledgeable about the therapeutic regimen and measures to increase general health	1. Teach patient a. Nature of COPD and need to follow prescribed therapy and activities. b. Home medication and treatment programs. c. Home exercise program. d. Avoidance of respiratory irritants and infections. e. Signs requiring medical attention. f. Professional and community resources. g. Measures to prevent infection. h. Need to consult with M.D. about flu immunization. i. Importance of a "smoke-free" home environment.

CHAPTER 10

Disorders of the Gastrointestinal System

Problems involving the gastrointestinal system include a wide variety of common and uncommon, acute and chronic disorders. Ingestion and digestion are essential to health and survival and are closely linked to enjoyment of life. They are also closely linked with cultural habits and values. Disorders involving them present challenging situations for medical and nursing management.

Disorders presented in this chapter include problems of both the upper and lower gastrointestinal tract, and encompass infections, obstructions, and tumors, as well as structural alterations. Figure 10-1 shows the anatomical structure of the digestive system.

DISORDERS OF THE UPPER GASTROINTESTINAL TRACT

ORAL CANCER

Cancers involving the lips, oral cavity, and the tongue represent 5% of all cancers in men and 3% of cancers in women. They are associated with heavy smoking and alcohol consumption. The mortality rate for cancer of the tongue and floor of the mouth is high due to the vascularity and extensive lymph drainage of the area.

Pathophysiology

Most forms of oral cancer are basically asymptomatic. Early malignant lesions such as leukoplakia (white patches on the tongue or mucosa) frequently become cancerous but leave only a small ulcer or growth. Parotid tumors often present as painless lumps. Minimal interference with function occurs in early stages.

Medical Management

Medical therapy usually is some combination of surgery, radiotherapy, and chemotherapy. The extent of surgery depends on the location and spread of the disease but usually includes wide excision that significantly interferes with major oral functions such as eating and speaking. Prosthetic reconstruction is a common adjunct to this type of surgery to gradually restore appearance and function.

Nursing Management
Assessment—subjective
History of symptoms and diagnosis
History of smoking and alcohol use
Patient's understanding of proposed surgery or treatment plan, including:
  Extent of tissue destruction
  Degree of interference with communication
  Loss or interference with eating function
  Planned method for nutrition postoperatively
Patient's stage of grief, attitude about altered body image

Assessment—objective
Presence of leukoplakia, ulcerated lesion, or palpable lump
General health and nutritional status

Nursing diagnoses
Diagnoses will depend on the nature and extent of proposed treatment but commonly include:
  Impaired verbal communication related to destruction of structures essential for speech
  Potential for ineffective individual coping related to alterations in eating, swallowing, and speaking functions

Alteration in nutrition, less than body requirements, related to structural alterations in mouth

Disturbance in self-concept (body image or self-esteem) related to visible structural changes in mouth and throat

Alteration in oral mucous membranes related to surgical wounds or effects of radiation and chemotherapy

Knowledge deficit related to techniques of feeding and mouth care for associated structural changes

Expected outcomes

Patient will maintain communication with staff and family and explore alternative methods to verbal communication.

Patient will acquire appropriate self-care skills and demonstrate positive coping with body changes.

Patient will ingest all needed fluid and nutrients and maintain a stable weight.

Patient will incorporate body changes into an altered but positive body image.

Patient's mouth and neck will heal without complications or skin breakdown.

Patient will be knowledgeable about self-care skills necessary to accomplish feeding and mouth care.

Nursing interventions

Preoperative

Teach patient about proposed surgery and its outcomes.

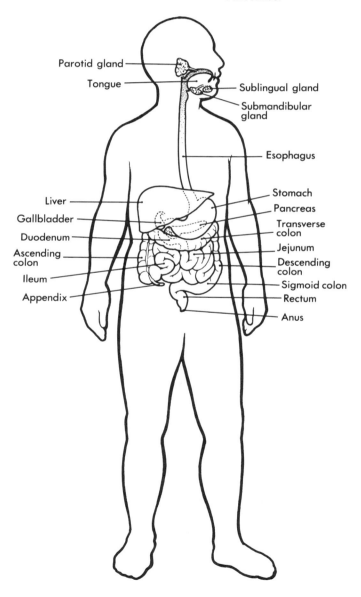

FIGURE 10-1 Digestive system.

Clarify misconceptions.

Ensure that patient's perceptions are accurate.

Encourage patient and family to verbalize their feelings and concerns about body changes.

Explain expected postoperative measures such as suctioning, nasogastric tube, drains.

Postoperative

Position patient to promote drainage of secretions from the mouth—usually in side-lying and then semi-Fowler's position when reactive.

Assist patient to remove saliva from mouth with suction, gauze wick, or emesis basin.

Provide constant monitoring if patient cannot swallow.

Assess for facial nerve damage or return of function— ask patient to raise eyebrows, frown, pucker lips.

Provide frequent oral hygiene care with mouth irrigations.

Use saline, water, or dilute hydrogen peroxide.

Teach patient technique for oral hygiene.

Provide nutrition through a liquid diet administered with a catheter, tube, or syringe.

Teach patient technique for feeding.

Advance patient to soft foods as healing progresses.

Provide privacy during feeding if patient prefers.

Teach patient to rinse mouth carefully after meals.

Establish effective communication with patient.

Use magic slate or pad and pencil.

Initiate speech retraining when healing occurs.

Teach patient to use throat and not lips for speech clarity.

Encourage patient to speak slowly.

Listen carefully and validate messages.

See Chapter 2 for appropriate interventions for patients receiving external or internal radiotherapy.

ALERT: Oral irradiation causes inflammation and tissue sloughing of mucous membranes, bad odor, and dry mouth. Meticulous oral hygiene and diet modifications are mandatory.

Put patient and family in contact with community agencies that can provide assistance.

Encourage patient to express feelings about surgery in order to reach grief resolution.

Evaluation

Patient is able to communicate needs accurately and maintains social interaction with family and friends.

Patient's surgical incisions heal without complications.

Patient demonstrates correct technique for mouth and incisional care and feeds self independently.

Patient successfully takes in prescribed diet and maintains a stable weight.

Patient demonstrates active coping and resumes familial roles.

Patient communicates acceptance of body changes and gradually resumes social and occupational roles.

ESOPHAGEAL DISORDERS

Esophageal disorders include several discrete and relatively unusual problems in which normal esophageal peristaltic function is disturbed. Table 10-1 defines some of these disorders and their treatment.

TABLE 10-1. Esophageal disorders

Disorder	Description	Treatment
Achalasia (cardio-spasm)	Absence of peristalsis in esophagus Failure of esophageal sphincter to relax after swallowing Esophagus dilates above the constriction Dysphagia is major symptom	Forceful dilation of the constricted sphincter Peristalsis is not restored
Esophageal diverticula	Bulging of esophageal mucosa through weakened portion of muscular layer Portions of ingested food may enter diverticula Causes regurgitation of food from diverticula	Surgical excision if symptoms severe
Esophageal tumors	Incidence higher in persons who have other esophageal problems and those with history of excessive alcohol intake Causes progressive dysphagia to solid food	Radiation therapy Surgical excision
Diaphragmatic hernia	Protrusion of part of the stomach through the diaphragm and into the thoracic cavity Precipitated by any condition increasing intraabdominal pressure Causes heartburn and reflux of gastric contents, especially when patient is in recumbent position	Minor problems treated with antacids, small frequent feedings, bland diet, and avoiding lifting Surgery to repair hernia via thoracic or abdominal route

PEPTIC ULCER DISEASE

A peptic ulcer is an ulceration involving the mucosa and deeper structures of the distal esophagus, stomach, or duodenum. Peptic ulcer is a common disorder among adults and affects men more often than women. Duodenal ulcers occur more often than gastric, especially in young adults.

Pathophysiology

Duodenal ulcers are related to an increase in acid secretion. Patients also demonstrate a markedly increased rate of gastric emptying that results in an increased amount of acid content entering the duodenum.

Gastric ulcers are not related to acid secretion or rate of gastric emptying. Ulceration appears to occur from decreased resistance of mucosa to acid.

Precipitating factors of diet, stress, medications, and heredity have been widely researched. Most of the findings are inconclusive but cigarette smoking, alcohol ingestion, and positive family history are related to ulcer development.

Medical Management

Medical therapy is usually employed to provide relief of symptoms and ulcer healing. Antacids are used to reduce gastric acidity by physical absorption or neutralization (see Table 10-2). A histamine antagonist (cimetidine) may be used to decrease secretion of acid by inhibiting action of histamine. Anticholinergics also decrease acid secretion and delay gastric emptying. A modified bland diet also may be prescribed.

ALERT: There is no evidence that modifying the diet accelerates healing of uncomplicated ulcers.

Rest, with cessation of normal activities, has been shown to be very effective in healing uncomplicated ulcers.

Surgery may be necessary if ulcers perforate, if they recur frequently, or if risk of cancer is high. Table 10-3 describes common types of ulcer surgery.

Nursing Management
Assessment—subjective

History of discomfort and home treatment attempted
Patient's description of pain:
  Onset: 1 to 2 hours after meals, often at night
  Type: aching, gnawing, or burning
  Location: epigastric, may radiate to back
  Relief: usually relieved by food or antacid
Patient's complaints of nausea or bloating
Smoking and alcohol history
Intake of potentially ulcerogenic drugs:
  Aspirin, steroids, antiinflammatory drugs
Family history of peptic ulcer
Personal and career stress levels

Assessment—objective

Guaiac-positive stools
Anemia
Hematemesis—frank GI bleeding
Signs of ulcer perforation:
  Rigid boardlike abdomen
  Decreased bowel sounds
  Signs of shock or sepsis
Positive results from upper GI series, gastroscopy, or gastric analysis

Nursing diagnoses
Diagnoses will depend on the severity of the ulcer but commonly include:
  Alteration in comfort—pain related to action of gastric secretions on the inflamed mucosa
  Knowledge deficit related to medications and diet modifications necessary to promote healing
  Nutrition, more than body requirements, related to the need to prevent ulcer pain through food ingestion
  Sleep pattern disturbance related to the occurrence of ulcer pain at night

Expected outcomes
Patient's discomfort will gradually decrease.
Patient will be knowledgeable concerning medications prescribed and life-style and diet modifications to promote healing.

TABLE 10-2 Antacids in common use

Trade Name	Composition	Comments
Maalox	Magnesium and aluminum hydroxide	Preferred antacid, good buffering Good taste Nonconstipating, low sodium
Mylanta	Magnesium and aluminum hydroxide Simethicone	Same as Maalox Antiflatulent
Amphogel	Aluminum hydroxide gel	Constipating Good antacid effects Contains sodium Can interfere with absorption of anticholinergics
Gelusil	Magnesium trisilicate Magnesium and aluminum hydroxide	Slower buffering effect Nonconstipating Gelatine effect in stomach coats and protects ulcer
Riopan	Magaldrate—chemical combination of magnesium and aluminum hydroxide	Rapid antacid effect High acid buffering No acid rebound Nonconstipating Low sodium

TABLE 10-3 Surgery used to treat ulcers

Procedure	Description	Procedure	Description
Vagotomy	Removes acid secreting stimulation and reduces responsiveness of stomach parietal cells; usually included in duodenal ulcer management. Types include: truncal (**A**); selective (**B**); proximal or parietal cell (**C**).	Subtotal gastrectomy	
		Billroth I	Removal of one half to two thirds of lower part of stomach and anastomosis of remaining segment to the duodenum (See **A** below.)
		Billroth II	Same procedure as Billroth I with anastomosis of remaining segment to the side of the proximal jejunum (See **B** below.)
		Gastrectomy	Removal of the entire stomach with anastomosis to duodenum or jejunum; presents many problems to patients and is usually done only for gastric cancer. (See **C** below.)

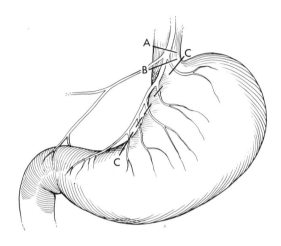

Procedure	Description
Pyloroplasty	Procedure to alter the pyloric outlet; usually to widen it to prevent gastric stasis after vagotomy. A longitudinal incision across pylorus is pulled apart and closed in a transverse position to widen pyloric outlet.

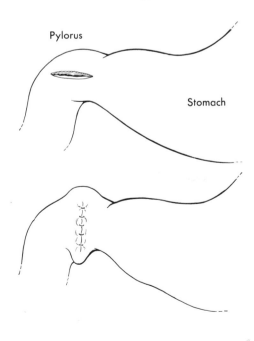

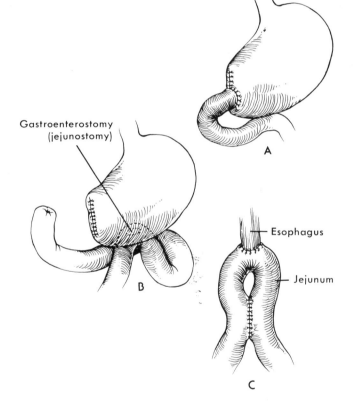

Illustrations from Phipps, W.J., Long, B.C., and Woods, N.F.: Medical-surgical nursing: concepts and clinical practice, ed. 2, St. Louis, 1983, The C.V. Mosby Co.

Patient will resume normal dietary patterns and maintain a stable weight.

Patient will enjoy restful, uninterrupted sleep.

Nursing interventions

Conservative treatment

Administer medications as prescribed.

Teach patient about side effects of antacids and their management.

Assess effectiveness of medications.

Teach patient proper timing of medications.

Give cimetidine 30 to 60 minutes before meals.

Give antacids 60 minutes after meals.

Teach patient to avoid medications known or suspected to be ulcerogenic, such as aspirin, steroids, antiinflammatory drugs.

Teach patient principles of diet modification. Patient should:

Eat bland diet if prescribed.

Avoid substances high in caffeine.

Avoid any foods that trigger ulcer pain.

Modify meal pattern to six small meals.

Avoid gastric overdistention which triggers reflux.

Teach patient importance of decreasing or eliminating cigarette smoking and alcohol intake.

Help patient to rest during ulcer attack.

Explore with patient life-style modification to reduce or better handle stress.

Preoperative

Provide appropriate patient teaching about proposed surgery and routines to be followed after the operation.

Postoperative

Initiate frequent position changes; use mid-Fowler's to high Fowler's position to facilitate chest excursion.

Encourage patient to cough and deep breathe.

Measure and observe nasogastric drainage frequently.

ALERT: Nastrogastric tubes are not routinely irrigated after stomach surgery. Clarify order before irrigating. Drainage should contain no fresh blood after first 12 hours.

Monitor for signs of leakage (peritonitis).

Monitor patient for signs of fluid and electrolyte imbalance.

Record intake and output accurately.

Introduce liquid and small amounts of bland food after nasogastric tube is removed—about 7 days after surgery.

Monitor for signs of early satiety and dumping syndrome (see box on p. 130)

Teach patient means of controlling symptoms.

Teach patient to monitor weight carefully and report signs of malabsorption and steatorrhea.

Teach patient to keep head elevated when lying down if reflux heartburn occurs.

DUMPING SYNDROME

Dumping syndrome is likely to occur following gastric resection but may occur with vagotomy, antrectomy, and gastroenterostomy procedures.

Early Dumping Syndrome:

Occurs within first hour after eating

Entrance of hyperosmolar food mixture into jejunum causes fluid to be drawn from the bloodstream to the jejunum

Symptoms: weakness, faintness, diaphoresis, palpitations, nausea, discomfort; diarrhea may follow

Late Dumping Syndrome:

Occurs between meals, 2 to 4 hours after eating

Sudden rise in blood sugar from hyperosmolar food mixture stimulates the release of insulin from the pancreas, triggering hypoglycemia

Symptoms: weakness, fatigue, diaphoresis, severe anxiety

Symptom Management:

Teach patient to eat meals low in carbohydrates, high in fats and proteins.

Teach patient to take fluids only between meals.

Teach patient to eat small, frequent meals.

Teach patient to lie down after eating.

Anticholinergic drugs may be used to control symptoms.

MANAGEMENT OF ULCER HEMORRHAGE (GI BLEEDING)

SYMPTOMS

Vomiting of blood (usually occurs with gastric ulcers)

Tarry stools (more common with duodenal)

Signs of early and progressive hypovolemic shock

Faint feeling, dizziness, thirst

Feelings of apprehension, restlessness

Dyspnea, pallor, rising pulse, falling blood pressure

INTERVENTIONS:

Place patient on bed rest.

Administer sedative to control restlessness if prescribed.

Monitor vital signs frequently (every 15 minutes).

Administer IV fluids and blood transfusions as prescribed.

Record accurate intake and output, assess response to treatment.

If bleeding is minor, administer milk and antacids hourly.

If bleeding is acute, irrigate through nasogastric tube with saline until clear.

Provide mouth care after patient vomits—a weak solution of hydrogen peroxide helps remove blood from oral mucous membranes.

Monitor stools for increasing blood content after episode.

Prepare patient for gastroscopy procedure if indicated.

Explain all procedures, keep calm, and reassure patient as much as possible.

Evaluation

Patient is free of ulcer pain.

Patient is knowledgeable about prescribed medications and has adjusted diet to eliminate substances that trigger ulcer pain.

Patient maintains a stable weight, shows no signs of malabsorption, and is able to control any symptoms of dumping syndrome.

Patient is able to enjoy uninterrupted sleep.

COMPLICATIONS OF PEPTIC ULCER

A peptic ulcer may perforate the stomach wall, obstruct the pyloric end of the stomach, or perforate a major blood vessel causing hemorrhage. Perforation and obstruction are usually treated surgically. Postoperative management for perforation involves supportive care for patient in severe shock. The mortality rate is quite high.

Peptic ulcers cause bleeding in about 15% to 20% of all cases. Management of this commonly occurring emergency is dealt with in the box on p. 130.

CANCER OF THE STOMACH

The incidence of stomach cancer has decreased significantly over the last 50 years but it remains a significant problem with a high mortality rate. It is a disease of later middle age affecting more men than women. The early symptoms are vague or nonexistent. Treatment involves subtotal or total gastrectomy followed by chemotherapy. Care is similar to that described for peptic ulcer disease.

DISORDERS OF THE LOWER GASTROINTESTINAL TRACT

INFLAMMATION
APPENDICITIS

Acute inflammation of the appendix occurs most commonly in people between 10 and 30 years, more often in males than females.

Pathophysiology

Occlusion of the lumen of the appendix by feces or kinking may impair the circulation and lower resistance to colon organisms. Mucosa becomes reddened, edematous, and often infected. Abscess, necrosis, or rupture can occur.

Medical Management

Removal of the appendix surgically is performed as quickly as the diagnosis can be established. It is an uncomplicated procedure with rapid recovery unless the appendix has abscessed or peritonitis is present.

Nursing Management
Assessment

Both subjective and objective factors should be assessed.

Subjective

History of sudden onset of right lower quadrant abdominal pain

Patient's complaints of:
Fever
Anorexia
Nausea or vomiting
Time of last food and fluid ingestion

Objective

Pain localizing at McBurney's point (halfway between umbilicus and crest of the right ileum)
Abdominal rigidity, rebound tendencies
Fever
Elevated white blood cell count, neutrophils over 75%

Nursing diagnoses

Alteration in comfort related to acute inflammation of appendix

Anxiety related to sudden onset of acute symptoms and need for emergency surgery

Potential fluid volume deficit related to NPO status and fever

Expected outcomes

Patient will be kept comfortable until surgical intervention can occur.

Patient will be knowledgeable about diagnostic workup and treatment as well as proposed surgery.

Patient will maintain a normal fluid and electrolyte balance.

Nursing interventions

Maintain patient on bed rest while diagnosis is established.

Give nothing by mouth and explain need for restriction to patient.

Monitor IV fluids carefully.
Record intake and output accurately.

Position patient for increased comfort and offer ice bag to abdomen for pain.

NOTE: Analgesics are generally withheld until diagnosis is confirmed.

Provide preoperative teaching and support to patient.

Post-op

Provide routine postsurgical care.

Encourage early ambulation.

Advance patient from liquid to diet as tolerated.

NOTE: Patients whose appendix ruptures and who develop peritonitis are seriously ill and will receive management similar to that offered to patients who experience perforation of a peptic ulcer.

Evaluation

Patient is free from pain and able to resume prior activity.

Patient does not develop complications in the postoperative period.

Patient maintains a stable fluid balance and resumes preillness food and fluid patterns.

CHRONIC INFLAMMATORY BOWEL DISORDERS

Crohn's disease and ulcerative colitis are two major inflammatory disorders of the large bowel. They tend to affect young adults. Specific causes have not been identified but both disorders follow recurrent patterns of exacerbation and remission and cause significant disruption to an individual's normal activity pattern. Table 10-4 compares some major aspects of both disorders.

Pathophysiology

Crohn's disease is characterized by ulcerations along the mucosa, thickening of the intestinal wall, and scar tissue formation. Ulcers commonly perforate and form fissures with the intestinal wall or hollow organ. Scar tissue interferes with normal bowel absorption. Lesions may occur in an ascending pattern throughout the bowel, often separated by patches of normal tissue.

Ulcerative colitis consists of mucosal ulcerations that begin in the rectosigmoid colon and spread upward through the colon. The ulcers may bleed or perforate. The bowel mucosa becomes edematous and thickened. The formation of scar tissue thickens the colon and causes loss of elasticity.

Medical Management

There is no specific treatment for Crohn's disease. The patient is offered symptomatic supportive care through diet modification and medications to provide comfort, decrease bowel motility, and prevent or treat local infection. Surgery may be necessary to treat obstruction or fistula formation.

The medical management of ulcerative colitis is directed toward treating infection, improving nutrition, and reducing bowel motility. Steroids may be administered to suppress bowel inflammation. Surgical intervention with total colectomy and permanent ileostomy is performed for acutely ill patients and those who suffer frequent exacerbations. Surgery cures the disease.

Nursing Management

Assessment—subjective

History of the disease and treatment

Patient's response to chronic disease

Patient's understanding of disease process, treatment plan, and precipitating factors if any

Diet pattern followed at home

Medications in use; patient's knowledge of action and side effects

Report of or signs of stress and anxiety

Patient's report of bowel pattern: frequency, consistency

Patient's report of pain or cramping

Patient's complaints of:
Fatigue
Anorexia, nausea

Problems with stool leakage

Assessment—objective

Body weight and recent changes

General appearance and health state

Presence of perianal excoriation

Stool assessment—presence of blood, pus, or fat

TABLE 10-4 Comparison of Crohn's disease and ulcerative colitis

	Crohn's Disease	Ulcerative Colitis
Age occurring	20–30 years 40–50 years	Young adults
Area affected	Mainly terminal ileum, cecum and ascending colon	Colon only, primarily the descending portion
Extent of involvement	Segmental areas of involvement	Continuous, diffuse areas of involvement
Character of stools	No blood; may contain fat, 3 to 4 semisoft stools per day	Blood present, frequent liquid stools
Complications	Fistulas; perianal disease; strictures; vitamin and iron deficiencies	Pseudopolyps, hemorrhage, cachexia, infrequently perforation
Etiology	Unknown—periods of exacerbation and remission	Unknown—periods of exacerbation and remission
Reasons for surgery	Fistulas; obstruction	Poor response to medical therapy, hemorrhage; perforation
Type of surgery	Colon resection with anastomosis	Total proctocolectomy with permanent ileostomy; continent ileostomy

Assessment of skin and mucous membranes for dehydration

Intake and output

Vital signs; fever

Positive results from stool analysis, proctoscopy or colonoscopy, barium enema

Nursing diagnoses

Diagnoses depend on stage and severity of the disorder but commonly include:

Activity intolerance related to extreme fatigue and debilitating effects of the disease

Alteration in bowel elimination (diarrhea) related to inflammation and ulceration of the bowel

Alteration in comfort—pain and cramping related to bowel ulceration and inflammation

Potential for ineffective individual coping related to chronic disabling effects of the disease

Actual or potential fluid volume deficit related to excessive GI losses through diarrhea

Alteration in nutrition, less than body requirements, related to inadequate intake and GI losses through diarrhea

Actual or potential impairment of skin integrity in perianal area related to excoriation from frequent diarrhea.

Expected outcomes

Patient's energy level will increase; patient will gradually resume normal activity pattern.

Patient will have less diarrhea and return to a nearly normal pattern of bowel elimination.

Patient will be relieved of discomfort of chronic diarrhea.

Patient will make a positive adjustment to chronic disease and maintain normal occupational and social activities.

Patient will return to a normal fluid and electrolyte balance.

Patient will gain weight to an appropriate level and select meals appropriate to dietary restrictions.

Patient will regain and maintain an intact skin.

CARE OF THE PATIENT WITH AN ILEOSTOMY

PREOPERATIVE CARE:

Teach patient in detail about the proposed surgery:
Size and appearance of stoma
Amount and consistency of drainage
Appliances used and their basic care
Encourage patient to ask questions and express feelings about major alteration in body appearance and function
Provide emotional support for stage of grief or acceptance patient exhibits
Provide for initiation of teaching and visits by enterostomal therapist
Therapist usually does stoma site selection

POSTOPERATIVE CARE:

Monitor fluid and electrolyte balance carefully:
Measure all output accurately
Maintain patency of IV lines and nasogastric drainage system
Observe for early signs of shock
Monitor stoma and suture line carefully:
Stoma should be pink–red; dark blue–red indicates impaired circulation and should be reported immediately
Note amount and type of drainage:
Mucus and serosanguineous discharge occurs for first 24–48 hours.
Liquid drainage occurs with returning peristalsis—may initially be as much as 1500 ml per day. Terminal ileum will begin absorption in about 2 weeks and drainage will then thicken.
Protect skin around stoma from fecal drainage:
Cleanse skin carefully and dry
Apply skin barrier
Change pouch as needed when leaking occurs—never simply add tape

Encourage patient to look at stoma and observe care.
Teach patient stoma management:
Teach technique for pouch application and skin care
Teach emptying and disposal or cleansing of pouch
Advance diet and fluids as prescribed:
Begin with bland low-residue diet
Avoid foods that cause increased gas or odor, such as corn, celery, cabbage, onions, and spiced foods
Teach patient that some foods and substances (seeds, kernels, enteric or slow-release medications) will pass through stoma unchanged.
Encourage patient to maintain an adequate fluid intake.
Discuss with patient modifications in life-style necessitated by ileostomy. Patient should:
Modify clothing.
Adjust recreational pursuits—contact sports should be avoided but most other activities may be resumed.
Make adaptations for traveling.
Hand carry all necessary ostomy supplies.
Use disposable equipment and take extra supplies.
Eat moderately—use restraint with new foods and water.
Put patient in touch with local ostomy associations.
Encourage patient to discuss concerns regarding resumption of sexual activity.
Teach patient importance of reporting any early signs of complications. Patient should be alert to:
Changes in color, consistency, or odor of stool.
Bleeding from stoma.
Persistent diarrhea or lack of stool.
Changes in stoma contour (prolapse or inversion) or signs of infection.
Skin irritation that doesn't respond to basic treatment.

Nursing interventions

Provide sufficient uninterrupted rest.
  Help patient to meet physical needs as indicated.
  Discuss appropriate relaxation and stress management.
  Space activities to avoid fatigue.
Avoid complications of bed rest.
  Provide regular skin care for cachectic patient.
  Protect bony prominences with sheepskin or pads.
  Provide perianal care when diarrhea is severe.
  Encourage regular use of sitz baths.
  Apply analgesic ointment (Nupercainal) to painful tissue.
Administer prescribed medications:
  Antibiotics (Azulfidine)
  Steroids (ACTH, prednisone)
  Antidiarrheals (Lomotil, paregoric)
  Antispasmodics (Pro-Banthine)
Teach patient about action and side effects of medications.
Monitor stools accurately: number, amount, and character.
Maintain accurate intake and output records, assess for dehydration.
Teach patient principles of diet modification if prescribed.
  Encourage patient to take oral nutrition.
  Encourage patient to explore use of high-protein, high-calorie, high-vitamin, low-residue diet if food tolerances permit.
Provide adequate fluids.
Make environment as pleasant as possible.
Offer ongoing emotional support to patient.
  Encourage patient to express feelings about disorder.
  Keep room as clean and odor free as possible.
  Empty bedpan promptly.
Provide appropriate care for patients undergoing total colectomy and ileostomy (see box on p. 133).

Evaluation

Patient has sufficient energy to perform all self-care activities and resume normal life-style.
Patient has normal pattern of bowel elimination and stabilizes colon output through ileostomy stoma.
Patient is free of cramping and discomfort.
Patient learns self-care management of ileostomy, establishes control over disease process, and resumes normal life-style.
Patient maintains a normal fluid and electrolyte balance.
Patient tolerates a normal diet and maintains desired weight.
Patient maintains an intact skin.

DIVERTICULITIS

Diverticula are small outpouchings of mucosa through defects in the muscular wall of the colon. This disorder occurs in late middle age and appears to be related to low intake of dietary fiber. Symptoms occur when diverticula become inflamed, causing painful spasms, or when complications develop such as perforation, obstruction, or hemorrhage.

Basic treatment consists of a diet high in fiber. Metamucil may also be prescribed to increase stool bulk. Antispasmodics (Pro-Banthine, Bentyl) may be prescribed during attacks of inflammation, along with analgesics and antibiotics. Colon resection surgery may be indicated for the patient who experiences complications.

BOWEL OBSTRUCTION

Obstruction of the movement of intestinal contents through the small or large intestine occurs from a wide variety of causes (see box below).

Pathophysiology

An increase in peristalsis occurs near the obstruction in an effort to move intestinal contents. As pressure increases, the proximal intestine dilates, smooth muscle becomes atonic, and peristalsis ceases.

CAUSES OF INTESTINAL OBSTRUCTION

MECHANICAL OBSTRUCTION:
Obstruction from causes that physically impede passage of intestinal contents:
  Adhesions
  Neoplasms
  Inflammatory bowel disease
  Foreign bodies, gallstones
  Fecal impaction
  Congenital strictures
  Radiation strictures
  Intussusception (telescoping of segment of bowel within itself)
  Volvulus (twisting of the bowel)

PARALYTIC OBSTRUCTION:
Peristalsis is inhibited from the effects of toxins or trauma on the autonomic control of intestinal motility. Frequently occurs from handling of the intestines during abdominal surgery. Passageway is open but peristalsis ceases. Causes include:
Abdominal surgery
Abdominal trauma
Hypokalemia
Myocardial infarction
Pneumonia
Spinal injuries
Peritonitis
Vascular insufficiency

Isotonic fluid then moves into the distended gut. The tissue becomes edematous and mucosal blood flow is decreased. Gas collects from air swallowing and the action of intestinal bacteria.

The end result may be the loss of large amounts of fluids and electrolytes with possible perforation or strangulation of the colon. The severity of the symptoms will depend on the site and degree of obstruction, and the amount of time that elapses before the patient seeks help.

Medical Management

Treatment of intestinal obstruction may include nasogastric intubation and decompression; fluid and electrolyte replacement; and surgical relief of the source of obstruction if necessary. The operative procedure will vary with the cause and location but may include release of adhesions, bowel resection, and temporary or permanent colostomy.

Nursing Management

Assessment—subjective
History and course of the symptoms
Location and severity of pain, cramping, tenderness
Patient's complaints of:
   Bloating or distention
   Nausea
Timing and consistency of latest bowel movement
Passage of flatus

Assessment—objective
Auscultation of the abdomen for:
   Loud high-pitched sounds early in obstruction
   Diminished or absent sounds late in obstruction
Vomiting
   Profuse, nonfecal if proximal small bowel
   Infrequent fecal type if distal bowel
Abdominal distention and girth
Signs of dehydration
Changes in vital signs
Abdominal x-ray studies showing air and fluid in the bowel and a gradually worsening electrolyte profile

Nursing diagnoses
Diagnoses may vary with cause and severity of obstruction but frequently include:
   Alteration in bowel elimination (absence of bowel motility) related to obstruction
   Alteration in comfort—pain related to pressure and accumulation of fluid and gas in the bowel
   Fluid volume deficit related to accumulation of excess fluid in the bowel
   Alteration in nutrition, less than body requirements, related to bowel obstruction and prolonged NPO period during treatment

Expected outcomes
Patient will return to a normal pattern of bowel elimination: obstruction will be relieved.
Patient will experience relief of pain and distention.
Patient will return to a normal fluid and electrolyte balance; intravascular volume will be restored.
Patient will return to a normal diet that meets daily nutritional requirements.

Nursing interventions
Maintain accurate intake and output records.
Assess for fluid and electrolyte imbalance.
Monitor IV fluids carefully.
Monitor vital signs for indications of shock, fluid overload, or peritonitis.
Provide good supportive care.
   Position patient comfortably and change positions frequently.
   Use Fowler's position to support ventilation.
   Assist patient as needed with activities of daily living.
   Provide regular skin care.
   Offer frequent, scrupulous mouth care, especially if patient is vomiting.
   Ensure adequate pulmonary ventilation; encourage deep breathing.
   Patient should avoid mouth breathing and air swallowing.
Auscultate for bowel sounds, passage of flatus.
Measure and record abdominal girth.
Maintain patency of intestinal tubes (see Table 10-5).

Evaluation
Patient has normal and regular patterns of bowel elimination.
Abdominal girth returns to normal.
Patient experiences no pain in the abdomen.
Patient has a normal fluid and electrolyte balance as evidenced by laboratory reports and intake and output balance.
Patient returns to a normal nutritional intake, regains lost weight, and meets body's basic nutritional needs.

HERNIA

A hernia is a protrusion of an organ or structure (usually the bowel) from its normal cavity through a congenital or acquired defect.

A reducible hernia can be returned by manipulation to its own cavity. An irreducible hernia cannot be returned to its own cavity. If the blood supply becomes occluded, the hernia is said to be strangulated.

Pathophysiology

Hernias may produce no symptoms beyond the palpable physical defect. Local irritation or pressure may cause pain. Severe pain is usually associated with strangulation, which may produce all of the problems of intestinal obstruction and necessitate emergency surgery.

Medical Management

The only cure for a hernia is surgical repair of the defect. Interim treatment with truss support may be used for patients who either refuse or are not candidates for surgery.

Nursing management

Assessment—subjective
History of the hernia:
 Onset, reducibility, change in size
Presence of pain or tenderness
Occupation and leisure activities that involve heavy lifting
Presence of smoking habit, allergies, upper respiratory infection that cause chronic coughing.

Assessment—objective
Appearance, size, tenderness of hernia
Lung sounds, presence of chronic cough

Nursing diagnoses
Alteration in comfort—pain related to tenderness of the hernia or postoperative incisional pain
Activity intolerance related to postoperative pain and edema at incisional site

Expected outcomes
Patient will have a decrease in pain and tenderness at hernia site.
Patient will gradually resume normal activity pattern and use good body mechanics when performing heavy lifting.

Nursing interventions
Report to physician presence of any respiratory disorder that may place extra strain on repair sutures.
Teach patient importance of ambulation and deep breathing since minimal postoperative coughing is preferred.
 Splint incisional area firmly if patient is coughing.
Patient should avoid any abdominal straining.
 Provide stool softeners or cathartics as needed.
Monitor postoperative voiding carefully.
 Assist patient out of bed to promote voiding.
Provide sufficient analgesia to enable patient to ambulate.
Provide icebags and scrotal support for inguinal hernias.
Monitor integrity and healing of the incision carefully.
Teach patient to refrain from driving and heavy lifting after discharge. Clarify specific physician's restrictions.
Reinforce and teach importance of using good body mechanics.

Evaluation
Patient experiences no residual pain or tenderness at hernia site.

TABLE 10-5 Use of intestinal tubes

Purpose	Types	Tube Use and Patient Care
To drain fluids and gas that accumulate above a mechanical obstruction and to decompress the bowel	Miller-Abbot (double-lumen tube). One lumen leads to the balloon and the other has openings for drainage or irrigation. Cantor (single-lumen tube). Cantor tube has only one opening used for drainage; balloon must be injected with mercury before insertion. Both tubes have balloons that, when inflated, act like a bolus of food, stimulating peristalsis and advancing along the intestinal tract. If peristalsis is absent, the weight of mercury in the balloon carries it forward.	Special care is taken during insertion as the presence of the balloon makes passage through the nose quite difficult. After tube passes into the stomach, its progression is aided by positioning the patient. Encourage patient to lie on right side for 2 hours. Patient switches to lying on back for 2 hours. Patient lies on left side for 2 hours. Walking about stimulates further movement by increasing peristalsis. Advance tube 7 to 10 cm (3 to 4 inches) at specified intervals to provide slack. Never tape tube in place until it reaches desired position. Pin excess tubing to clothing. Provide comfort measures for nose and throat. Irrigate tube for patency if ordered—return aspiration is often not feasible. If tube is well advanced in bowel, light food and fluid may be permitted. Monitor patient for return of bowel sounds, passage of flatus, or spontaneous bowel movement.

Patient resumes prior activities and utilizes good principles of body mechanics in moving and lifting.

CANCER OF THE BOWEL

Malignant tumors of the colon and rectum are among the most common cancers affecting adults of both sexes. These cancers represent a serious health problem, affecting over 110,000 persons per year. Their cause remains unknown but both environmental and genetic factors are implicated. Diets low in dietary fiber appear to be related.

Pathophysiology

Colon cancer may develop as a polyplike lesion or as a ringlike wall mass that encircles the lumen of the colon. Polyps may ulcerate but rarely obstruct. In the descending and rectosigmoid portion of the colon, the constricting tumor may present with symptoms of bowel obstruction. Specific symptoms vary with position and type of tumor growth pattern. The tumor may alter bowel elimination patterns, trigger nausea or vomiting, or produce blood in the stool. Diagnosis is confirmed by proctoscopy or biopsy.

COLOSTOMY IRRIGATION

Position patient on toilet, or on padded chair next to toilet if perineal wound has not healed.
Remove old pouch.
Clean skin and stoma with water.
Apply irrigating sleeve and belt.
Fill bag with desired amount of warm water (250 to 1000 ml).
Hang bag so bottom of bag is at shoulder height.
Remove air from tubing.
Gently insert irrigating cone snugly into stoma, holding it parallel to floor.
Let water run in slowly until patient identifies need to expel stool.
Remove cone and allow solution to drain into container.
When most of stool is expelled (about 15 min), rinse sleeve with water and close up bottom end.
Encourage activity to complete bowel emptying (about 30–45 min).
Remove sleeve and apply clean pouch:
1. Trace pattern ⅛ inch larger than the stoma on paper side of the skin barrier (Stomadhesive, Hollihesive, Reliaseal, Colly Seal).
2. Cut hole on pattern line and round the edges.
3. Trace pattern on pattern side of the pouch, making it slightly larger than hole for the skin barrier.
4. Cut hole on pattern line and round the edges.
5. Remove paper backing from pouch and apply to shiny side of the skin barrier.
6. Warm skin barrier slightly, remove paper backing, and press and seal to dry clean skin around the stoma.

Medical Management

The treatment of colon cancer is surgical with removal of the tumor, surrounding colon, and lymph nodes. If possible, the remaining portions of the bowel are anastomosed. Usually tumors of the middle and lower portion of the rectum necessitate formation of a permanent colostomy. Preoperative work-up includes an extremely thorough bowel prep with laxatives, antibiotics, and enemas to empty and cleanse the bowel.

Nursing Management

The nursing management associated with bowel cancer is very similar to that described for intestinal obstruction in general. Preoperative and postoperative care for a patient with a colostomy also closely follows that outlined for the ileostomy patient. Problems with altered body image are often more severe for bowel cancer patients because they have little time to comprehend and internalize the implications of the diagnosis and treatment. Depending on the location of the colostomy, irrigation may be prescribed to facilitate management. This procedure is outlined in the box on p. 137. General principles of care for a patient with bowel surgery are outlined in the box on p. 137.

CARE OF THE PATIENT HAVING BOWEL SURGERY

PREOPERATIVE CARE:
Give patient low-residue diet during workup period.
Give patient clear liquids for day prior to surgery.
Administer prescribed laxatives and enemas.
Administer prescribed bowel cleansing antibiotics.
Provide adequate perianal cleansing and ointments.
Reinforce teaching about proposed surgery and postoperative routines and equipment.

POSTOPERATIVE CARE:
Encourage maximum possible activity, coughing, and deep breathing.
Maintain patency of IV and drainage apparatus.
Monitor intake and output accurately; assess for signs of fluid imbalance.
Monitor for signs of returning peristalsis—bowel sounds, flatus.
Provide good oral hygiene, keep nose and mouth well lubricated.

MEASURES SPECIFIC TO ABDOMINAL PERINEAL RESECTION:
Monitor perineal dressings; initial drainage is profuse.
Reinforce or change dressings as ordered, wound is often open.
Encourage leg exercises as risk of thrombophlebitis is high.
Maintain patency of drainage tubes and suction if present.
Initiate normal saline perineal irrigations as prescribed. Hold dressings in place with T-binders.
Substitute sitz baths for irrigations when patient is fully ambulatory.
Help patient to find comfortable positions for rest and sleep—usually side-lying position is best tolerated.

ANORECTAL LESIONS

Common anorectal lesions are described in Table 10-6. Of these, hemorrhoids are the most frequently occurring and cause a great deal of pain and discomfort. Causes that have been identified include heredity, prolonged sitting or standing, chronic constipation, and any situation that increases intraabdominal pressure such as pregnancy, cirrhosis, or CHF.

Pathophysiology

Congestion in the hemorrhoidal plexus leads to varicosities in the lower rectum or the anus. Internal hemorrhoids (above the internal sphincter) often bleed on defecation. External hemorrhoids (outside the anal sphincter) bleed relatively rarely and seldom cause pain unless a vein ruptures and causes a thrombosis.

Medical Management

A variety of treatments are available for hemorrhoids. Local conservative treatment is usually managed independently by the patient and involves some combination of warm or ice compresses, analgesic ointments, sitz baths, and stool softeners. Sclerosing substances may be injected into internal hemorrhoids. Rubber band ligation or standard surgical ligation may also be performed.

Nursing Management
Assessment—subjective
History of condition
Self-treatment methods used
Medications in use
Normal diet and exercise pattern
Amount and severity of pain and bleeding
Normal defecation pattern

Assessment—objective
Appearance of stool
Presence of blood in stool

Nursing diagnoses
Alteration in bowel elimination (constipation) related to fear and pain associated with defecation
Alteration in comfort—pain related to defecation or postsurgical incisional discomfort
Knowledge deficit related to the effects of diet and exercise on normal bowel patterns

Expected outcomes
Patient will reestablish a regular pattern of bowel elimination without pain or bleeding.
Patient will not have pain or discomfort with defecation.
Patient will be knowledgeable about diet and exercise effects on patterns of bowel elimination and modify patterns to enhance regular elimination.

Nursing interventions
Preoperative
Administer laxatives or enema as prescribed.
Encourage normal intake of food or low-residue diet.
Teach use of sitz bath for postoperative period.
Teach patient about surgical procedure and management of pain and elimination in the postoperative period.
Postoperative
Administer pain medication liberally as prescribed.
Assist patient to position of comfort.
  Patient should avoid sitting and supine position.
Monitor rectal area for signs of bleeding.
  Carefully inspect dressings if in use.

TABLE 10-6 Common anorectal lesions

Lesion	Description	Signs and Symptoms	Medical Treatment
Anal fissure	Slitlike ulceration in epithelium of anal canal	Pain with defecation; bleeding; constipation	Stool softeners; analgesic ointments; sitz baths; surgical removal of fissure if medical therapy ineffective
Anal abscess	Abscess in tissue around anus	Persistent throbbing anal pain with walking, sitting, defecation; systemic signs of infection	Incision and drainage of abscess
Anal fistula	Hollow track leading through anal tissue from anorectal canal through skin near anus	Purulent discharge near anus	Fistulectomy or fistulotomy
Hemorrhoids	Varicosities of lower rectum and anus	Bleeding with defecation; pain if thrombosed	Analgesic ointments for mild discomfort; injection, ligation, or hemorrhoidectomy for severe discomfort

From Phipps, W.J., Long, B.C., and Woods, N.F.: Medical-surgical nursing: concepts and clinical practice, ed. 2, St. Louis, 1983, The C.V. Mosby Co.

Monitor for adequate urinary elimination.

Encourage patient to be out of bed to void.

Administer ice packs, warm compresses, or ointments as prescribed.

Initiate use of sitz baths three or four times daily.

Monitor patient for hypotension during first sitz bath.

Administer stool softeners, mineral oil, or bulk formers to assist in stool passage.

Provide analgesia and monitor patient for fainting during first bowel movement.

Encourage use of sitz bath after defecation.

Provide discharge teaching about promoting proper bowel function. Patient should:

Ingest high fiber diet.

Keep fluid intake high.

Engage in regular moderate exercise.

Respond promptly to defecation stimulus.

Continue use of stool softeners if indicated.

Evaluation

Patient establishes pattern of regular bowel elimination, passes soft formed stool without straining.

Patient passes stool without pain or bleeding.

Patient eats a diet with adequate fiber, maintains a liberal fluid intake, and exercises regularly.

BIBLIOGRAPHY

Almy, T.P., and Howell, D.A.: Diverticular disease of the colon, N. Engl. J. Med. 302:324-330, 1980.

Broadwell, D.C., and Jackson, B.S.: Principles of ostomy care, St. Louis, 1982, The C.V. Mosby Co.

Burkhart, C.: Upper GI hemorrhage: the clinical picture, Am. J. Nurs. 81:1817-1820, 1981.

Cancer of the colon and rectum, CA 30:208-215, 1980.

Daly, D.M.: Oral cancer: everyday concerns, Am. J. Nurs. 79:1415-1419, 1979.

Given, B., and Simmons, S.: Gastroenterology in clinical nursing, ed. 3, St. Louis, 1979, The C.V. Mosby Co.

Kratzer, J.B., and Rauschenberger, D.S.: What to teach your patient about his duodenal ulcer, Nurs. 78 8(1):54-56, 1978.

Literte, J.W.: Nursing care of patients with intestinal obstruction, Am. J. Nurs. 77:1003-1006, 1977.

McNamara, J.P.: Esophageal cancer, Nurs. 82 12(3):64-65, 1982.

Stromberg, M.F., and Stromberg, P.: Test your knowledge of caring for the patient with peptic ulcer, Nurs. 81 11(5):66-69, 1981.

Trowbridge, J., and Carl, W.: Oral care of the patient having head and neck irradiation, Am. J. Nurs. 75:2146-2149, 1975.

Wilpizeski, M.D.: Helping the ostomate return to normal life, Nurs. 81 11(3):60-64, 1981.

NURSING CARE PLAN

PEPTIC ULCER

Nursing Diagnoses	Expected Patient Outcomes	Nursing Interventions
Alteration in comfort—pain related to the action of gastric secretions on the inflamed mucosa	Patient's pain decreases or resolves	1. Give prescribed medications: a. Antacids: 1 and 3 hrs after meals and at bedtime for best effect; may be given as often as every 30 min for severe pain b. H₂ blockers: cimetidine with meals and at bedtime, ranitidine at bedtime c. Sucralfate: 1 hr before meals and at bedtime d. Do not give antacids concurrently with cimetidine or sucralfate. 2. Avoid substances high in caffeine. 3. Eliminate foods that trigger gastric pain. 4. Eliminate smoking and alcohol intake. 5. Use a 5–6 meal pattern. 6. Assist patient to rest.
Potential for injury related to ulcer perforation or hemorrhage	Patient does not experience bleeding	1. Monitor patient for signs of complications: a. Signs of overt bleeding: hematemesis, tarry stools b. Signs of shock c. Signs of perforation: severe sharp abdominal pain 2. If signs of complications occur, give patient nothing by mouth and prepare to insert NG tube for lavage. 3. Eliminate ulcerogenic medications if possible: aspirin, antiinflammatories, steroids
Ineffective individual coping related to life stresses	Patient is able to understand and identify stressors and effectively problem solve to reduce them	1. Assist patient to identify: a. Any present stressors in daily life b. Feelings and responses to identified stressors c. Usual coping mechanisms d. Individuals who can serve as support persons when new stressors occur 2. Assist patient to explore alternative ways of coping. 3. Teach patient stress management techniques, such as relaxation response, as appropriate. 4. Encourage activities that promote relaxation (recreation, hobbies). 5. Assist patient to: a. Identify specific health-risking behaviors that may aggravate the ulcer (such as smoking, caffeine, alcohol, stressful situations) b. Explore ways of modifying the behaviors, such as ways to stop smoking or drinking, or to avoid certain stressful situations 6. Encourage health-seeking behaviors, such as good nutrition and adequate activity and rest.
Knowledge deficit related to medications and diet modifications necessary to promote healing	Patient is knowledgeable concerning prescribed medications and diet modifications necessary to promote healing.	1. Teach patient: a. Nature of peptic ulcers b. Factors that contribute to healing and decreased occurrence of ulcers c. Medication regimens d. Methods to reduce stress and promote relaxation e. Need to report symptoms of bleeding, perforation and pyloric obstruction to physician immediately

NURSING CARE PLAN

ULCERATIVE COLITIS

Nursing Diagnoses	Expected Patient Outcomes	Nursing Interventions
Alteration in nutrition: less than body requirements related to inadequate intake and losses throuth diarrhea	Patient's weight stabilizes at an appropriate level Patient selects meals appropriate to dietary restrictions	1. Give prescribed feedings during acute episode. 2. If elemental feedings are required, chill the fluids and offer a variety of flavors. 3. Provide a high-protein, high-carbohydrate diet after acute episode subsides. Offer supplemental vitamins. 4. Identify foods, such as foods high in fats or very high in fiber, spicy foods, or milk products, that are poorly tolerated by patient and eliminate these foods from the diet. 5. Use measures to encourage increased food intake (pleasant environment, reduction of stress at mealtime, between-meal snacks). 6. Give prescribed vitamins. 7. Monitor weight 2 to 3 times a week.
Actual or potential fluid volume deficit related to excessive GI losses	Patient maintains a balance of intake and output	1. Monitor intake and output daily. 2. Encourage fluids to 2500 ml/day if patient is on oral diet. 3. Assess skin turgor and status of mucous membranes daily. 4. Give mouth care as needed to keep membranes moist and encourage eating.
Alteration in bowel elimination: diarrhea related to inflammation and ulceration of the bowel	Patient passes soft, formed stools without cramping or urgency	1. Monitor stools for characteristics and frequency. 2. Give prescribed antiinflammatory medications (sulfasalazine, corticosteroids) and monitor for side effects. 3. Give prescribed bulk hydrophilic agents (Metamucil). 4. Give prescribed antidiarrheals as needed.
Alteration in comfort: pain and abdominal cramping related to bowel inflammation and perianal irritation	Patient is relieved of abdominal discomfort	1. Facilitate easy patient access to toilet, commode, or bedpan (abdominal cramping is relieved by bowel movements). Empty promptly. 2. Provide soft toilet tissue or medicated wipes (Tucks). 3. Keep anal area clean with mild soap and water and dry well. Apply ointments for comfort. 4. Provide sitz baths for rectal comfort, as necessary. 5. Protect and massage pressure areas developing from prolonged toilet/bedpan sitting. Keep sheepskin or eggcrate mattress on bed. 6. Use room deodorizers, as needed. 7. Examine anus at intervals for signs of perianal fissures.

Potential for ineffective individual coping related to chronic disabling effects of disease	Patient makes a positive adjustment to chronicity of disease and maintains usual occupational and social roles	1. Assess patient's knowledge of disorder and provide information as needed.
		2. Schedule regular time periods to interact with patient and begin to develop a trust relationship.
		3. Give patient opportunities to express feelings about condition (frustration, depression, anger) and identify content related to these feelings.
		4. Help patient identify:
		  a. Life stressors and usual response to the stressors
		  b. Usual coping mechanisms and alternative methods of coping
		5. Encourage patient to participate in planning activities and assuming self-care.
		6. Give family opportunities to identify their feelings about the patient's condition and related behavior.

Continued.

NURSING CARE PLAN

ULCERATIVE COLITIS—cont'd

Nursing Diagnoses	Expected Patient Outcomes	Nursing Interventions
Activity intolerance related to extreme fatigue and debilitating effects of the disease	Patient will experience and increasing energy level and gradually resume a normal activity pattern	1. Encourage rest during exacerbations to decrease peristalsis. 2. Space activities to conserve energy. 3. Provide privacy and quiet for uninterrupted rest. 4. Assist with ADL as needed. 5. Encourage patient to gradually resume responsibility for self-care as condition improves. 6. Discuss need for independence with family.

CHAPTER 11

Disorders of the Liver, Biliary System, and Pancreas

The liver, biliary system, and pancreas are affected by a variety of pathologic processes, many of which are chronic in nature and require significant adjustments in life-style. They include disorders caused by infectious organisms as well as those that result from changes in structure or function.

LIVER DISORDERS

The liver is subject to a wide variety of disorders ranging from trauma and abscess through infection and cancer. The two most common disorders, hepatitis and cirrhosis, will be the focus of this presentation. Figure 11-1 shows portal circulation.

HEPATITIS

Hepatitis is an acute liver inflammation. It can be caused by viruses, bacteria, or toxic injury to the liver. There are some pathologic differences, but the management of the different types of hepatitis is very similar. Hepatitis represents a significant health problem both in the United States and worldwide.

Type A viral hepatitis primarily affects children and young adults. The route of infection is primarily oral-fecal through contaminated food or water. It has an abrupt, often febrile onset and usually resolves without complications.

Type B viral hepatitis affects all age groups. The route of infection is primarily parenteral through contaminated blood or blood products, but direct and sexual transmission can occur. It runs a more protracted course and may lead to chronic disease.

Non-A–Non-B viral hepatitis affects all age groups but primarily adults. The route of infection is parenteral through contaminated blood or blood products. It has an insidious onset and may lead to chronic liver disease. Table 11-1 details the specific differences between these three major forms.

Pathophysiology

Viral hepatitis causes diffuse inflammatory infiltration of hepatic tissue with local necrosis. The pathologic process is evenly distributed throughout the liver. Inflammatory destruction and regeneration occur almost simultaneously. Bile flow is interrupted, antigen-antibody complexes activate the complement system, bilirubin diffuses into the tissues and is excreted by the kidney, bile salts accumulate under the skin, and hepatomegaly and splenomegaly occur.

Medical Management

There is no specific medical therapy for hepatitis. Treatment is aimed at providing sufficient rest and nutrition to allow the body to return to normal. Although the disease usually persists for 2 to 4 months, recovery is usually complete.

Nursing Management

Assessment—subjective

History of symptoms

History of exposure to hepatotoxic agents, jaundiced persons, injections, or blood transfusions

Preicteric stage

Patient's complaints of:

Headache

Fever

Chills

Severe anorexia, nausea, and vomiting

Severe fatigue and malaise

Arthralgia and liver tenderness

Pruritus (itching)

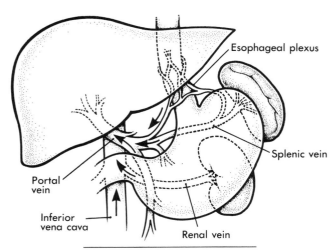

FIGURE 11-1 Portal circulation.

Assessment—objective

Icteric phase

Elevated temperature

Yellow sclera and skin

Dark amber urine

Clay colored stools

Hepatomegaly and acute tenderness

Skin rashes

Abnormal liver function tests—SGOT (serum glutamic oxidase transaminase), SGPT (serum glutamic pyruvate transaminase), direct and indirect bilirubin

Nursing diagnoses

Diagnoses will vary depending on the severity and stage of the disease, but commonly include:

Activity intolerance related to extreme fatigue

Alteration in comfort related to abdominal distention, liver tenderness, and pruritus

Deficit in diversional activity related to bed rest and the protracted course of the disease

Alteration in nutrition, less than body requirements, related to pronounced anorexia and nausea

Potential impairment of skin integrity related to severe pruritus

Expected outcomes

Patient will gradually resume a normal activity level and cease to feel fatigued.

Patient will not experience pruritus or abdominal discomfort.

Patient will receive appropriate meaningful stimulation and not be troubled by boredom or depression.

Patient will resume a normal nutritional intake that meets all basic body needs.

Patient will maintain an intact skin.

Nursing interventions

Maintain patient on bed rest during acute phase.

Caution patient to resume activity very gradually.

ALERT: Relapses are believed to be frequently related to too rapid increases in activity.

Promote patient comfort while on bed rest.

Provide frequent position changes.

Keep environment quiet.

Encourage the restriction of visitors during acute phase.

Space care activities and assist patient with activities of daily living as needed.

Encourage oral fluid intake (to 3000 ml/day).

Use IV supplement if nausea or vomiting is severe.

Maintain accurate intake and output records.

Discuss food preferences with patient.

Fruit juices, carbonated beverages, and hard candy are well tolerated.

Diet high in protein and carbohydrates but low in fats is optimal.

Provide frequent mouth care—keep environment pleasant and odor free.

Provide or encourage good skin care.

Implement measures to treat pruritus.

Give tepid water baths; avoid use of heat and rubbing as they increase vasodilation and itching sensation.

Encourage patient to keep nails trimmed short.

Administer medications if prescribed—antiemetics, antihistamines, vitamins.

Maintain appropriate precautions.

Provide separate toilet facilities.

Use disposable dishes and utensils.

Take special precautions with excreta, blood, and blood drawing equipment.

Avoid direct contact.

Provide diversionary activities to prevent boredom.

Teach patient importance of continuing to restrict activity during home convalescence.

Teach family measures for continuing care at home.

Describe symptoms indicative of relapse.

Evaluation

Patient maintains limited activity until liver enzymes return to normal, then gradually resumes all pre-illness activities.

Patient experiences no discomfort or pruritus.

TABLE 11-1 Characteristics of different types of viral hepatitis

Characteristic	Hepatitis A	Hepatitis B	Hepatitis non-A, non-B
Previous names	Infectious Epidemic Short-incubation	Serum Homologous serum Long-incubation	None
Onset	Abrupt, febrile	Insidious, seldom febrile	Insidious, often nonicteric
Incubation period			
Onset	10–40 days	45–180 days	14–150 days
Average	30	90	50
Incidence	50% of cases	25% of cases	25% of cases
Primary sources	Fecally contaminated food, water, milk, shell-fish	Blood, serum, plasma	Blood, serum, plasma
Primary route of infection	Fecal-oral	Percutaneous, sexual	Percutaneous, sexual
Mortality	Less than 0.5%	1%-5%	1%-3%
Populations: Posttransfusion	No	10% of cases	90% of cases
Age	Younger	Older	Older
High risk	Low income, overcrowded, institutionalized	Health-care workers, patients and staff in dialysis units, laboratory workers, homosexuals, drug users	Recipients of blood transfusions or blood components
Carrier state	Does not occur	Occurs	Occurs
Prophylaxis	Gamma globulin (ISG) ameliorates severity	Hepatitis B immune globulin (HBIG) at 1 wk, repeated at 1 mo reduces risk of infection Hepatitis B vaccine (HbVac)	Not available
Major preventive measures	Sanitation controls (food, water, milk, sewage), pollution control of lakes and rivers; enteric precautions with diagnosed cases	Screening of blood donors for HBsAg or history of jaundice; use of volunteers who donate blood rather than those who receive pay Use of disposable and individual equipment for parenteral administration Avoidance of blood products from pooled sources Blood/body secretions precautions with diagnosed cases	

From Long, B.C., and Phipps, W.J.: Essentials of medical-surgical nursing: a nursing process approach, St. Louis, 1985, The C.V. Mosby Co.

Patient maintains social interactions and avoids boredom and depression.

Patient eats a normal diet and meets all basic nutritional needs.

Patient's skin is intact and without abrasions.

CIRRHOSIS

Cirrhosis is a term applied to several diseases that are characterized by diffuse liver inflammation and fibrosis leading to severe structural changes and significant loss of liver function. Table 11-2 describes the common forms of cirrhosis. Laënnec's cirrhosis, the most common variety in the United States, tends to affect more men than women and is closely associated with malnutrition, particularly in conjunction with alcoholism.

Pathophysiology

The basic process of cirrhosis is liver cell death, scar tissue formation, and regeneration of cells that distorts structure and produces circulatory changes. The signs and symptoms are the result of progressive loss of normal metabolic functions. The proliferation of fibrous tissue causes obstruction of the portal vein. The body attempts to circumvent the obstruction by establishing collateral

TABLE 11-2 Types of cirrhosis

Type	Etiology	Description
Laënnec's cirrhosis (nutritional, portal, or alcoholic cirrhosis)	Alcoholism, malnutrition	Massive collagen formation; liver in early fatty stage is large and firm; in late state is small and nodular
Postnecrotic cirrhosis	Massive necrosis from hepatotoxins, usually viral hepatitis	Liver is decreased in size with nodules and fibrous tissue
Biliary cirrhosis	Biliary obstruction in liver and common bile duct	Chronic impairment of bile drainage; liver is first large, then becomes firm and nodular; jaundice is a major symptom
Cardiac cirrhosis	Right side congestive heart failure (CHF)	Liver is swollen and changes are reversible if CHF treated effectively; some fibrosis with long-standing CHF
Nonspecific, metabolic cirrhosis	Metabolic problems, infectious diseases, infiltrative diseases, gastrointestinal diseases	Portal and liver fibrosis may develop; liver is enlarged and firm

From Long, B.C., and Phipps, W.J.: Essentials of medical-surgical nursing: a nursing process approach, St. Louis, 1985, The C.V. Mosby Co.

circulation. Early degenerative changes produce general gastrointestinal symptoms. Later symptoms include jaundice, ascites, and edema.

Medical Management
There is no specific treatment for cirrhosis. The emphasis is on supportive care and preventing further damage to the liver. Therapy includes diet modification, balance of rest and exercise, supplemental vitamins, and treatment of specific complications. Liver biopsy is felt to be essential for establishing a definitive diagnosis. The box on p. 147 outlines the care associated with a liver biopsy.

Nursing Management
  Assessment—subjective
  Early phase
  Patient's complaint of:
    Weight loss
    Anorexia and indigestion
    Intestinal dysfunction
    Pain, particularly in right upper quadrant
  History and severity of symptoms
  History of other health problems
  Normal dietary pattern
  History of alcohol intake
  Later phase
  Patient's complaint of:
    Easy bruising
    Hair loss—axilla, pubic area
    Menstrual irregularities or impotence

  Assessment—objective
  Later phase
  Jaundice
  Ascites—increased abdominal girth

Peripheral edema
Presence of dilated visible abdominal veins
Hemorrhoids
Palmar erythema (red palms)
Spider angiomas (tiny, red, pulsating arterioles)
Gynecomastia (breast development in males)
Decreasing level of consciousness
Abnormal liver function tests
Anemia leukopenia and thrombocytopenia

Nursing diagnoses
Diagnoses depend on stage and severity of the disorder, but commonly include:
  Activity intolerance related to chronic fatigue, anemia, weight of ascites, and peripheral edema
  Alteration in comfort related to liver inflammation and ascites
  Alteration in fluid volume (excess) related to increased intraabdominal pressure and decreased osmotic gradient
  Potential for injury related to thrombocytopenia and leukopenia
  Noncompliance with diet modification and prohibition concerning alcohol intake
  Alteration in nutrition, less than body requirements, related to fatigue and anorexia
  Disturbance in self-concept (body image) related to jaundice and ascites
  Potential impairment of skin integrity related to decreased activity, ascites, and peripheral edema

Expected outcomes
Patient will have sufficient energy to maintain independence in self-care activities.

CARE OF THE PATIENT HAVING A LIVER BIOPSY

PROCEDURE:
A specially designed needle is inserted through the chest or abdominal wall into the liver and a small piece of tissue is removed for study.

PREPROCEDURE CARE:
Be sure that patient understands the nature and risks of the test; informed consent is frequently required.
Explain the need to hold breath during the procedure to stabilize the liver.
Check prothrombin levels; administer supplemental vitamin K as ordered.

POSTPROCEDURE CARE:
Maintain patient on bed rest for 8 to 24 hours.
Turn patient on right side for first few hours with pillows or sandbags against the abdomen to provide pressure.
Monitor patient carefully for signs of hemorrhage.
Check vital signs and do site inspection every 15 minutes for 1 hour.
Continue checking vital signs and site every 30 minutes and then hourly for remaining 24 hours.

Patient will be free of pain.
Patient will not have bleeding or infection related to depressed blood values of white cells and platelets.
Patient will make a positive adjustment to disease and express desire to comply with treatment regimen.
Patient will reestablish a normal fluid and electrolyte balance.
Patient will eat sufficient nutrients to meet the body's basic needs.
Patient will adapt to changes in appearance and continue to maintain social contacts.
Patient will maintain an intact skin.

Nursing interventions
Encourage patient to balance rest and activity.
  Encourage moderate planned exercise within patient's tolerance.
  Encourage patient to remain independent in activities of daily living.
Patient should avoid exposure to infections and toxins.
  Alcohol is contraindicated.
Work with patient to modify diet yet include food preferences. Diet should include:
  Sufficient protein to meet body repair needs (approximately 40 g)
  Carbohydrates for energy
  Low fat
Make environment pleasant to encourage patient to eat.
  Try frequent small feedings.

Administer vitamins as prescribed.
Discuss measures to increase compliance with treatment regimen.
  Remind patient that controlling disease will be a lifelong process.
Implement measures to control pruritus.
Provide or encourage good skin care.
Encourage patient to verbalize concerns over changes in body image and function.
Teach patient bleeding precautions to be observed if patient is thrombocytopenic. Patient should:
  Use gentle mouth care and soft toothbrush.
  Avoid use of straight razor.
  Avoid trauma.
  Report presence of blood in stools or urine.
  Maintain pressure over venipuncture sites for several minutes.
Keep accurate intake and output records.
  Check weight and abdominal girth daily.

Evaluation
Patient maintains independence in the activities of daily living and resumes some preillness social activities.
Patient is free of discomforting disease symptoms.
Patient is free of fluid overload; electrolyte values are within normal limits.
Patient is free of infection and does not experience bleeding.
Patient expresses desire to understand and comply with treatment regimen and can discuss diet and activity modifications.
Patient maintains a stable weight and is able to eat a healthy diet within prescribed restrictions.
Patient integrates body changes and continues normal pattern of social interactions.
Patient maintains an intact skin.

COMPLICATIONS OF CIRRHOSIS

Complications tend to appear in patients with long-standing chronic liver disease. Common serious complications include ascites, portal hypertension–esophageal varices, and hepatic encephalopathy.

ASCITES

The mechanisms of ascites are poorly understood but seem to be related to:
  Decreased synthesis of albumin necessary for adequate colloid osmotic pressure
  Increased portal vein pressure, which moves fluid into the peritoneal space
  Increased serum aldosterone level
  A vicious cycle is established as escaped albumin further aggravates the osmotic balance. Fluid is retained in the abdomen and throughout the body.

Medical Management

Restriction of sodium significantly limits the formation of ascitic fluid. Sodium is usually restricted to 1 g. Fluid restrictions may be as severe as 500 ml/day. Bed rest facilitates reabsorption of fluid.

If conservative measures fail, then diuretics may be administered with a potassium supplement. Lasix is the most frequently prescribed diuretic. Albumin may be administered to retain adequate vascular volume. If other measures fail, a peritoneojugular shunt may be placed. Special attention must be paid to positioning, skin care, and pulmonary ventilation for patients with massive edema.

PORTAL HYPERTENSION–ESOPHAGEAL VARICES

Portal hypertension occurs when peripheral resistance is increased from vessel damage within the liver. Obstruc-

tion causes backup of blood in the veins and development of collateral circulation. Varices in the esophageal veins commonly develop. Bleeding of these varicosities may be spontaneous or precipitated by straining, coughing, or sneezing. Severe hematemesis and resultant shock are not uncommon.

Medical Management

Treatment for bleeding varices consists of restoring blood volume and controlling the bleeding through gastric lavage and injection of Pitressin to reduce portal pressure and blood flow. Esophagogastric tamponade with a Sengstaken-Blakemore tube is the most widely used intervention for massive bleeding. See the box on p. 148 for specific care related to this procedure. Figure 11-2 shows the Sengstaken-Blakemore tube.

HEPATIC ENCEPHALOPATHY (COMA)

Hepatic coma is a form of metabolic encephalopathy of the brain associated with liver failure. It is believed to be precipitated by factors that increase the ammonia level or depress liver function. In liver failure, ammonia (a waste product of the breakdown of protein in the intestine) is not converted to urea and accumulates in the blood. It adversely affects the brain and the patient exhibits changes in level of consciousness:

Impaired attention span
Irritability and restlessness
Apathy, loss of interest

CARE OF THE PATIENT WITH A SENGSTAKEN-BLAKEMORE TUBE

DESCRIPTION OF TUBE:

The esophagogastric tube has three lumens and two balloons:
Nasogastric suction lumen
Lumen to inflate gastric balloon
Lumen to inflate esophageal balloon
Gastric balloon
Esophageal balloon

PATIENT CARE:

Monitor output from tube.
Correct balloon inflation will exceed portal pressure and cause esophageal bleeding to stop.
Stomach may be lavaged with ice water to provide vasoconstriction as well as pressure.
All blood must be removed from stomach to prevent its breakdown to ammonia in intestine, which can lead to hepatic coma.
Monitor patient carefully for respiratory problems.
Any shift in the tube can cause obstruction of the airway.
Patient cannot swallow around the tube and may aspirate secretions.
Provide emesis basin and tissues to handle saliva.
Use suction if needed.
Provide mouth and nasal care frequently.
Administer blood or IV fluids to counter shock.
Monitor vital signs frequently.
Provide supplemental oxygen as ordered.
Administer medications as prescribed.
Magnesium sulfate is used to hasten excretion of blood in GI tract.
Antibiotics lessen bacterial action on blood in GI tract.
Antacids reduce acidity and prevent esophageal reflux.
Administer enemas as prescribed to cleanse GI tract of blood.
Provide comfort measures and support to patient.
Esophageal balloon is left inflated for a maximum of 48 hours.
Gastric balloon must be deflated regularly to prevent erosion and ulceration.

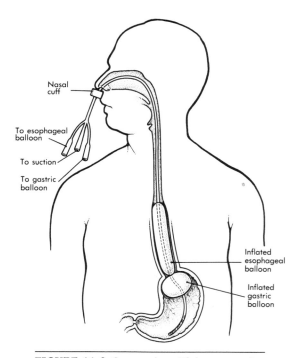

FIGURE 11-2 Sengstaken-Blakemore tube.

Medical Management

Treatment centers around identifying and reversing the precipitating cause. Strain on the liver is reduced by: eliminating protein in the diet temporarily, administering antibiotics to reduce ammonia-forming bacteria in the bowel, and administering enemas or cathartics to empty the bowel and prevent ammonia formation. Lactulose may also be given to decrease ammonia formation. General supportive care is maintained with special attention to the prevention of infection.

BILIARY DISORDERS

The biliary system consists of the gallbladder and its associated ductal system. The principal disorders are cholecystitis (inflammation of the gallbladder) and cholelithiasis (presence of stones in the biliary tract). These are common disorders affecting adults of both sexes in the United States.

CHOLECYSTITIS/CHOLELITHIASIS

Cholecystitis and cholelithiasis are frequently encountered together. Stone formation may be preceded by inflammation or follow it in a chronic form. These disorders tend to occur in middle age and afflict women more frequently than men. Inflammation tends to be associated with sedentary life-styles and obesity.

Pathophysiology

In acute cholecystitis, the gallbladder is very enlarged and becomes thickened and edematous. A reaction is triggered by retained bile that may impair circulation and produce ischemia. In an acute attack the patient is extremely ill with nausea, vomiting, and severe abdominal pain.

Three specific factors contribute to the development of gallstones: metabolic factors, stasis, and inflammation. An increase in bile salts, bile pigment, or cholesterol may cause precipitation of the substance. About 90% of gallstones are cholesterol stones. Stasis leads to water absorption and increases the risk of precipitation. Inflammation alters the bile constituents and may reduce the solubility of cholesterol.

Stones may lodge anywhere in the system. Biliary colic is caused by spasm of the bile ducts as they attempt to move the stone. Diagnosis is usually confirmed by cholecystogram or cholangiogram. Figure 11-3 shows common sites for gallstones.

Medical Management

The treatment of choice for cholecystitis is surgery. Medical therapy may be attempted until acute infection subsides. This involves antibiotics, nothing by mouth, analgesics, and IV fluids. A nasogastric tube is used if vomiting persists. Although measures to dissolve stones are attempted, the basic treatment for cholelithiasis is also surgical. Conservative treatment is again commonly employed until the patient's condition has stabilized. Table 11-3 outlines various surgeries of the biliary tract.

Nursing Management
Assessment—subjective
History of the problem and symptoms
History of fat intolerance, heartburn, dyspepsia
Patient's complaints of:
    Mild to severe pain and right upper quadrant tenderness
    Nausea and vomiting
Normal dietary pattern

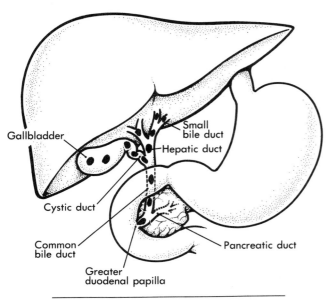

FIGURE 11-3 Common sites for gallstones.

TABLE 11-3 Surgeries of the biliary tract

Term	Description
Cholecystectomy	Removal of gallbladder
Cholecystostomy	Creation of an opening into gallbladder for drainage
Choledochotomy	Incision into common bile duct
Choledocholithotomy	Incision into common bile duct to remove a stone
Choledochoduodenostomy	Anastomosis of common bile duct with duodenum
Choledochojejunostomy	Anastomosis of common bile duct with jejunum
Cholecystogastrostomy	Anastomosis of gallbladder with stomach

From Long, B.C., and Phipps, W.J.: Essentials of medical-surgical nursing: a nursing process approach. St. Louis, 1985, The C.V. Mosby Co.

Assessment—objective
Fever
Jaundice
Leukocytosis
Tenderness and rigidity in right upper quadrant
Color of urine or stool (dark urine and clay-colored
   stools indicate obstruction)

Nursing diagnoses
Diagnoses will depend on the severity of the disorder and
approach used to manage it. Diagnoses may include:
   Alteration in comfort—pain related to inflammation or
      obstruction within the gallbladder
   Alteration in nutrition, more or less than body require-
      ments, related to pain and vomiting or obesity.
   Potential impairment of skin integrity related to severe
      pruritus or postoperative wound drainage.
   Knowledge deficit related to adoption of low fat diet.

Expected outcomes
   Patient will experience decreasing levels of pain and
      tenderness.
   Patient will reestablish an adequate nutrient intake
      within the framework of suggested restrictions.
   Patient will maintain an intact skin.
   Patient will be knowledgeable about diet modifications
      to be followed after discharge.
   Patient who is treated surgically will recover without
      complications.

Nursing interventions
During acute phase
Administer medications as prescribed for pain.
   ALERT: Demerol is administered rather than morphine
      because it does not cause spasm in sphincter of
      Oddi.
   Assess for effectiveness.
Offer comfort measures.
   Provide position changes, skin care, fresh linen.
Give patient nothing by mouth.
   Keep accurate intake and output records and mon-
      itor IV infusion.
   Provide oral care.
   Maintain patency of nasogastric tube if used.
   Administer antiemetics if ordered.
Offer measures to relieve itching.
Monitor stools and urine for signs of bile obstruction.
Assess patient for jaundice.
Monitor vital signs for infection.
Administer anticholinergics and vitamins as pre-
   scribed.
Teach patient principles of low fat diet.
   Suggest use of smaller frequent meals.
   Plan diet for patient to reduce weight if needed.

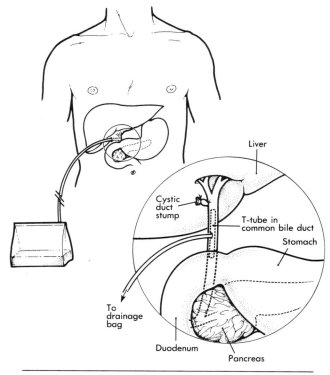

FIGURE 11-4 T-tube insertion into common bile duct.

Preoperative
Teach patient deep breathing and coughing.
   NOTE: High abdominal incision makes respiratory hy-
      giene difficult in postoperative period.
Prepare patient for postoperative routine.
   Explain use of nasogastric tube or T-tube.
Postoperative
Administer routine postoperative care.
Provide adequate pain relief to enable good ventilation.
   Patient should cough and deep breathe every 1 to 2
      hours.
   Change patient's position frequently.
   Keep patient in low Fowler's position to reduce pres-
      sure on diaphragm.
Maintain NPO until peristalsis resumes.
Maintain patency of nasogastric tube if used.
Encourage ambulation.
Advance diet from clear liquids to regular or low fat.
   Assess patient's response and tolerance.
   Teach principles of low fat diet if indicated.
Change dressing as needed.
   Keep skin clean from irritating bile.
Maintain patency of T-tube if used (see Figure 11-4
   and box on p. 151).

Evaluation
Patient experiences no gallbladder-related pain or tenderness.

CARE OF THE PATIENT WITH A T TUBE

PURPOSE:
To ensure patency of the common bile duct after surgical exploration. Edema produced by surgical probing can produce obstruction.

ASSOCIATED NURSING INTERVENTIONS:
Attach tube to closed gravity drainage.
  Never irrigate or clamp tube without direct order.
Avoid pulling or kinking tube; teach patient not to lie on it.
Monitor and record amount and color of drainage each shift.
  Initial output will be 500–1000 ml/day and gradually taper off.
  Report presence of blood in drainage.
Change dressings as needed.
  Cleanse surrounding skin of bile to avoid irritation.
Assess patient's response to before-meal clamping regimen if ordered.
Assess stools and urine for indications of returning bile flow normalcy.

Patient maintains an adequate nutrient intake, chooses foods appropriate to well-balanced, regular or low-fat diet, and reduces to or maintains weight at desired level.

Patient is able to discuss food groups to be reduced or eliminated to maintain a low fat diet.

Patient's incision and drainage tube sites heal without complications; pruritus is gone.

Postsurgical patient heals without complications and returns to normal life-style.

EXOCRINE PANCREATIC DISORDERS
PANCREATITIS

Acute and chronic pancreatitis are the most common disorders affecting the exocrine functions of the pancreas. (Endocrine disorders are discussed in Chapter 12.) Exocrine disorders are serious inflammatory disorders that occur infrequently in the middle-aged population. Acute pancreatitis carries a significant mortality rate. Normal pancreatic function usually returns after resolution of acute pancreatitis, whereas chronic pancreatitis causes permanent damage.

Pathophysiology
Acute pancreatitis has been found to be related to biliary tract disease and alcohol abuse although the relationships have not been identified. Many forms are idiopathic. The mechanism by which pancreatitis is triggered is also unknown although it is theorized that toxins, ischemia, or reflux of duodenal contents may precipitate the disorder. Autodigestion occurs from the apparent activation of pancreatic enzymes within the pancreas itself. Autodigestion results in edema, hemorrhage, vascular damage, and coagulation and fat necrosis.

Acute pancreatitis has three grades of severity, reflecting the primary pathologic process:
  Edematous: mild form, usually self-limiting
  Hemorrhagic: interstitial bleeding in the gland
  Necrotizing: rapid necrotic destruction of tissue

Distention and inflammation of the pancreatic capsule, obstruction of bile flow, hemorrhage, and fluid exudation into the peritoneum create the classic symptoms of intense pain, nausea and vomiting, fluid and electrolyte imbalance, peritonitis, and shock. Serum amylase and lipase levels frequently rise significantly.

The clinical picture and pathophysiology for chronic pancreatitis are similar, but the disease process does not fully resolve. Both exocrine and endocrine functions are disturbed, producing diabetes, malabsorption, and malnutrition.

Medical Management
Treatment is aimed at resting the injured pancreas while treating the major symptoms and reversing shock. Management of pain is a primary consideration. The patient is given nothing by mouth until inflammation resolves and may receive TPN (total parenteral nutrition). Intestinal tubes may be used to reverse paralytic ileus. Careful attention is paid to preventing or treating developing infection.

Long-term management is aimed at preventing future attacks through use of a bland, low-fat diet and frequent small meals. The patient should avoid alcohol and may receive vitamin supplements and antacids to decrease pancreatic stimulation.

Nursing Management
Assessment—subjective
History of biliary disease
Pattern of alcohol use
Patient's complaints of:
  Sudden onset pain (acute, constant, widespread in abdomen, radiating to back, flanks, and substernal area)
  Nausea and vomiting
  Difficulty in breathing

Assessment—objective
Fever
Jaundice
Cyanosis
Signs of incipient shock:
  Altered level of consciousness, restlessness
  Tachycardia, hypotension
  Poor skin turgor, clammy or dry mucous membranes
Abdominal tenderness and rigidity

Decreased bowel sounds
Decreased breath sounds
Presence of elevated amylase and lipase levels; elevated white blood cells, serum bilirubin, and glucose; decreased calcium

Nursing diagnoses
Diagnoses may vary depending on the severity of the disorder, but will commonly include:
Alteration in comfort—severe pain related to inflammation and obstruction within the pancreas
Actual or potential fluid volume deficit related to prolonged vomiting and decreased vascular volume
Alteration in nutrition, less than body requirements, related to nausea, vomiting, or malabsorption
Impaired gas exchange related to decreased chest excursion and pain
Knowledge deficit related to diet modifications appropriate to decrease pancreatic activity
Potential for infection related to decreased respiratory excursion or necrotic tissue in pancreas

Expected outcomes
Patient will experience decreasing pain.
Patient's fluid and electrolyte balance will be restored to normal limits.
Patient will have basic nutritional needs met and gradually resume eating.
Patient will be assisted to maintain adequate chest excursion and gas exchange.
Patient will be knowledgeable about diet and life-style modifications appropriate to preventing recurrent attacks of pancreatitis.
Patient is free of preventable infection.

Nursing interventions
Administer prescribed pain medication liberally.
Demerol is usually used because it is not spasmogenic.
Position patient to achieve greatest comfort.
Suggest sitting with trunk flexed.
Suggest side-lying position with knees to chest.
Monitor intake and output accurately.
Administer IV fluids as ordered.
Assess patient for dehydration, incipient shock.
Monitor vital signs frequently.
Give patient nothing by mouth.
Offer frequent mouth care.
Maintain patency of nasogastric tube or intestinal tubes.
Administer antispasmodic drugs (Banthine, Pro-Banthine) as prescribed.
Administer antacid drugs as prescribed.
Assist patient to deep breathe and cough every 2 hours.
Auscultate breath sounds.

Assess for signs of infection.
Check urine or blood for glucose every 4 to 6 hours.
Observe for signs of hypocalcemia.
Assess patient for response to oral feedings when initiated.
Advance to low-fat, bland diet with 5 to 6 meals daily.
Teach patient principles of low fat and bland diet.
Teach patient to avoid alcohol and rich foods after discharge.
Teach patient signs and symptoms to be reported:
Recurrence of pain, nausea or vomiting
Change in bowel pattern, weight loss
Teach patient about medications ordered for chronic disease:
Pancreatic enzymes given with meals
Bile salts
Oral hypoglycemics or insulin

Evaluation
Patient is free of pain.
Patient's fluid and electrolyte balance is stable as demonstrated by intake and output measures and laboratory reports.
Patient's baseline nutritional needs were met during acute phase; patient is able to ingest low fat, bland diet without pain or nausea and maintains optimum weight.
Patient's lungs are clear to auscultation; patient is free of infection or atelectasis.
Patient modifies diet and life-style to meet needs of therapy regimen and can state rationale for restrictions.
Patient is free of infection or abscess; pancreatitis resolves.

BIBLIOGRAPHY

Fredette, S.L.: When the liver fails, Am. J. Nurs. 84:64-67, 1984.
Guenter, P., and Slocum, B.: Hepatic disease: nutritional implications, Nurs. Clin. North Am. 18(1):71-80, 1983.
Howes, R.M.: Our approach to acute pancreatitis, Resident Staff Phys. 23(3):51-56, 1977.
Klopp, A.: Shunting malignant ascites, Am. J. Nurs. 84:212-213, 1984.
Peterson, A.: Acute viral hepatitis, Nurse Pract. 13(4):9-11, 1979.
Quinless, F.: Portal hypertension; physiology, signs and symptoms, Nurs. 84 14(1):52-53, 1984.
Sherlock, S.: Diseases of the liver and biliary system, ed. 6, Philadelphia, 1981, F.A. Davis Co.
Taylor, D.L.: Gallstones: physiology, signs and symptoms, Nurs. 83, 13(6):44-45, 1983.
Taylor, D.L.: Jaundice: physiology, signs and symptoms, Nurs. 83 13(8):52-54, 1983.
Thompson, M.A.: Managing the patient with liver dysfunction, Nurs. 81 11(11):100-107, 1981.

NURSING CARE PLAN

CIRRHOSIS

Nursing Diagnoses	Expected Patient Outcomes	Nursing Interventions
Activity intolerance related to chronic fatigue, anemia, and weight of ascites	Patient has sufficient energy to remain independent in self care activities	1. Encourage bedrest during acute phase. 2. Encourage increasing activity interspaced with rest periods as tolerated. 3. Intervene if patient shows fatigue after prolonged visits by family and/or friends. 4. Encourage patient to remain independent in ADL
Alteration in nutrition, less than body requirements related to fatigue and anorexia	Patient ingests sufficient balanced nutrients to meet the body's basic needs	1. Assess nutrient intake. 2. Teach patient how to plan and implement a well-balanced, high-carbohydrate diet that limits fat and total protein. 3. Encourage use of salt substitute or alternative seasonings. 4. Give antiemetics and mouth care if nausea is present. Make environment pleasant. 5. Suggest small frequent meals. 6. Administer vitamins as prescribed.
Alteration in fluid volume—excess related to increased intraabdominal pressure and decreased osmotic gradient	Patient's fluid and electrolyte values return to normal Patient maintains a stable weight without evidence of edema	1. Monitor for signs of peripheral edema; measure abdominal girth and weigh daily. 2. Monitor intake and output until excess fluid is excreted. 3. Teach patient rationale for sodium restriction. 4. Give prescribed medications (diuretics, salt-free albumin infusions). 5. Restrict fluids if prescribed; provide fluids that are best tolerated and space these fluids throughout day.
Potential impairment of skin integrity related to decreased activity, ascites, and edema	Patient's skin remains intact	1. Assess skin daily for signs of pressure or breakdown. 2. Prevent skin breakdown during bedrest. Keep skin clean and moisturized.
Alteration in comfort related to liver inflammation and pruritus	Patient will be free of abdominal discomfort and itching	1. Avoid heat and heavy clothing or linens; provide a cool environment. 2. Apply antipruritic lotion to skin after bathing. 3. Give prescribed antihistamines. 4. Use diversional activities. 5. Keep fingernails cut short. 6. If patient must scratch, provide a soft cloth to prevent excoriations. 7. Keep patient with ascites in a high Fowler's position. 8. Support abdomen when positioned on side.

Potential for injury related to thrombocytopenia and leukopenia	Patient will not experience bleeding or infection from depressed blood values	1. Monitor for signs of infection. Assess lungs.
		2. Encourage pulmonary hygiene.
		3. Use sterile technique for all intrusive procedures.
		4. Restrict patient exposure to persons with infections.
		5. Monitor for bleeding:
		  a. Urine and stool for blood.
		  b. Skin and mucous membranes for signs of bleeding.
		6. Avoid injections, if possible; apply pressure at all puncture sites for several minutes.
		7. Give prescribed vitamin K.
		8. Teach patient to use soft toothbrush and to avoid use of straight razor.

Continued.

NURSING CARE PLAN

CIRRHOSIS—cont'd

Nursing Diagnoses	Expected Patient Outcomes	Nursing Interventions
Disturbance in self-concept related to jaundice and ascites	Patient will adapt to changes in appearance and maintain social patterns	1. Encourage patient to participate in goal setting and decision making. 2. Help patient identify personal strengths and give positive feedback. 3. Assist family to understand patient's need for a positive self-concept and how they can help. 4. Encourage patient to verbalize concerns over body image changes. 5. Assist patient to explore ways to diminish overt signs of jaundice and ascites and thus help body image.

Knowledge deficit related to treatment regimen and needed lifestyle modifications	Patient is knowledgeable about the disease and expresses the desire to comply with the treatment regimen	1. Teach patient:
		  a. Basis of symptoms and therapeutic regimen.
		  b. Dietary and fluid restrictions.
		  c. Medication therapy.
		  d. Avoidance of infection and substances toxic to liver.
		  e. Importance of avoiding alcohol use.
		  f. Signs requiring immediate medical follow-up.
		  g. Importance of compliance as disease requires life long management.

NURSING CARE PLAN

CHOLECYSTECTOMY WITH EXPLORATION OF COMMON BILE DUCT

Nursing Diagnoses	Expected Patient Outcomes	Nursing Interventions
Ineffective breathing patterns related to pain and splinting of high abdominal incision	Patient's lungs are clear to auscultation and chest movements are symmetrical	1. Monitor respirations and breath sounds (especially RLL) every 2 to 4 hours for 24 hours, then every 4 hours while awake until patient is ambulating well. 2. Place patient in low-Fowler's position and encourage patient to change position frequently. 3. Encourage deep breathing and coughing exercises at least every 1 to 2 hours for 24 hours, then every 2 to 4 hours while awake until patient is ambulating well. 4. Give analgesics prior to ambulation. 5. Splint incision to encourage deep coughing. 6. Encourage use of incentive spirometer. 7. Encourage ambulation as permitted.

NURSING CARE PLAN

CHOLECYSTECTOMY WITH EXPLORATION
OF COMMON BILE DUCT—cont'd

Nursing Diagnoses	Expected Patient Outcomes	Nursing Interventions

Potential for injury related to accidental obstruction of bile drainage	Patient does not experience obstruction or dislodgement of T-tube drainage	1. Maintain patency of T-tube:
		  a. Connect tube to closed gravity drainage.
		  b. Provide sufficient tubing to facilitate patient mobility.
		  c. Explain to patient importance of avoiding kinks, clamping or pulling of tube.
		2. Monitor amount and color of drainage from T-tube.
		3. Monitor color of urine and stool.
		4. Report signs of peritonitis (abdominal pain or rigidity, fever) immediately.
		5. If clamping of T-tube is prescribed before removal, monitor patient for signs of distress; if this occurs, unclamp tube and notify physician.

Alteration in comfort: pain related to high abdominal incision	Patient experiences decreasing levels of pain	1. Assess type and quality of pain. 2. Give analgesics liberally for 48 to 72 hours after surgery. Demerol is the drug of choice. 3. If nasogastric tube is present, give mouth and nose care as needed. 4. Encourage activity. 5. Use other pain-relieving measures, as appropriate. 6. Employ measures to control itching.

Potential impairment of skin integrity related to wound drainage	Skin remains intact—incision heals without complications	1. Assess skin around incision and stab wound with each dressing change.
		2. Change dressings as needed to maintain a dry dressing
		  a. Use Montgomery straps if frequent changes are necessary.
		  b. Use soap and water to remove bile drainage from skin.

Knowledge deficit related to necessary diet modifications and care after discharge	Patient is knowledgeable about diet and self-care requirements after discharge	1. Teach patient:
		  a. Techniques of dressing change if drainage is still occurring at time of discharge.
		  b. Any prescribed dietary changes such as low fat or low calories.
		  c. Signs to report to physician (excessive drainage, jaundice, light-colored stools).
		  d. Resumption of normal activities by 4 weeks, but avoiding heavy activity until 6 weeks.

CHAPTER 12

Endocrine Disorders

An alteration in the function of the endocrine glands may result in a wide variety of signs and symptoms because of the diversity of physiologic functions that are under hormonal control. Disorders may be primary or secondary to disorders present elsewhere in the body or system. Some of the disorders occur frequently while others are relatively rare. This chapter will discuss the major disorders of hyperfunctioning or hypofunctioning of the endocrine glands. Figure 12-1 shows the anatomical structure of the endocrine system.

ANTERIOR PITUITARY DISORDERS

The largest section of the pituitary is the anterior portion, which plays a major role in regulating the functioning of the individual endocrine glands. Table 12-1 lists the major hormones of the anterior pituitary and their functions. Dysfunctions may be related to individual hormones or combinations of them. Table 12-2 presents various anterior pituitary disorders and their distinguishing characteristics.

HYPERPITUITARISM

The most common cause of hyperpituitarism is pituitary adenoma. The adenomas are frequently classified according to the type of hormone they secrete. Adenomas cause symptoms related to the hypersecretion of hormones or from pressure on surrounding neurologic tissue.

Pathophysiology
Hypersecretion of adrenocorticotropic hormone (ACTH), prolactin, and thyroid stimulating hormone (TSH) is commonly identified during a workup for adrenal, menstrual, or thyroid dysfunction.

Excess growth hormone produces the unique problems of giantism in children and acromegaly in adults. Bony enlargement is most apparent in the hands, nose, and mandible. Soft tissue enlargement also occurs with coarsening of the facial features—nose, lips, and cheeks. Visceral enlargement also may occur. Prominent muscular development is present with an initial increase in strength followed by progressive weakness.

An increase in metabolic rate causes excessive sweating and skin coarsening. Growth hormone excess precipitates other endocrine abnormalities. Patients frequently wait to seek help until symptoms of intracranial pressure occur. Tests for hormonal level will reveal excess growth hormone; CT scans are used to confirm presence and size of the adenoma growth.

Medical Management
Treatment is aimed at decreasing abnormal hormone levels and removing the adenoma. Bromocriptine may be used to suppress growth hormone secretion but destruction or removal of the adenoma by surgery or irradiation is the treatment of choice. Surgery may involve craniotomy if the tumor spread is excessive, or a transsphenoidal approach, in which the sella turcica is entered from below through the sphenoid sinus. The patient will require either temporary or long-term replacement of anterior pituitary hormones after surgery.

Nursing Management
Assessment—subjective
History of symptoms: progression, severity
History of cardiovascular problems
Patient's understanding of diagnosis and treatment plan
Patient's complaints of:
    Visual changes or deficits
    Changes in hat, shoe, or glove size
    Muscle weakness

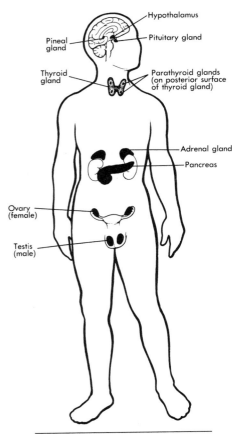

FIGURE 12-1 Endocrine system.

Headache
Changes in facial appearance
Persistent sweating

Assessment—objective
Coarse facial features, enlarged tongue, abnormal
body proportions
Husky voice
Warm, moist, coarse skin
Elevated blood pressure
Signs of diabetes
Early signs of increasing intracranial pressure
Height and weight changes

Nursing diagnoses
Diagnoses depend on the severity of the disorder, but
commonly include:
Knowledge deficit related to etiology and management
of endocrine disorders
Disturbance in self-concept (body image) related to
growth hormone excess changes
Visual sensory perceptual alteration related to pressure
of tumor on the optic nerve
Fluid volume deficit related to diabetes insipidus in
the postoperative period

TABLE 12-1 Hormones of the anterior pituitary gland

Hormone	Functions
Thyroid stimulating hormone (TSH)	Stimulates thyroid to secrete thyroxin
Adrenocorticotropic hormone (ACTH)	Stimulates adrenal cortex to secrete cortisol
Gonadotropic hormones	
Luteinizing hormone (LH)	Induces ovulation and stimulates formation of corpus luteum and progesterone secretion in female
Follicle-stimulating hormone (FSH)	Stimulates follicle growth in ovary and secretion of estrogen in female
Interstitial cell–stimulating hormone (ICSH)	Stimulates secretion of testosterone in male
Growth hormone (GH) (somatotropin-STH)	Stimulates body growth; influences protein, carbohydrate, and fat metabolism
Prolactin	Stimulates mammary gland development

From Long, B.C., and Phipps, W.J.: Essentials of medical-surgical
nursing: a nursing process approach, St. Louis, 1985, The C.V.
Mosby Co.

Expected outcomes
Patient will be knowledgeable about the disorder and
be able to describe the treatment plan and temporary and permanent deficits.
Patient will be assisted in resolving feelings about
changed body appearance into a positive self-concept
Patient will learn how to compensate for any permanent changes in visual perception to maintain a safe
environment
Patient with diabetes insipidus will reestablish a normal intake and output balance.

Nursing interventions
Preoperative
Teach patient about proposed surgical procedure.
Explain that there is no external incision with transsphenoidal approach.
Explain that a fascia graft is taken from leg to patch
dura mater.
Explain that soft tissue changes will gradually decrease but most of the bony changes are irreversible.
Teach patient rationale for temporary or long-term hormone replacement.
Postoperative: Transsphenoidal approach
NOTE: See Chapter 3 for discussion of care of the craniotomy patient.
Assess for cerebrospinal fluid (CSF) leakage—should
seal within a few days.

TABLE 12-2 Anterior pituitary dysfunction

Alteration in Secretion	Etiology	Signs and Symptoms	Medical Management
Growth hormone (GH) excess	*Primary* Pituitary tumors Pituitary hyperplasia	Gigantism in children Acromegaly in adults: 　Growth of soft tissues, cartilages, bones 　Enlargement and coarsening of facial features 　Enlarged tongue 　Visceral enlargement (liver, spleen, heart, kidneys) 　Warm, moist, coarse skin 　Husky voice 　Increased sweating 　Hypertension 　Prominent muscle development 　Insulin resistance	Removal of tumor: 　adenectomy, hypophysectomy Medications that suppress GH: estrogen, medroxyprogesterone, chlorpromazine, bromocriptine mesylate
GH deficit	*Primary* Hemorrhage Aneurysm Infection Granuloma Trauma Congenital tumor	Dwarfism in children Sensitivity to insulin Fasting hypoglycemia Hypoglycemia	Growth hormone replacement in children
ACTH excess	*Primary* Pituitary tumors Pituitary hyperplasia *Secondary* Nonpituitary-secreting tumor Stimulation of the hypothalamus *Iatrogenic* Bilateral adrenalectomy	Similar to Cushing's syndrome (adrenocortical excess)	Pituitary ablation: 　adenectomy, radiation, hypophysectomy Surgical removal of ectopic source of ACTH
ACTH deficit	*Primary* Same as GH deficiency *Iatrogenic*	Similar to Addison's disease (adrenocortical deficit) Asthenia (weakness)	Cortisone or cortisone derivative

Check patient's complaint of postnasal drip or frequent swallowing.
Test drainage for halo ring formation on gauze pad or positive glucose test.
Instruct patient not to:
Cough, sneeze, blow nose.
Bend over.
Strain at isometric exercise or stool.
Maintain patient on bed rest with head of bed elevated if CSF leak is severe.
Monitor patient for signs of meningitis.
Encourage frequent oral hygiene.
Patient should use saline rinse, mouthwash, toothettes.
ALERT: Patient should not brush teeth at first as this may disrupt the suture line.
Provide oxygen or humidity if prescribed.
Monitor for signs of diabetes insipidus.

Observe for polydipsia and polyuria.
Watch for dilute urine with 1.000 to 1.005 specific gravity.
Keep accurate intake and output records.
Maintain adequate fluid at bedside.
Teach patient correct use of vasopressin (Pitressin) if diabetes insipidus is not self-limiting or if there is inadequate fluid replacement.
Teach patient about medications prescribed for temporary or long-term replacement: cortisol, gonadotropins, or thyroid replacement.
Explain to patient importance of long-term follow-up and regular checkups.

Evaluation
Patient is knowledgeable about residual hormone deficits and can discuss purpose, schedule, and side effects of prescribed medications.

TABLE 12-2 Anterior pituitary dysfunction—cont'd

Alteration in Secretion	Etiology	Signs and Symptoms	Medical Management
	Suppression of hypo-thalamic-pituitary axis by endogenous corticosteroids	Nausea, vomiting Hypotension Hypoglycemia Hyponatremia Hyperkalemia	
TSH excess	*Primary* Pituitary tumor Pituitary hyperplasia	Same as hyperthyroidism (thyroid hormone excess)	Hypophysectomy
TSH deficit	Same as GH deficit	Same as hypothyroidism (thyroid hormone deficit) Cretinism in newborn Myxedema in adult	Thyroid hormone replacement
Prolactin excess	*Primary* Pituitary tumor *Secondary* Hypothalamic dysfunction *Iatrogenic* Side effect of certain drugs	Amenorrhea, galactorrhea, depressed libido, infertility, impotency, change in secondary sex characteristics	Pituitary surgery Drugs to suppress prolactin (bromocriptine)
Prolactin deficit Gonadotropic hormone excess	Same as GH deficit	Failure of lactation post partum Precocious sexual development in children Changes in secondary sex characteristics Hirsutism	
Gonadotropic hormone deficit	Same as GH deficit	Delayed sexual development in children In adults: female: amenorrhea, infertility male: impotency In both: changes in secondary sex characteristics	Replacement of sex hormones in cyclic pattern

From Long, B.C., and Phipps, W.J.: Essentials of medical-surgical nursing: a nursing process approach, St. Louis, 1985, The C.V. Mosby Co.

Patient resolves feelings about altered body image and speaks positively about self and body; patient resumes former social activity pattern.

Patient has adequate visual perception and maintains a safe environment.

Patient compensates for diabetes insipidus by increasing fluid intake; patient maintains normal fluid and electrolyte balance.

HYPOPITUITARISM

Hypopituitarism may result from vascular lesions, developmental disorders, trauma or surgery, and tumors. It may involve only one or all of the hormones of the anterior pituitary. Deficits in growth hormone and gonadotropins appear first. The clinical picture will vary with specific hormones, severity of the deficits and the age of the patient. Treatment involves identifying and replacing the deficient hormones and careful long-term follow-up.

POSTERIOR PITUITARY DISORDERS

The posterior pituitary secretes two hormones: oxytocin and antidiuretic hormone (ADH). The primary disorders of the posterior pituitary involve excesses and deficits of ADH secretion.

ADH EXCESS: SYNDROME OF INAPPROPRIATE ADH (SIADH)

Inappropriate ADH syndrome involves a continual release of hormone that is unrelated to serum osmolality. Water is retained, extracellular fluid volume expands, and dilutional hyponatremia occurs. The syndrome is associated with diseases of the nervous system, extreme stressors, and, most commonly, oat cell carcinoma of the lung, where the cells actually secrete ADH.

The patient retains water and exhibits the weakness, lethargy, and central nervous system changes characteristic of hyponatremia (see Chapter 1). Treatment is directed at the specific cause. Water retention is managed by water restriction of 800 to 1000 ml per day, combined with the administration of hypertonic saline if the patient's condition worsens. The syndrome is usually self-limiting, and responds promptly to treatment.

ADH DEFICIT: DIABETES INSIPIDUS

True diabetes insipidus in which the posterior pituitary fails to secrete ADH is quite rare, but the symptoms are seen fairly commonly after trauma, with pituitary tumor, or after hypophysectomy. Without ADH to stimulate reabsorption from the renal tubules, as much as 15 L of fluid may be excreted daily, with the potential for serious fluid and electrolyte imbalance. If fluid is not replaced, dehydration and vascular collapse occur rapidly.

Treatment is aimed at correcting the underlying condition if possible, and providing adequate hormone replacement. Initial therapy will begin with intramuscular administration of vasopressin (Pitressin). If long-term management is needed, a synthetic solution of vasopressin is administered by nasal spray or drops. Associated nursing interventions are included in the discussion of anterior hyperpituitarism.

THYROID GLAND DISORDERS

HYPERTHYROIDISM

Excess thyroid function results from excessive secretion of thyroxine (T_4) or triiodothyronine (T_3). It is a common disorder which primarily affects women aged 20 to 40. Hyperthyroidism occurs in several forms, all of which share similar clinical symptoms. The two most common forms are Graves' disease and toxic nodular goiter. Graves' disease is more prevalent.

Pathophysiology

The etiology of hyperthyroidism is unknown, although Graves' disease appears to have an autoimmune basis and follows a pattern of exacerbation and remission, which may be stress related. It seems to have a genetic component. The excess thyroid hormone produces increased metabolic rate, increased cardiac and respiratory stimulation, and increased nervous system activity (see Table 12-3 for thyroid hormone functions).

Graves' disease is characterized by a triad of goiter, hyperthyroidism, and exophthalmos. The mechanism behind exophthalmos is poorly understood, but increased deposits of fats and fluids in the tissues behind the eye lead to protrusion of the eye and even incomplete eye closure, which can cause serious damage.

Medical Management

Therapy is aimed at reducing thyroid hormone levels and treating other signs and symptoms. This may be done by using antithyroid drugs, removing thyroid tissue through

TABLE 12-3 Functions of the thyroid gland hormones

Hormone	Functions
Thyroxine (T_4) and triiodothyronine (T_3)	Regulates protein, fat, and carbohydrate catabolism in all cells Regulates metabolic rate of all cells Regulates body heat production Insulin antagonist Necessary for muscle tone and vigor Maintains cardiac rate, force, and output Maintains secretion of gastrointestinal tract Affects respiratory rate and oxygen utilization Maintains calcium mobilization Affects RBC production Stimulates lipid turnover, free fatty acid release, and cholesterol synthesis
Thyrocalcitonin	Lowers serum calcium and phosphorus levels by inhibiting osteoclastic activity Decreases calcium and phosphorus absorption in gastrointestinal tract

From Long, B.C., and Phipps, W.J.: Essentials of medical-surgical nursing: a nursing process approach, St. Louis, 1985, The C.V. Mosby Co.

surgery, or destroying thyroid tissue by radioactive iodine. Drug therapy is the preferred method of treatment unless the patient fails to respond, experiences drug toxicity, or develops a large goiter. Subtotal thyroidectomy is preferred for young patients, whereas radioactive iodine may be used for older adults. Table 12-4 lists drugs frequently used to treat hyperthyroidism.

Nursing Management
Assessment—subjective
History of symptoms and severity
Family history of thyroid disease
Patient's complaints of:
  Nervousness and irritability
  Exaggerated emotions and mood swings
  Heat intolerance
  Palpitations
  Fatigue and weakness
  Increased hunger plus weight loss
  Angina pain
  Menstrual irregularities

Assessment—objective
Body weight and proportions
Skin appearance and texture:
  Presence of sweating or reddening
Tachycardia; signs of CHF

TABLE 12-4 Drugs used in the treatment of hyperthyroidism

Drug	Actions
Antithyroid Drugs	
Propylthiouracil Methimazole	Block thyroid hormone synthesis; slow-acting drugs that may take 2 to 4 weeks to produce noticeable improvement
Iodine Preparations	
Lugol's solution	Block the synthesis and release of thyroid hormone, producing rapid reduction in metabolic rate; do not have a sustained effect, but reduce gland vascularity and are frequently given preoperatively
Beta Adrenergic Blockers	
Propranolol (Inderal)	Used to treat tachycardia, arrhythmia, and angina symptoms which may accompany hyperthyroidism; is used for all patients in thyroid storm

Fine tremors
Exophthalmos; lid lag; lid retraction
Goiter; thyroid bruit
Elevated T_3, T_4, and PBI test results

Nursing diagnoses

Diagnoses will depend on the severity of the disease and its treatment but commonly include:
  Activity intolerance related to easy fatigability of muscles
  Alteration in nutrition, less than body requirements, related to excess metabolic rate
  Sleep pattern disturbance related to irritability and hyperactivity
  Disturbance in self-concept (body image) related to the occurrence of goiter or exophthalmos
  Anxiety and nervousness related to excess nervous system activity

Expected outcomes

Patient will regain muscle strength and endurance and resume preillness activity pattern.
Patient will ingest sufficient nutrients to meet body needs and maintain desired weight.
Patient will sleep uninterrupted at night for at least 6 hours.
Patient will incorporate body changes into an altered but positive self-concept.
Patient will feel in control of body and environment.

CARE OF THE PATIENT AFTER THYROIDECTOMY

MONITORING FOR COMPLICATIONS:

Check for signs of:
  Hemorrhage:
    Bleeding on dressings behind neck and on pillow
    Increased difficulty in swallowing
    Choking sensation
  Vocal cord edema:
    Hoarseness
    Dyspnea
  Laryngeal nerve damage:
    Difficulty in speaking, hoarseness
    Shortness of breath; obstruction; crowing sound
  Injury to parathyroid glands:
    Hypocalcemia; tetany
    Numbness and tingling in fingertips and around lips
ALERT: It is imperative to have a tracheostomy set and calcium gluconate available at the bedside in case of complications.

GENERAL CARE:

Introduce diet with caution, supervise swallowing.
  Advance diet as tolerated.
Maintain patient in semi-Fowler's position to avoid stress on sutures.
Use a humidifier if indicated.
Encourage activity.
  After 5 to 7 days, initiate range of motion exercises for the neck.
Teach patient about any drugs required after discharge.

Nursing interventions

Establish a calm, quiet environment.
  Keep temperature cool.
  Assign patient to room away from major activities.
Assist patient to plan activities to foster rest.
Patient should avoid activities needing fine coordination.
Assist patient to understand physiologic basis for nervousness and moods.
Provide high-calorie, high-protein diet.
  Keep snacks at bedside.
  Maintain adequate fluid intake.
  Patient should avoid caffeinated substances.
Chart daily weights.
Provide care for exophthalmos.
  Protect cornea from ulceration and infection; patch eye if needed.
  Administer methylcellulose eye drops for comfort.
  Teach patient to use sunglasses outdoors for protection from wind, sun, and dust.
  Encourage patient to verbalize feelings about altered appearance.
Teach patient about radioactive iodine treatment if prescribed.
  Radiation precautions are not usually required.

Response to treatment is delayed—may take 2 to 3 months.

Treatment will be administered orally.

Treatment may induce hypothyroidism in future.

Administer and teach patient about prescribed medications (see Table 12-4).

Provide preoperative teaching if surgery is scheduled.

Teach patient importance of supporting head with hands post-op to prevent stress on sutures.

Explain to patient that talking may be difficult initially. (The box on p. 161 presents postoperative care associated with thyroidectomy.)

Teach patient importance of ongoing medical supervision.

Evaluation

Patient has increased muscle strength and endurance, resumes preillness exercise and activity pattern.

Patient establishes and maintains desired weight, adjusts intake to meet decreased metabolic needs.

Patient enjoys restful sleep pattern.

Patient speaks positively of self and accepts changes in appearance.

Patient is not anxious, feels in control of body and environment.

HYPOTHYROIDISM

Hypothyroidism is a metabolic state resulting from deficient thyroid hormone, which may occur at any age. It may result from a congenital deficiency (cretinism), iodine deficiency, or drugs, but the most common cause is surgical or radioactive destruction of the gland. Myxedema is a severe adult form of hypothyroidism that has a significant mortality.

Early signs of hypothyroidism are vague, with cold intolerance, constipation, and menstrual disorders occurring commonly. Sluggishness, weight gain, and sleepiness are also common. As the disease progresses, the patient exhibits slowed intellectual functioning, dry skin, and diminished reflexes. The patient with advanced myxedema may lapse into coma.

Treatment involves lifelong replacement of deficient thyroid hormone: Synthroid, Cytomel, Trionine, and Euthroid are among the drugs in use. Relief of symptoms begins within 2 to 3 days of therapy.

PARATHYROID DYSFUNCTION

The parathyroid glands secrete parathyroid hormone (PTH), which maintains serum calcium and phosphorus levels by controlling bone resorption, gastrointestinal absorption, and urinary excretion of these minerals.

HYPERPARATHYROIDISM

The most common cause of primary hyperparathyroidism is benign neoplasm. It tends to occur in adults aged 30 to 60. It may also result from chronic hypocalcemia associated with renal disease or malabsorption.

Pathophysiology

Hypersecretion of parathyroid hormone produces an elevated serum calcium level and a decreased phosphorus level. The increased calcium can cause bone destruction leading to pathologic fracture. The serum calcium excess can predispose the patient to kidney stones and produces gastrointestinal symptoms and mental changes varying from confusion and depression to outright psychosis. Relatively small elevations in calcium may cause major mental changes, particularly in the elderly. Calcium imbalance is discussed in Chapter 1.

Medical Management

Surgery, usually the removal of three glands and a portion of the fourth, is the treatment of choice for most patients with primary hyperparathyroidism. The electrolyte imbalance must be corrected prior to surgery, however. This is usually accomplished by rehydration and physiologic flushing with isotonic sodium chloride, combined with a diuretic to enhance calcium excretion. Mithracin may be used to lower serum calcium in patients whose renal or cardiovascular function is inadequate to handle high volume sodium chloride flushing.

Nursing Management
Assessment—subjective
Subjective

History and severity of presenting symptoms

History of renal or cardiovascular disease

History of renal stones

Normal dietary pattern

Patient's complaints of:

Anorexia, nausea, or vomiting

Fatigue and muscle weakness

Bone pain

Polyuria, polydipsia, and constipation

Alteration in mental status or personality, such as depression, stupor, behavior changes

Objective

Intake and output balance

Depressed reflexes

Elevated serum calcium levels, decreased phosphorus levels

Mental status evaluation

Nursing diagnoses

Diagnoses may vary with the severity of the disorder, but commonly include:

Alteration in bowel elimination (constipation) related to decreased gastrointestinal functioning

Alteration in comfort—bone pain related to demineralization, or nausea and vomiting related to decreased gastrointestinal functioning

Alteration in nutrition, less than body requirements, related to anorexia and nausea

Alteration in thought processes related to effects of calcium on cerebral tissue

Potential fluid volume deficit related to excess urination and nausea

Expected outcomes

Patient will return to a normal bowel elimination pattern.

Patient will experience decreasing bone pain and be relieved of the symptoms of nausea and vomiting.

Patient will resume a normal dietary pattern adequate to meet basic body needs.

Patient will return to preillness level of mental functioning and exhibit no ongoing depression or behavioral changes.

Patient will be restored to a normal fluid volume balance.

Nursing interventions

Monitor intake and output accurately.

Maintain IV fluids as ordered.

Assess for signs of renal stones.

Help patient balance rest and activity to preserve energy.

Assist patient with activities of daily living as needed.

Teach patient rationale for low-calcium diet.

Encourage use of acid ash diet or ascorbic acid supplements in diet to acidify urine.

Encourage patient to drink large amounts of fluid.

Modify environment to make it as pleasant and odor free as possible.

Encourage frequent mouth care.

Offer small frequent feedings.

Teach patient importance of fiber and bulk in diet and adequate fluids to prevent constipation.

Administer prescribed medications, such as stool softeners or antiemetics.

Maintain environmental safety.

Keep side rails up; supervise ambulation.

Assess patient's mental status regularly.

Provide encouragement and stimulation.

Administer analgesics as ordered; position patient for comfort.

Teach patient about proposed surgery and postoperative routine.

Provide standard postoperative care for parathyroidectomy, which is essentially the same as that for thyroidectomy patients.

ALERT: The serum calcium level will decrease within 24 hours and the patient must be assessed carefully for signs of tetany until parathyroid function returns to normal. Calcium replacement will be given until function normalizes.

Evaluation

Patient has a normal bowel elimination pattern and passes soft stool regularly without need for laxatives or stool softeners.

Patient experiences no further bone pain and is able to resume former activities.

Patient is free of nausea and eats a normal diet; patient modifies diet appropriately if indicated to enrich or restrict calcium content.

Patient's mental status is at preillness levels; patient returns to normal social activities without ongoing depression or behavior changes.

Patient has a normal fluid balance and experiences no inappropriate thirst or urination.

Patient is knowledgeable about any prescribed medications and recognizes the importance of ongoing medical supervision.

HYPOPARATHYROIDISM

Hypoparathyroidism is a metabolic disorder that results in hypocalcemia. It commonly occurs after thyroid or parathyroid surgery, but may be idiopathic. It can produce serious effects as decreased calcium leads to neuromuscular irritability, tetany, largyngeal stridor, and cardiac arrhythmias.

Treatment involves the early identification of symptoms so prompt intervention is possible. Calcium gluconate is given intravenously for immediate replacement. Vitamin D and calcium salts are prescribed and the patient is taught to follow a vitamin D–rich diet and to recognize the early signs of calcium deficiency.

ADRENAL GLAND DISORDERS

Dysfunction of the adrenal gland may result from hypersecretion or hyposecretion by either the cortex or the medulla. Table 12-5 lists the hormones secreted by the adrenal gland and their functions.

HYPERSECRETION OF THE ADRENAL CORTEX: CORTISOL EXCESS

Hypersecretion of the adrenal cortex may result from:

Excess ACTH production by the pituitary

TABLE 12-5 Hormones of the adrenal gland

Portion of Gland	Hormones	Functions
Adrenal cortex	Glucocorticoids (cortisol)	Overall effect is to maintain blood glucose level by increasing gluconeogenesis; decrease rate of glucose utilization by cells
		Increase protein catabolism
		Promote lipolysis
		Promote sodium and water retention
		Antiinflammatory
		Degrade collagen
		Decrease T-lymphocyte participation in cellular-mediated immunity by decreasing circulating level of T-lymphocytes
		Increase neutrophils by increasing release and decreasing destruction
		Decreases new antibody release
		Decrease eosinophils, basophils, and monocytes
		Decrease scar tissue formation
		Increase RBC formation and possibly increase platelet formation
		Increase gastric acid and pepsin production
		Maintain emotional stability
	Mineralocorticoids (aldosterone)	Major stimulus in renin-angiotensin system
		Primarily responsible for maintenance of normovolemic state by increasing sodium and water retention in distal tubules
		Cause potassium excretion
		Cause increased excretion of ammonium and magnesium ions
	Androgens	Same functions as gonadal sex hormones
Adrenal medulla	Epinephrine and norepinephrine	Necessary for maintenance of neuroendocrine integrating functions of body
		Elevate blood pressure, increase heart rate, and cause vasoconstriction
		Stimulate conversion of glycogen to glucose for emergency fuel
		Stimulate gluconeogenesis
		Increase lipolysis

Modified from Long, B.C., and Phipps, W.J.: Essentials of medical-surgical nursing: a nursing process approach, St. Louis, 1985, The C.V. Mosby Co.

Adrenocortical hyperplasia from an ectopic ACTH source

Primary hyperplasia from adenoma or carcinoma or Cushing's syndrome

An iatrogenic Cushing's syndrome is a common complication of treatment with corticosteroids. Cushing's syndrome is seen most frequently in middle-aged women.

Pathophysiology

The effects of cortisol excess produce widespread changes in body appearance and function. These changes are presented in Table 12-6. The metabolic dysfunctions place the patient at higher risk for several chronic illnesses: peptic ulcer, osteoporosis, psychoses, hypertension, and diabetes mellitus.

Aldosterone excess will produce hypokalemia, hypernatremia, and hypertension from fluid volume excess. Excess androgen will result in masculinizing effects in the female.

Medical Management

Effective treatment is dependent on the cause of hypersecretion. Surgical adrenalectomy will be performed if a tumor is found. The patient may receive medications to block cortisol synthesis, such as mitotane, aminoglutethimide, or metyrapone during radiation therapy to the pituitary or when surgery is not feasible. Bilateral adrenalectomy necessitates lifelong hormone replacement. Skilled supportive care is mandatory while hormonal balance is reestablished.

Nursing Management
Assessment—subjective
History and severity of symptoms
Patient's perception of the problem
Perceived changes in body appearance: skin, hair
Patient's complaints of:
    Fatigue: onset, severity, interference with activities of daily living
    Edema or weight gain
    Indigestion
    Mood swings or instability
    Menstrual irregularities
Recent infections
Normal dietary pattern
Medications in use
History of other chronic health problems

TABLE 12-6 Effects of excess adrenocortical secretion

Characteristic	Hormone and Effect
	Cortisol
Appearance	Moon face
	Deposits of adipose tissue on back of neck and shoulders
	Truncal obesity
Muscles and bones	Thin extremities from muscle wasting
	Easy fatigability
	Osteoporosis
Skin	Thinning of the skin
	Pale purplish striae
	Bruises and petechiae
	Flushed face
Cardiovascular	Excess fluid volume
	Hypertension
Gastrointestinal	Increased secretion of HCL
Metabolism	Hyperglycemia
Immune system	Inhibition of immune response and inflammation
Emotions	Euphoria or irritability
	Excitability or depression
	Aldosterone
Fluid and electrolytes	Severe sodium and water retention
	Severe hypokalemia
	Androgens
Skin	Hirsutism in females
Reproductive	Menstrual irregularities

Assessment—objective
Daily weights
Vital sign patterns
Intake and output balance
Urine and blood glucose levels
Body appearance (see Table 12-6)
Energy level, self-care abilities
Skin integrity
Laboratory values showing increased cortisol; hypokalemia

Nursing diagnoses
Diagnoses may vary according to the severity of the disorder but commonly include:
Activity intolerance related to muscle fatigability
Fluid volume excess related to sodium and water retention
Potential for injury and infection related to skin changes and decreased immune response
Knowledge deficit related to mechanisms of the disorder and measures to control symptoms
Alteration in nutrition, more than body requirements, related to decreased activity, increased appetite, and altered gastrointestinal function
Alteration in self-concept (body image) related to changes in appearance
Anxiety related to the physical and emotional changes produced by excess glucocorticoids

Expected outcomes
Patient will balance rest and activity while muscle strength and endurance improve.
Patient will maintain a stable weight and show no signs of peripheral edema.
Patient will take measures to avoid exposure to infection.
Patient will be knowledgeable about disorder and treatment and comply with treatment regimen.
Patient will adjust diet pattern to compensate for hyperglycemia and fluid excess characteristic of the disease.
Patient will maintain a positive self-concept while waiting for physical changes to reverse or lessen.
Patient will maintain positive control and coping during diagnostic and treatment period.

Nursing interventions
Monitor vital signs frequently.
   Assess patient for early signs of infection.
Maintain accurate intake and output records.
Measure blood glucose and urinary sugar and acetone as ordered.
Protect patient from staff, other patients, and visitors with infections.
Teach patient importance of good hygiene.
Teach patient principles of, and purpose of, diet modification. Diet should be:
   Low in calories
   High in protein
   Low in sodium
   High in potassium
Administer antacids as prescribed.
Encourage patient to verbalize feelings about body changes.
   Provide ongoing support.
Balance rest and activity.
   Encourage patient to take short walks to combat osteoporosis.
   Assist patient with activities of daily living as needed.
   Keep environmental stimuli at low levels.
   Decrease physical and emotional stressors where possible.
Assist patient to control and understand mood swings.
Teach patient about widespread disease effects and proposed treatment.
Monitor patient for edema or early symptoms of CHF and hypertension.

Teach patient with iatrogenic Cushing's syndrome measures that will minimize effects of steroid therapy:

Modify diet.

Use good hygiene.

Patient should avoid infection.

Teach patient signs and symptoms of complications.

NOTE: Interventions for patients being treated with adrenalectomy are outlined in the box below.

Evaluation

Patient is able to engage in normal activities without the onset of fatigue.

Patient exhibits no signs of fluid excess; blood pressure is in normal range.

Patient maintains scrupulous personal hygiene and is free of preventable infection.

Patient is knowledgeable about the disease and treatment and can discuss prescribed diet and medication regimen.

Patient follows a controlled-calorie, low-sodium diet and is able to maintain a stable weight.

Patient has an improving self-concept as body appearance returns to preillness state.

Patient is free of anxiety and is knowledgeable about long-term disease management.

CARE OF THE PATIENT EXPERIENCING ADRENALECTOMY

PREOPERATIVE:

Teach patient about proposed surgery and care routines to be followed postoperative.

Teach usual coughing and deep breathing exercises.

POSTOPERATIVE:

Monitor vital signs frequently as adrenal function tends to be very labile.

Vasopressors may be needed.

Maintain infusions of steroids as prescribed.

Maintain accurate records for:

Intake and output, blood glucose, urine glucose, and ketones.

Observe patient for signs of hypoglycemia.

Monitor for signs of adrenal crisis.

Monitor adequacy of urine output regularly.

Introduce activity gradually and assess patient's response.

Maintain adequate pain relief to facilitate coughing.

Initiate teaching concerning medication regimen prescribed:

Medication may be needed for lifelong replacement.

Close supervision is needed during initial months to adjust dose.

Patient should be alert for signs of hormone excess or deficit.

Patient should be cognizant of situations that will increase need for hormone, such as physical or emotional stress or illness.

HYPOSECRETION OF THE ADRENAL CORTEX

A decrease in adrenocortical secretions may result from a primary deficiency of the cortex (Addison's disease), or a secondary failure resulting from pituitary insufficiency or suppression of adrenal function from the administration of exogenous steroids. Deficiencies in glucocorticoids lead to impairments in metabolism and an inability to maintain a normal glucose level. Deficiencies in mineralocorticoids produce fluid and electrolyte problems. Early symptoms are often vague and insidious. Table 12-7 lists the common symptoms of deficiency. Adrenocortical hormones are essential to life and must be replaced.

Adrenal crisis (Addisonian crisis) is a sudden, life-threatening condition that may be precipitated by the

TABLE 12-7 Signs of adrenal insufficiency

Characteristic	Signs and Symptoms
Appearance	Patient has lost weight; appears fatigued
Skin	Bronze coloration of skin and mucous membranes from increased levels of melanocyte stimulating hormone
Cardiovascular	Hypotension
	Tendency to develop shock
Gastrointestinal	Anorexia
	Cramping abdominal pain
	Diarrhea
	Nausea and vomiting
Metabolism	Hypoglycemia
Fluid and electrolytes	Hyponatremia
	Hyperkalemia
	Dehydration

TEACHING FOR PATIENT REQUIRING CORTISOL REPLACEMENT

Never omit a dose of the drug.

Notify physician if a dose is not taken or not retained.

Wear an identification bracelet.

Carry information concerning:

Name and dosage of drug to be given in case of an emergency

Name and phone number of physician to be notified in an emergency

Carry an emergency supply of a rapid-acting cortisone preparation with directions for use (e.g., hydrocortisone 100 mg in a sterile syringe).

Report to physician any signs and symptoms of adrenocortical deficiency.

Avoid undue stress, when possible.

Notify physician when illness, injury, or emotional crises occur.

Maintain regular medical follow-up.

From Long, B.C., and Phipps, W.J.: Essentials of medical-surgical nursing: a nursing process approach, St. Louis, 1985, The C.V. Mosby Co.

sudden cessation of steroid therapy or situations that create a sudden need for more cortisol than is available. The syndrome is characterized by hypotension, cardiovascular collapse (shock), hyperpyrexia (extremely high fever), hypoglycemia, and hyponatremia.

Adrenal insufficiency is treated by administration of the deficient hormones. Patients must be helped to understand the serious nature of the disorder and the importance of taking their medications regularly and avoiding situations of undue stress. The box on p. 166 outlines teaching principles for patients receiving cortisol replacement.

HYPERSECRETION OF THE ADRENAL MEDULLA: PHEOCHROMOCYTOMA

Pheochromocytoma is a rare catecholamine-producing tumor that occurs in individuals in middle age. It is usually unilateral and benign. It produces malignant hypertension that may be labile or persistently elevated. Diagnosis is usually made during a workup for refractory hypertension.

Initial treatment is aimed at controlling blood pressure. Surgical resection of the tumor is the treatment of choice for a stabilized patient. Blood pressure instability is a common problem in the postoperative period and the patient requires careful monitoring. The remainder of the care is similar to that for any adrenalectomy patient. Most individuals have a complete recovery.

PANCREATIC HORMONE DYSFUNCTION: DIABETES MELLITUS

Diabetes is a complex chronic disease involving disorders in carbohydrate, fat, and protein metabolism. It is one of the most common diseases and, despite extensive research, remains a major cause of death and disability. Although it occurs at all ages, diabetes occurs most commonly in adults over 40. The incidence rate increases steadily with age. Although the cause remains unknown, diabetes is believed to be a group of disorders with various precipitating causes. Viral, autoimmune, socioeconomic, and environmental factors are all suspected of playing a part. The current classification system for diabetes is presented in Table 12-8.

Pathophysiology

The primary function of insulin is to promote the transport of serum glucose across the cell membrane where

TABLE 12-8 Diagnoses of diabetes mellitus and other categories of glucose intolerance

Disorder	Description	Criteria for Diagnosis
Diabetes mellitus Insulin dependent (IDDM), Type I; previously called juvenile-onset	Insulin deficient due to islet cell loss; often associated with specific HLA types, predisposition to viral insulitis or autoimmune phenomena; *ketosis prone;* occurs at any age, common in youth	Unequivocal elevation of plasma glucose ($\geq$200 mg/dl) and classic symptoms of diabetes (polydipsia, polyuria, polyphagia, weight loss) Fasting plasma glucose $\geq$140 mg/dl on two occasions Fasting plasma glucose <140 mg/dl and 2-h plasma glucose $\geq$200 mg/dl with one intervening value $\geq$200 mg/dl following a 75-g glucose load (OGTT)
Noninsulin dependent (NIDDM), Type II; previously called maturity-onset	*Ketosis resistant;* more frequent in adults but occurs at any age; majority of patients are overweight; familial tendencies; may require insulin for hyperglycemia during stress	
Gestational diabetes (GDM), Type III	Glucose intolerance with recognition of onset during pregnancy; after pregnancy ends, patient may have normal glucose tolerance or may be classified Type I or Type II	Two or more of following plasma glucose concentrations met or exceeded using a 100 g glucose load: fasting plasma glucose 105 mg/dl; 1-h 190 mg/dl; 2-h 165 mg/dl; 3-h 145 mg/dl
Diabetes associated with certain conditions or syndromes, Type IV	Hyperglycemia occurring in relation to other disease states: pancreatic disease, drugs or chemicals, endocrinopathies, insulin receptor disorders, certain genetic syndromes	
Impaired glucose tolerance	Abnormality in glucose levels; intermediate between normal and overt diabetes; may progress to diabetes, improve to normal, or remain unchanged	Fasting plasma glucose <140 mg/dl and 2-h plasma glucose $\geq$140 mg/dl and <200 mg/dl with one intervening value $\geq$200 mg/dl following a 75 g glucose load

Modified from C.R. Shuman and I.L. Spratt; Office guide to diagnosis and classification of diabetes mellitus and other categories of glucose intolerance, Diabetes Care 4(2):335, 1981. With permission from the American Diabetes Association, Inc.

it may be used for energy, stored as glycogen, or converted into fat. In diabetes there is a discrepancy between the amount of insulin available to the tissues and the amount required by the body.

Hyperglycemia develops as the serum glucose increases beyond the 110 mg/100 ml normal limit. When the glucose level exceeds the renal threshold (usually about 180 mg/100 ml), glucose is excreted in the urine, producing glycosuria. Since glucose is hyperosmolar, it carries large amounts of water and electrolytes with it, producing polyuria, which can lead to dehydration and electrolyte imbalance. This fluid loss triggers thirst in the patient and polydipsia.

Since the glucose is not entering the cells, a cellular starvation occurs, leading to increased mobilization of fats and proteins for energy. Ketone bodies, the acidic metabolites of fats, accumulate in the blood, causing ketosis and ketonuria. This inefficient energy source produces weakness and hunger in the patient, resulting in polyphagia (excessive eating).

The individual with diabetes is susceptible to a number of long-term complications resulting from macrocirculatory and microcirculatory changes and neuropathies.

Macrovascular changes
Diabetics develop the same atherosclerotic vessel changes as do nondiabetics, but the incidence and severity of the changes are both earlier and more rapid. These macrovascular changes significantly increase the risk for coronary artery disease, cerebrovascular disease, and hypertension, and contribute to the development of peripheral vascular disease.

Microvascular changes
Microvascular changes appear to be related to thickening of the capillary basement membranes. Renal structure and function are particularly affected. The vessels in the eye also are affected. Microvascular changes contribute to widespread peripheral vascular disease.

Neuropathy
Changes in nerve structure and function are pervasive among diabetics. The sensory fibers are usually affected first and then motor functions. These changes contribute to the severity of peripheral vascular disease.

Other changes
Diabetics are more susceptible to infection because of the accumulation of glucose in the skin and impairments in the response of white blood cells in a glucose-rich environment.

Medical Management
The goal of therapy is the control of diabetes to delay or prevent the development of complications. Adjusting to

and controlling the disease requires a carefully planned program, including:
1. *Diet*. A diabetic's diet is calculated to distribute nutrients effectively over a 24 hour period. Carbohydrates account for about 45% of the daily calories, proteins 10% to 20%, and fats about 35%. The ADA exchange system diet has been most commonly utilized.
2. *Medications*. Subcutaneous insulin administration is used for all Type I diabetics. Oral hypoglycemic agents may be prescribed for Type II diabetics who cannot be managed by diet and weight control alone (see Tables 12-9 and 12-10).
3. *Exercise*. A regular planned activity and exercise program maximizes general health and glucose utilization.
4. *Teaching and support*. An individualized approach to teaching is used to maximize the individual's knowledge of the disorder and thus enhance intelligent self-management.

Nursing Management
Assessment—subjective (Newly diagnosed patient)
Presence of classic signs of hyperglycemia:
 Polyuria
 Polydipsia, polyphagia (excessive eating)

TABLE 12-9 Hypoglycemic agents *(insulins)*

Type of Insulin	Time of Onset (hr)	Peak of Action (hr)	Duration of Action (hr)
Rapid acting			
Regular	<1	2–4	4–6
Crystalline zinc	<1	2–4	5–8
Semilente	<1	4–7	12–16
Intermediate acting			
NPH	1–2	8–12	18–24
Globin zinc	2–4	6–10	12–18
Lente	1–4	8–12	18–24
Slow acting			
Protamine zinc	4–8	16–18	36+
Ultralente	4–8	16–18	36+

TABLE 12-10 Oral hypoglycemic agents

Name	Usual Daily Dose	Doses per Day
Acetohexamide (Dymelor)	250 mg–1.5 g	1–2
Chlorpropamide (Diabinese)	100–500 mg	1
Tolazamide (Tolinase)	100 mg–1 g	1–2
Tolbutamide (Orinase)	0.5 mg–2 g	2–3 after meals

From Long, B.C., and Phipps, W.J.: Essentials of medical-surgical nursing: a nursing process approach, St. Louis, 1985, The C.V. Mosby Co.

Weight loss

Fatigue

Presence of other chronic diseases involving the kidneys, blood vessels, or metabolism

Presence or history of obesity

Current dietary pattern

Assessment—subjective (Formerly diagnosed patient)

Knowledge of and attitude toward diabetes

Normal dietary pattern

  Patient's knowledge of prescribed diet

Presence of paresthesias or pruritus

Hypoglycemic agents in use

Self-care knowledge and skills:

  Insulin administration/site rotation

  Blood or urine testing and record keeping

  Foot care

  Use of ADA exchange system

  Knowledge of hypoglycemia and ketoacidosis and their prevention and treatment

  Knowledge of need to adjust regimen with illness or exercise

Assessment—objective

Body weight

Vital signs

Blood and urine glucose concentrations

Skin turgor and condition of mucous membranes

Urine volume and specific gravity

Intake and output balance

Assessment for ketoacidosis if applicable (see box on p. 173)

Neurovascular changes in lower extremities:

  Peripheral pulses

  Temperature of extremities

  Skin appearance: color, intactness, and texture

Nursing diagnoses

Diagnoses depend on the recency of diagnosis and the extent of complications, but commonly include:

  Actual or potential fluid volume deficit related to the hyperosmolar fluid loss that occurs with hyperglycemia

  Potential for injury and infection related to circulatory and nerve impairment in the extremities

  Potential for noncompliance related to the diet and life-style modifications prescribed for diabetes treatment

  Alteration in nutrition, potential for less than or more than body requirements, related to impaired glucose utilization or the presence of obesity

  Tactile sensory perceptual alteration related to paresthesias and peripheral neuropathies

  Knowledge deficit related to the self-care skills necessary for successful self-management of diabetes

  Potential for ineffective individual coping related to the

life-style changes mandated by the treatment of diabetes

Expected outcomes

Patient will return to a normal fluid and hydration status as blood glucose is normalized.

Patient will practice scrupulous hygiene and foot care to prevent the development of extremity complications.

Patient will maintain effective control of diabetes and maintain a normal occupational and social life-style.

Patient will maintain desired weight and meet body's nutritional needs through proper diet and medication usage.

Patient will take measures to compensate for sensory losses in the extremities to prevent injury.

Patient will have adequate knowledge of diabetes and its treatment and demonstrate the necessary self-care skills.

Patient will demonstrate positive coping behaviors and meet age-specific developmental tasks while maintaining effective disease control.

Nursing interventions

Diet

Initiate diet teaching (see the box below for guidelines).

Patient's diet plan should take into consideration:

  Personal and cultural preferences where possible,

  Life-style and occupational considerations,

  Exercise and activity pattern,

  Timing of medication usage.

Teach patient to calculate menus using the ADA exchange system (see Tables 12-11 and 12-12 for examples).

Teach patient about the relationship of exercise to diet.

DIETARY RECOMMENDATIONS FOR DIABETIC PATIENT

Calorie allotment should be sufficient to promote normal growth and development in the child and maintenance of ideal weight in the adult.

Most of the carbohydrate calories should come from starches. Sharp limitations are placed on refined sugars.

The amount of saturated fat in use should be less than 10%.

Consistency in the timing and distribution of nutrients and meals is very important in Type I diabetes.

Achieving and maintaining desired weight is very important in Type II diabetes.

Special or "dietetic" foods are not required; their content should be analyzed carefully if they are used.

Small amounts of alcohol may be planned into the diet if this will help to foster patient's adjustment and compliance.

TABLE 12-11 Use of the Exchange System for meal planning

Food Product	CHO (gm)	Fat (gm)	Equivalents
Milk and milk products	12	Trace	1 C skim or nonfat milk 1 C yogurt $\frac{1}{2}$ C evaporated milk
Vegetable			
Nonstarchy	5	2	$\frac{1}{2}$ C asparagus, carrots, eggplant, collards, tomatoes, and such
"Free" (lettuce, endive)			As desired
Fruit	10	—	1 small apple $\frac{1}{3}$ C apple sauce $\frac{1}{2}$ banana $\frac{1}{2}$ grapefruit
Breads and starchy vegetables	15	2	1 slice bread $\frac{1}{2}$ bagel 1 tortilla (6 in) $\frac{1}{2}$ hamburger bun 2 graham crackers 15 potato chips $\frac{3}{4}$ C unsweetened cereal
Meat			
Lean	—	3	$\frac{1}{4}$ C cottage cheese (dry) 1 oz lean beef or fish $\frac{1}{4}$ C tuna
Moderate fat	—	15	1 oz ground beef (15% fat) or boiled ham $\frac{1}{2}$ C cottage cheese (creamed) 2 tbs peanut butter
High fat	—	20	1 oz ground beef (20% fat) Pork ribs or deviled ham 1 oz cheddar cheese 1 oz frankfurter
Fats	—	5	1 tsp margarine or butter 1 strip crisp bacon 1 tbs French dressing
Other	—	—	Calorie-free beverages, unsweetened gelatin, and such: as desired

Exercise decreases the need for insulin and increases the need for food.

A rapid-acting glucose source should be taken and carried prior to planned strenuous exercise.

Exercise should be planned to avoid the period of peak insulin action if possible (see Table 12-9).

Teach patient how to adapt diet during gastrointestinal upset or illness (see Table 12-9).

Encourage patient to verbalize and discuss perceived effects of diet restrictions on normal desired lifestyle.

Medications

Teach patient and family about prescribed insulin.

Explain onset, peak, and duration of action.

Explain that food must be taken within the time of onset for insulin prescribed.

Explain importance of planning a snack for time of peak action of insulin.

Explain importance of bedtime snack for patients on long-acting insulin to provide glucose coverage for the night.

Teach patient relationship of insulin need and illness.

Insulin needs are greater during illness; patient should never skip a dose.

Patient should adjust diet to liquids if necessary but maintain intake.

Patient should increase frequency of blood and urine testing and contact physician if hyperglycemia worsens.

Teach patient the proper preparation and administration of insulin (see box on p. 173).

Encourage patient to utilize all available sites to avoid the development of lipodystrophies (see Figure 12-2 for acceptable insulin sites).

Teach use of insulin pump if prescribed:

Blood glucose must be monitored frequently.

Explain technique for needle changing (every 2 to 3 days).

Describe delivery rate setting and adjustment.

Patient should be monitored for complications.

Testing

Teach patient technique of blood or urine testing:

Describe method to use and number of times it should be done per day.

Explain importance of accurate record keeping.

TABLE 12-12 Sample of two menu plans using the exchange list*

Exchanges	Menu 1	Menu 2
	Breakfast	**Breakfast**
1 Fruit	½ Glass orange juice	¼ Cantaloupe
1 Milk (low fat)	1 Glass skim milk	1 Glass skim milk
1 Meat	1 Egg poached	1 Scrambled egg
3 Bread	2 Toast, ½ C oatmeal	1 English muffin, ½ C bran flakes
2 Fat	1½ Tsp margarine	1½ Tsp margarine
	Lunch	**Lunch**
1 Fruit	1 Peach	½ Banana
1 Milk (low fat)	1 Glass skim milk	1 Glass skim milk
2 Meat	Tuna salad sandwich (¼ C tuna with celery, 2 slices	1 McDonald's cheeseburger (2 bread, 2 meat, 1 fat)
2 Bread	bread, 3 tsp mayonnaise, and lettuce)	1 Lettuce salad with 2 Tbsp French dressing
	Afternoon snack	**Afternoon snack**
1 Bread	6 Thin round crackers	Pretzels
1 Fruit	1 Apple	Grapes
	Dinner	**Dinner**
1 Fruit	¾ C strawberries	½ C pineapple
2 Vegetable B	1 C green beans	Sliced tomatoes
4 Meat	4 Oz round steak	4 Oz ham (boiled)
1 Milk (low fat)	1 Glass skim milk	1 Glass skim milk
2 Bread	1 Small baked potato	2 slices bread
	1 Roll	
3 Fats	1 Tbsp sour cream/2½ tsp butter	1 Tsp mayonnaise
	Evening snack	**Evening snack**
1 Bread	3 Rye wafers	6 Salt crackers
1 Meat	1 Oz low-fat cheese	¼ C low-fat cottage cheese

Modified from American Diabetes Association, Inc.: American Diabetes Association and National Institute of Health, U.S. Public Health Service exchange lists for meal planning, Chicago, 1976, The Association; from Long, B.C., and Phipps, W.J.: *Essentials of medical-surgical nursing: a nursing process approach,* St. Louis, 1985, The C.V. Mosby Co.
*Diet distributed over three meals and two snacks. Diet based on 2000 calories with 45% CHO (225 g); 35% fats (78 g); and 20% proteins (100 g).

Explain importance of recording urine results by percent since the scales vary with different brands of equipment.

Explain how to interpret the results.

Tell when to notify the physician.

Explain importance of increasing the frequency of testing during illness.

Hygiene
Teach patient importance of scrupulous hygiene.

Explain importance of meticulous care for even minor trauma to skin.

Describe methods for prevention of peripheral vascular disease (see box on p. 173 for foot care principles).

Adjustment
Encourage patient to discuss feelings and frustrations about treatment regimen.

Include appropriate family members in teaching sessions.

Explain importance of wearing Medic Alert tag or bracelet.

Support and reinforce all positive coping behaviors.

Support involvement in self-help groups.

Complications
Teach patient to recognize signs of hypoglycemia (see box on p. 173).

Hypoglycemia is usually related to too much insulin or exercise, and too little food.

Reverse effects with a rapidly absorbed glucose source, such as:

½ cup juice or cola

4 cubes or 2 packets sugar

2 squares graham crackers

When symptoms resolve, offer additional food, either a scheduled meal or a complex carbohydrate and protein.

Teach patient to recognize symptoms of ketoacidosis (see box on p. 173).

Ketoacidosis is usually related to insufficient insulin, too much food, or the presence of illness or infection, which increases insulin requirements.

Treatment requires hospitalization.

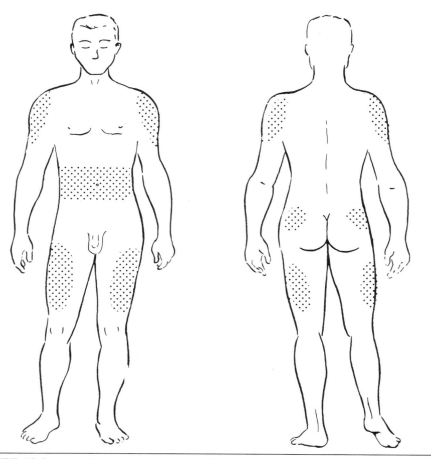

FIGURE 12-2 Arms, legs, buttocks, or abdomen can be used for insulin injection. A different site (indicated by each dot) should be used for each injection. (From Phipps, W.J., Long, B.C., and Woods, N.F.: Medical-surgical nursing: concepts and clinical practice, ed. 2, St. Louis, 1983, The C.V. Mosby Co.)

Provide fluid and electrolyte replacement.
Adjust insulin dosage if appropriate (usually low dose IV infusion).
Provide scrupulous monitoring.
Note: Another complication, hyperglycemic hyperosmolar nonketotic coma (HHNC), may occur in Type II diabetics or in elderly persons with no history of diabetes. The signs and symptoms and treatment principles for HHNC are outlined in the box on p. 173. This complication has a high mortality.

Evaluation
Patient maintains an adequate fluid and electrolyte balance and maintains blood glucose within desired levels.
Patient can discuss importance of good hygiene to prevent complications and practices good preventive foot care.
Patient maintains good control of diabetes while participating fully in occupational, social, and recreational pursuits.

Patient can describe basic prescribed meal plan, chooses and follows a balanced diet, makes correct adjustments to maintain control while traveling or eating out; maintains desired weight; and properly adjusts diet to changes in activity and occurrence of illness.
Patient compensates for sensory losses in extremities by practicing preventive foot care and inspection; patient scrupulously treats all skin abrasions.
Patient is knowledgeable about diabetes and its complications; correctly prepares and administers insulin; rotates injection sites; stores equipment and insulin properly; correctly and consistently tests urine or blood and maintains accurate records; can identify signs of hypoglycemia and ketoacidosis; states correct treatment to follow; wears Medic Alert tag; and receives adequate medical supervision.
Patient demonstrates effective coping behaviors and expresses desire and commitment to maintain adequate disease control.

GUIDELINES FOR INSULIN ADMINISTRATION

Always use an insulin syringe calibrated in the same unit/ml scale that matches the scale of the insulin.

Select insulin according to type, strength, species, and brand name as specified by the prescription.

Rotate or gently roll the bottle if it is other than regular or globin insulin.

Examine *intermediate* and *long-acting* insulin vials: for appearance and expiration dates; do not use unless solution is cloudy.

Check for and remove any air bubbles after insulin is drawn into the syringe (do not use an air bubble to clear the needle after injection).

When mixing insulins, do not vary the sequence in which two insulins are drawn into the same syringe; usually air is injected into both bottles (regular and intermediate); the insulin is withdrawn first from the regular vial and then from the longer acting insulin vial.

Use a needle insertion site that has not been used in the past month.

Insert the needle into fatty tissue *closer to muscle than to skin* using a 90 degree angle if fat pad is adequate.

It is no longer considered necessary to refrigerate insulin in current use. Unused insulin should be kept in refrigerator.

From Long, B.C., and Phipps, W.J.: Essentials of medical-surgical nursing: a nursing process approach, St. Louis, 1985, The C.V. Mosby Co.

GUIDELINES FOR DIABETIC FOOT CARE

Wear well-fitting shoes and clean stockings at all times when ambulating and never walk barefooted.

Bathe feet daily and dry them well, paying particular attention to areas between the toes. Keep skin softened.

Do not self-treat calluses, corns, or ingrown toenails; a podiatrist should be consulted if these are present.

Bath water should be 29.5–32° C (85–90° F) and should be tested with a bath thermometer or the elbow before immersing the feet.

Heating pads and hot water bottles should be avoided.

Measures that help increase circulation to the lower extremities should be instituted:

Avoid smoking.

Avoid crossing legs when sitting.

Protect extremities when exposed to cold.

Avoid immersing feet in cold water.

Use socks or stockings that do not apply pressure to the legs at specific sites.

Institute a regimen of regular exercise.

Inspect feet daily and report any cuts, cracks, redness, blisters, or other signs of trauma so early treatment can be instituted.

From Long, B.C., and Phipps, W.J.: Essentials of medical-surgical nursing: a nursing process approach, St. Louis, 1985, The C.V. Mosby Co.

SIGNS AND SYMPTOMS OF HYPOGLYCEMIA

SYMPATHETIC NERVOUS SYSTEM ACTIVITY (usually precedes CNS manifestations):

Pallor	*Perspiration
Piloerection	Hunger
Tachycardia	Palpitation
*Nervousness	Irritability
*Weakness	Trembling

CENTRAL NERVOUS SYSTEM ACTIVITY:

Headache	Blurred vision
Diplopia (double vision)	Incoherent speech
Emotional changes	Fatigue
*Mental confusion	Numbness of lips, tongue
Convulsions	Coma

*Four most commonly reported by patients (Paulk, 1983).
From Long, B.C., and Phipps, W.J.: Essentials of medical-surgical nursing: a nursing process approach, St. Louis, 1985, The C.V. Mosby Co.

SIGNS AND SYMPTOMS OF KETOACIDOSIS

Onset is slow.

SYMPTOMS:

Increased thirst
*Nausea and vomiting, anorexia
Abdominal cramping
*Lethargy

SIGNS:

Increased temperature
*Kussmaul breathing (deep and rapid)
*Fruity acetone odor to breath
*Hot, dry, flushed skin
Loss of skin turgor
Decreasing level of consciousness to coma

*Classic signs and symptoms

SIGNS AND TREATMENT OF HYPERGLYCEMIC, HYPEROSMOLAR, NONKETOTIC COMA (HHNC)

SIGNS:	TREATMENT:
Fluid deficit	IV fluid and electrolyte replacement
Dehydration	Small amounts of insulin
Hypotension	Careful monitoring of:
Anuria	Intake and output
Circulatory collapse	Vital signs
Elevated body temperature	Level of consciousness
Neurologic changes	Electrolytes
Sensory deficits	Vascular response to fluid
Motor deficits	
Focal seizures	
Aphasia	
Coma	

REFERENCES

Anderson, J.W., *et al.*: Fiber and diabetes (review), Diab. Care 2:369-379, 1979.

Paulk, L.H.: Hypoglycemic reactions: from the diabetic's perspective, unpublished thesis, Kent, Ohio, 1983, Kent State University.

BIBLIOGRAPHY

Camunas, C.: Pheochromocytoma, Am. J. Nurs. 83:887-891, 1983.

Danowski, T.S., *et al.*: Diabetic complications and their prevention or reversal, Diab. Care 3:94-99, 1980.

Diabetes mellitus, Volume V, New York, 1981, American Diabetes Association.

Evangelisti, J.T., *et al.*: Thyroid storm: a nursing crisis, Heart and Lung 12:184-194, 1983.

Fairchild, R.S.: Diabetes insipidus: a review, Crit. Care Q. 2:111-118, 1980.

Geola, F., and Chopra, I.: Hyperthyroidism and hypothyroidism, Med. Times 108:64-69, 73-74, 1980.

Gotch, P.M.: Teaching patients about adrenal corticosteroids, Am. J. Nurs. 81:78-85, 1981.

Guthrie, D.W., and Guthrie, R.A.: Nursing management of diabetes mellitus, ed. 2, St. Louis, 1982, The C.V. Mosby Co.

Hamburger, S., and Rush, D.: Syndrome of inappropriate secretion of antidiuretic hormone, Crit. Care Q. 2:119-129, 1980.

Hoffman, J.T., and Newby, T.B.: Hypercalcemia in primary hyperparathyroidism, Nurs. Clin. North Am. 15:469-480, 1980.

McFadden, E.A., Zaloga, G.P., and Chernow, B.: Hypocalcemia: a medical emergency, Am. J. Nurs. 83:227-230, 1983.

Nemeroff, D.R.: Transphenoidal hypophysectomy, J. Neurosurg. Nurs. 13:303-312, 1981.

Sanford, S.J.: Dysfunction of the adrenal gland: physiologic considerations and nursing problems, Nurs. Clin. North Am. 15:481-498, 1980.

Sneid, D.S.: Hyperosmolar hyperglycemic nonketotic coma, Crit. Care Q. 2:29-43, 1980.

Urbanic, R.C., and Mazzaferri, E.L.: Thyrotoxic crisis and myxedema coma, Heart and Lung 7:435-447, 1978.

Wake, M.M., and Brensinger, J.F.: The nurse's role in hypothyroidism, Nurs. Clin. North Am. 15:453-467, 1980.

NURSING CARE PLAN

HYPERTHYROIDISM

Nursing Diagnoses	Expected Patient Outcomes	Nursing Interventions
Anxiety and nervousness related to excess nervous system activity	Patient understands reason for change in behavior Emotional lability is minimized Patient feels in control of environment	1. Discuss reasons for emotional lability. 2. Maintain calm, relaxed environment. 3. Encourage visitors who promote relaxation. 4. Provide privacy (such as single room). 5. Explain all interventions. 6. Avoid stimulants such as coffee, tea, cola, alcohol. 7. Help patient identify previous successful coping mechanism or explore new mechanisms. 8. Avoid activities requiring fine motor coordination. 9. Decrease known stressors, explain planned interventions, and listen to patient's concerns. Administer prescribed drugs and document therapeutic response.
Alteration in nutrition less than body requirements, related to excess metabolic rate	Patient ingests sufficient nutrients to meet body needs and maintain desired weight	1. Monitor weight every other day or weekly. 2. Help patient plan for high-calorie, high-protein, high-carbohydrate diet, selecting foods from all food groups. 3. Suggest six small meals/day or between meal snacks. Keep snacks at bedside. 4. Use supplements such as Ensure if necessary. 5. Encourage adequate fluid intake to replace losses.

Potential for visual sensory deficit related to eye changes of exophthalmos	Patient employs measures to prevent eye damage	1. Assess visual acuity, ability to close eyes, photophobia.
		2. Protect eyes from irritants:
		   a. Use patches or glasses for excess light or wind or if eyes cannot completely close.
		   b. Use artificial tears if prescribed.
		   c. Elevate head of bed at night.
		3. Encourage patient to restrict dietary sodium.

Alteration in comfort related to heat intolerance, diaphoresis, or palpitations	Patient's metabolic rate decreases to normal	1. Control environmental temperature for comfort (fans may be helpful). 2. Suggest patient take frequent showers. 3. Encourage adequate fluid intake to replace losses. 4. Instruct patient to report any symptoms of palpitations, chest pain, dizziness, dyspnea.
Activity intolerance related to easily fatigued muscles	Patient will regain muscle strength and endurance and resume preillness activity pattern	1. Assess activity schedule. 2. Suggest ways to modify fatiguing activities. 3. Identify activities that can be done by others until condition is controlled. 4. Balance periods of activity with rest. 5. Encourage activities that promote sleep at night.
Disturbance in self-concept related to the occurrence of goiter or exophthalmos	Patient will incorporate body changes into an altered but positive self-concept	1. Encourage patient to verbalize feelings about altered appearance. 2. Provide patient with factual information about the degree of reversibility of symptoms. 3. Support positive coping efforts. 4. Teach patient about self-care.

CHAPTER 13

Disorders of the Urinary System

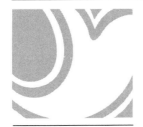

The kidneys and other structures of the urinary system play a major role in regulating the body's internal environment. Functions include: regulating the fluid and electrolyte balance, excreting metabolic wastes, maintaining the acid-base balance, producing or modifying the level of hormones responsible for regulation of blood pressure, metabolism of calcium, and synthesis of red blood cells.

Renal disease may cause extensive disruption in body chemistry and significantly impair health. Some of the more common disorders are those resulting from infection or obstruction. Figure 13-1 shows the anatomical structure of the urinary system.

URINARY TRACT INFECTIONS

Infections within the urinary tract, both acute and chronic, are common health problems, especially in women. They may occur at any point in the system. Individuals who experience urinary retention or stasis or the intrusion of a foreign body such as a catheter or stone are particularly susceptible. The two most common forms of infection are cystitis and pyelonephritis.

Pathophysiology

Cystitis involves infection of the bladder or urethra. Bacterial contamination from the rectum or during intercourse is frequently a predisposing factor. Inflammation of the bladder wall creates the classic symptoms.

Pyelonephritis involves infection of the kidney tissue and may occur when bacteria ascend the urinary tract following cystitis. It may be acute or chronic and may cause symptoms quite similar to those of cystitis. Infection usually starts in the medulla and spreads to the cortex and may produce kidney fibrosis and scarring during healing. In rare cases it may advance to renal failure.

Medical Management

The treatment of cystitis and pyelonephritis revolves around identification of the infecting organism through urine cultures and elimination of the infection with appropriate antibiotic therapy. Follow-up cultures are indicated in pyelonephritis to identify and treat chronic forms. Medications commonly prescribed include sulfonamides (Gantrisin, Bactrim, Septra), antiseptics (Neg-Gram, Furadantin, Mandelamine), systemic antibiotics (ampicillin, cephalosporins, aminoglycosides), and urinary analgesics (Pyridium).

Nursing Management

Assessment—subjective

History of urinary tract infection

History of chronic disease or other urinary tract disease

History of renal stones, prostatic enlargement, stasis, or intrusive procedure

Patient's complaint of:

Dysuria (painful urination): urgency, frequency, burning sensation

Fatigue or malaise

Flank pain or tenderness (pyelonephritis)

Use of bubble baths, contraceptive jellies, underwear without cotton panels

Assessment—objective

Hematuria (blood in urine)

Urine sample: odor, cloudiness, pH

Chills and fever

Positive lab reports from urine culture, elevated white blood cell count

Nursing diagnoses

Frequently encountered diagnoses include:

Alteration in comfort—pain and burning on urination related to bladder inflammation and irritation

Alteration in patterns of urinary elimination related to urgency and frequency

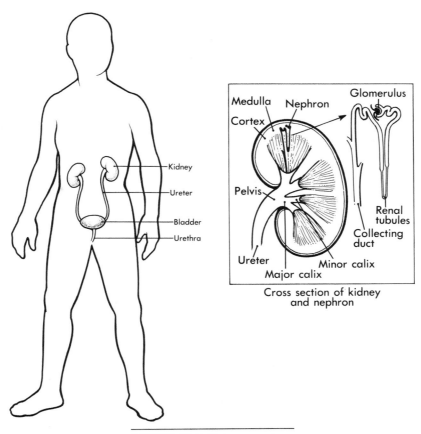

FIGURE 13-1 Urinary system.

Knowledge deficit related to health promotional activities that prevent the recurrence of urinary tract infection

Expected outcomes

Patient's symptoms will gradually decrease.

Patient will reestablish a normal urination schedule.

Patient will be knowledgeable about measures that can help prevent recurrences of urinary tract infection.

Nursing interventions

Administer prescribed medication.

Teach patient importance of taking full course of antibiotics.

Maintain high fluid intake (either orally, intravenously, or both) during infection.

    Give 3000 to 4000 ml per day if not contraindicated.

Encourage patient to take warm sitz baths for comfort.

Monitor patient's temperature until infection is resolved.

Encourage rest during acute phase.

Teach patient health promotion activities.

    Explain importance of scrupulous perineal hygiene.

        Patient should wipe carefully from front to back.

        Patient should empty bladder and cleanse before and after intercourse.

    Patient should avoid use of bubble baths and contraceptive jellies.

    Explain importance of maintaining high fluid intake (approximately 3 L daily).

    Patient should modify diet to ensure urinary acidity (fish and poultry, whole grains).

    Patient should monitor urine pH regularly.

    Explain importance of responding promptly to urge to void. Empty bladder q 2-3 hrs.

    Describe signs and symptoms of reinfection.

Evaluation

Patient is free of symptoms of burning and urgency.

Patient empties bladder at regular intervals but does not have urinary frequency.

Patient maintains an adequate fluid intake, practices optimal hygiene, and is free of recurrent infection.

OBSTRUCTIVE DISORDERS

RENAL CALCULI

Urinary stones may develop at any level in the urinary system but are most commonly found within the kidney.

Stones are crystallizations of minerals around an organic base. Calcium stones account for about 75% of stones. No cause can be found in many cases, but urinary tract infection, alkaline urine, and urinary stasis are precipitating factors for stone development.

Pathophysiology
Renal calculi produce urinary tract problems that reflect the stones' size and position. Large stones may produce obstruction of urine flow, pressure destruction of kidney tissue, and infection. Small stones may be successfully excreted from the urinary tract, but cause severe local pain spasm, and inflammation in the process. Rough stone edges may cause hematuria.

Medical Management
Since about 90% of renal calculi are passed spontaneously, the patient receives symptomatic support with hydration and analgesics. Larger stones may need to be removed surgically by
  Ureterolithotomy—removal of stones blocking a ureter
  Pyelolithotomy—removal of a stone from the renal pelvis
  Nephrolithotomy—removal of a stone from the kidney parenchyma
Extracorporeal shock wave lithotripsy is a new, successful alternative to surgery for some patients with large stones.

Nursing Management
Assessment—subjective
Patient's complaints of:
  Pain
    Constant, dull pain if stone in kidney
    Excruciating pain if stone in ureter; pain may radiate to genitals or thigh
  Nausea and vomiting
Prior history of stones or urinary tract infection
Family history of stones

Assessment—objective
Hematuria
Changes in vital signs—fever or mild shock
Positive results from IVP

Nursing diagnoses
Alteration in comfort—intense pain related to spasm and pressure in kidney or ureter
Alteration in patterns of urinary elimination related to symptoms of dysuria
Knowledge deficit related to measures to prevent recurrence

Expected outcomes
Patient's pain will decrease; nausea and vomiting will be relieved.

Patient will return to a normal pattern of urinary elimination.
Patient will be knowledgeable concerning measures that can prevent the reoccurrence of calculi.

Nursing interventions
Administer analgesics liberally as prescribed.
Assess effectiveness of pain relief.
Instruct patient to strain all urine.
Force fluids orally, or administer intravenously to at least 3000–4000 ml daily.
Encourage patient to ambulate as tolerated.
Monitor intake and output.
Assess urine for blood.
Teach patient measures to prevent reoccurrence of stones.
  Patient should maintain high daily fluid intake.
  Patient should engage in active exercise and avoid immobility.
  Patient should modify diet if appropriate. Possible modifications include:
    Restrict calcium, found in milk and milk products, beans, dried fruit, chocolate, and cocoa

---

CARE OF THE PATIENT FOLLOWING UROLOGIC SURGERY

PREOPERATIVE:
Reinforce teaching about procedure and aftercare as needed.
Teach coughing and deep breathing methods.
  Emphasize importance of effective coughing to patients with high flank incision since the incision's proximity to diaphragm will make coughing difficult.

POSTOPERATIVE:
Provide adequate analgesia to facilitate deep breathing and coughing.
  Use incentive spirometer every 2 hours.
Monitor urine output every 1 to 2 hours.
  Record output separately for each drainage tube.
  Estimate urine drainage on dressings.
  Observe urine's color and consistency.
Weigh patient daily.
Encourage patient to ambulate if ureteral catheters are not in place.
Assess patient for return of bowel sounds, passage of flatus.
Ensure IV hydration until patient tolerates taking food and fluids orally.
Monitor patient carefully for signs of bleeding.
  Risk is high if parenchyma has been incised.
  Risk is greatest on day of surgery and 8 to 12 days after surgery.
Change dressing aseptically frequently to keep site of incision dry.
  Stoma bags may be utilized for large amounts of drainage.
  Keep skin clean and odor free.
Maintain patency of all drainage tubes.
  Position patient so kinking or obstruction does not occur.
  Never clamp or irrigate ureteral catheters or nephrostomy tubes.

Restrict oxalate found in coffee, tea, chocolate, spinach, beans.

Restrict purines, found in organ meats, legumes, sardines, herring, moderate amounts in most meats.

Take measures to acidify the urine, by eating meat and fish, whole grains, cheese, cranberries.

Monitor urine pH at regular intervals.

Explain purpose and side effects of prescribed medications.

Provide appropriate preoperative teaching if surgery is planned.

(Care of the patient following kidney surgery is outlined in the box on p. 178.)

Evaluation

Patient passes stone and is free of pain, nausea, and tenderness.

Patient voids at regular intervals and is free of hematuria or dysuria.

Patient can discuss appropriate diet modification for type of stone; patient understands importance of hydration and exercise to avoid reoccurrence.

Patient who is treated surgically recovers without complications.

RENAL NEOPLASMS

Tumors of the urinary system affect both the kidney and bladder. Nephrectomy is the treatment of choice for renal tumors and the associated care is similar to that provided for other renal or abdominal surgery. Bladder cancer is a problem of increasing significance. It affects individuals in late middle age, men most commonly, and is associated with cigarette smoking and chronic exposure to certain chemicals and dyes.

Pathophysiology

Most bladder tumors begin as benign papillomas and occur in multiple locations. Most arise from transitional epithelium cell types. Painless hematuria is a common early sign. Advanced disease may cause infection, fistula development, or ureteral obstruction leading to renal failure.

Medical Management

All benign papillomas are treated as premalignant and removed through cystoscopic resection and fulguration. More radical procedures—up to full cystectomy and urinary diversion—are employed for recurrent or highly invasive disease. Radiation and chemotherapy may be used to augment treatment.

Table 13-1 outlines less commonly occurring conditions affecting urinary system functioning and their medical management.

Nursing Management

Primary nursing management revolves around care of the patient following urinary diversion. This is outlined in the box on p. 180.

TABLE 13-1 Conditions affecting urinary system function

Condition	Description	Signs and Symptoms	Medical Management
Glomerulonephritis Acute Chronic	An inflammatory process involving the glomerulus, which results from a disordered immune response: Poststreptococcal reaction Autoantibody production to glomerular basement membrane Most patients experience complete recovery. Some go on into renal failure.	Glomerular porosity increases, causing proteinuria and hematuria Scarring produces gradual loss of glomerular function Fluid retention may cause massive edema and hypertension	Treatment is based on relief of symptoms and management of renal failure Maintain patient on bed rest. Restrict sodium, fluids. Administer diuretics. Administer antihypertensives. Provide high-carbohydrate, low-protein diet.
Nephrosis (nephrotic syndrome)	A clinical syndrome that may result from many causes; basement membrane becomes very porous, allowing massive excretion of protein in the urine.	Massive proteinuria and pitting edema Albuminuria	Administer diuretics. Provide low-sodium, high-protein diet. Corticosteroid therapy is effective for certain causes.
Polycystic kidney disease	Adult form is an autosomal dominant disorder that becomes symptomatic in middle age. Kidney is filled with thin-walled cysts that enlarge and destroy surrounding tissue. Eventually progresses to renal failure.	Steady dull flank pain from enlarged kidneys Hematuria if cysts rupture Episodes of infection	There is no specific treatment. Goals are to prevent development of infection or treat promptly. Supportive care is offered as gradual renal failure occurs. Nephrectomy is often needed.

CARE OF THE PATIENT WITH A URINARY DIVERSION (ILEAL CONDUIT)

DESCRIPTION OF OPERATION:

Ureters are excised from the bladder and transplanted into a section of ileum resected from the intestinal tract with blood supply intact. One end is closed and the other brought to the surface of the abdomen to form a stoma to drain urine.

PREOPERATIVE CARE:

Provide accurate information about procedure and care.
Provide introduction to self-care materials if patient exhibits readiness.
Introduce stomal therapist to begin teaching plan.
Encourage patient to verbalize feelings about change in body image and function.
Initiate bowel preparation as ordered.
    Provide clear liquids.
    Administer enemas and intestinal antibiotics.

POSTOPERATIVE CARE:

Use standard interventions to identify and prevent complications.
Provide TED stockings; encourage patient to do range of motion exercises, make position changes, and ambulate as permitted to prevent thrombophlebitis (risk is high after pelvic surgery).
    Assess for Homans' sign every shift.
Maintain patency of nasogastric tube until peristalsis returns (3 to 5 days).
    Auscultate abdomen for bowel sounds.
Observe stoma for complications.
    Stoma should be healthy red in color.
    Observe for bleeding or erosion.
    Assess surrounding skin.
Maintain high fluid intake.
    Urine will contain mucus from bowel.
    Empty bag every 2 hours; attach to Foley drainage bag at night
Provide meticulous care to surrounding skin.
    Ensure proper fit of appliance.
    Maintain an acid pH.
    Teach patient skills for self-care of appliance.
Encourage patient to verbalize feelings about surgery.
    Discuss impact of surgery on work, leisure, clothes, and sexual activity.
Put patient in touch with support groups and agencies in the community to facilitate adjustment.

RENAL FAILURE

Renal failure is a state of severe impairment or total lack of renal function. The patient is unable to excrete waste products and maintain the fluid and electrolyte balance.

ACUTE RENAL FAILURE

Acute failure is a sudden and frequently reversible decrease or cessation of kidney function. It generally follows contact with a nephrotoxic agent, trauma, or surgical

CAUSES OF ACUTE RENAL FAILURE

TOXIC SUBSTANCES

Solvents (carbon tetrachloride, methanol, ethylene glycol)
Heavy metals (lead, arsenic, mercury)
Antibiotics (kanamycin, gentamicin, polymyxin B, amphotericin B, colistin, neomycin, phenazopyridine)
Pesticides
Mushrooms

ISCHEMIA

Hypovolemia
Blood loss (surgery, trauma)
Plasma loss (burns, surgery, acute pancreatitis)
Sodium and water loss (prolonged diarrhea or vomiting, gastrointestinal tract drainage, sustained high fever)
Cardiac failure
Myocardial infarction
Cardiac arrhythmias
Congestive heart failure
Septic shock
Bilateral occlusion of renal arteries

OTHER FACTORS

Acute glomerular disease
Acute, severe infection of kidney tissue
Hemoglobinuria (from hemolysis, for example, a transfusion reaction)
Myoglobinuria (from massive muscle insult, for example, a crush injury)
Mechanical obstructions in the urinary tract

Modified from Phipps, W.J., Long, B.C. and Woods, N.F.: Medical-surgical nursing: concepts and clinical practice, ed. 2, St. Louis, 1983, The C.V. Mosby Co.

procedures. The box above lists some of the common causes.

Pathophysiology

Renal ischemia occurs when blood flow to the kidneys is decreased. The kidney responds with vasoconstriction, which further reduces blood flow and worsens ischemia. Prolonged ischemia produces death of renal tubular tissue and triggers the failure. Acute failure commonly occurs in three phases:

Oliguric phase. Output falls to 400 ml or less per day, reflecting damage to nephrons. Urine is also dilute because of the tubules' loss of concentrating ability.

Diuretic phase. Second phase begins in days or weeks. Increasing output indicates healing of the nephrons. Inability to excrete wastes or concentrate urine reflects continued tubular damage.

Recovery phase. Recovery may take months as kidneys gradually return to normal or near normal levels of functioning.

Table 13-2 lists the major symptoms of and physiologic changes occurring in renal failure.

TABLE 13-2 Symptoms caused by physiologic changes in acute renal failure

Symptoms	Physiologic Effects	Findings
Oliguric Phase		
Nausea; vomiting, drowsiness; confusion; coma; GI bleeding; asterixis; pericarditis	Inability to excrete metabolic wastes	Increased serum urea nitrogen and creatinine levels
Nausea; vomiting; cardiac arrhythmias; Kussmaul's breathing; drowsiness; confusion; coma	Inability to regulate electrolytes	Hyperkalemia; hyponatremia; acidosis
Edema; congestive heart failure; pulmonary edema; hypertension	Inability to excrete fluid loads	Fluid overload; hypervolemia
Diuretic Phase		
Urinary output of up to 4 to 5 L/day: postural hypotension; tachycardia	Increased production of urine	Hypovolemia; loss of sodium and potassium in urine
Increasing mental alertness and activity	Slowly increasing excretion of metabolic wastes	Initially, high BUN (fluid loss greater than solute loss); gradual return of BUN to normal

From Long, B.C., and Phipps, W.J.: Essentials of medical-surgical nursing: a nursing process approach, St. Louis, 1985, The C.V. Mosby Co.

Medical Management

The treatment of acute renal failure is specific to the problems of each stage. In the oliguric phase, dialysis is used to control and excrete rising metabolic wastes. Diet is modified to reduce protein and provide carbohydrates for energy. Careful monitoring is employed to maintain appropriate electrolyte levels; the patient should be observed for signs of fluid overload and other complications.

In the diuretic phase, fluid replacement may be necessary to prevent dehydration. Dialysis is continued as needed to maintain acceptable levels of electrolytes and excretion of wastes until adequate kidney function returns.

Nursing Management
Assessment—subjective (Onset of failure)
History of precipitating factors
Patient's complaints of:
    Change in voiding pattern
    Abrupt weight gain, edema
    Shortness of breath
    Weakness, fatigue, nausea
    Confusion or drowsiness

Assessment—objective
Signs of fluid overload
    CHF, pulmonary edema
    Hypertension
    Edema
Accurate intake and output records
    Low specific gravity of urine
Level of consciousness
Laboratory reports demonstrating hyperkalemia, ele-
vated creatinine and BUN (blood urea nitrogen), metabolic acidosis, hyponatremia

Nursing diagnoses
Diagnoses will depend on the extent and duration of failure and the adequacy of therapy. Common diagnoses include:
    Alteration in fluid volume—excess related to failure of the renal regulatory mechanism
    Potential impairment of skin integrity related to alterations in skin turgor associated with edema
    Alteration in patterns of urinary elimination related to falling urine production
    Alteration in thought processes related to the accumulation of waste products
    Alteration in comfort related to nausea, thirst, or pain

Expected outcomes
Patient's thirst and nausea will decrease.
Patient will maintain a fluid and electrolyte balance that is within an acceptable range.
Patient will maintain an intact skin; edema will decrease.
Patient will return to normal urinary elimination patterns without need for dialysis.
Patient will be fully oriented and able to problem-solve effectively.

Nursing interventions
Oliguric phase
Fluid and electrolytes
Maintain accurate intake and output records.
Restrict fluids as prescribed (usually 500 cc plus output).

Plan with patient to distribute fluids effectively throughout the day.

Teach the rationale and importance of fluid restrictions.

Employ comfort measures for thirst (mouth care, ice chips, moist cloth for mouth).

Assess status of edema.

Weigh patient daily.

Monitor vital signs frequently.

Assess for signs of sodium and potassium imbalance.

Teach patient rationale for dialysis and mechanisms of action.

Monitor patency of vascular access site.

Diet

Maintain flow of patient's IV at prescribed rate.

Explore use of simple foods rich in carbohydrates as tolerated.

Add high biologic value protein to diet to prevent tissue wasting as tolerated.

Administer antiemetics if prescribed.

Activity and comfort

Promote maximal rest to lower metabolic load.

Assist patient with activities of daily living as needed.

Encourage use of deep breathing during immobility.

Turn patient frequently and provide excellent skin care.

Encourage patient to ambulate as condition stabilizes.

Maintain safe environment during period of lethargy.

Use side rails and check patient frequently.

Administer measures to combat pruritus.

Protect patient from exposure to infection.

Monitor patient's level of consciousness frequently.

Keep patient oriented to environment and reassure patient about reversible nature of mental changes.

Diuretic phase

Maintain interventions outlined above.

Monitor patient for fluid and electrolyte depletion.

Monitor output hourly.

Assess skin turgor and mucous membranes.

Provide replacement fluid as prescribed.

Teach patient rationale for ongoing dialysis in face of rising urine output.

Teach patient about diet restrictions and medications for long-term rehabilitation and explain importance of avoiding infection.

Evaluation

Patient is relieved of anorexia and nausea through dialysis or returning renal function; patient eats diet within ongoing restrictions.

Patient follows prescribed fluid restriction, lab reports and clinical signs demonstrate an adequate fluid and electrolyte balance.

Patient's skin is intact; edema is minimal or absent; pruritus is relieved.

Patient experiences a gradual return of renal function, has a normal pattern of urinary elimination, and no longer needs dialysis.

Patient returns to preillness levels of intellectual functioning and personality.

CHRONIC RENAL FAILURE

The development of chronic failure is usually a slow process, occurring over a period of years. Recurrent infections, obstruction, and blood vessel destruction from diabetes and hypertension are common predisposing causes. Repeated episodes of tissue death and scarring may trigger insufficiency and finally total failure.

Pathophysiology

In chronic failure the nephrons are selectively destroyed. Intact nephron units hypertrophy and allow the kidney to compensate until about 75% of the nephrons are destroyed. Initially the heavy solute load may trigger an osmotic diuresis but eventually, with the loss of more nephrons, oliguria and retention of waste products occur. Table 13-3 summarizes the effects of chronic failure on various organ systems.

Medical Management

In early stages the failure may be controlled by strictly limiting the intake of fluid and substances that require kidney excretion. Most patients progress to the point at which dialysis or transplantation are essential to preserve life.

Nursing Management

Assessment—subjective

History/duration of disease and its treatment

Knowledge of disease and treatment

Medications in use and patient's knowledge of their purpose

Usual dietary patterns

Impact of disease and treatment on preferred life-style

Effect of disease on relationships, sexual functioning

Patient's complaints of:

Lethargy, fatigue, irritability, or depression

Headaches and anorexia

Paresthesias, muscle twitching, pruritus

Weight loss

Bone pain with ambulation, neuropathies

Assessment—objective

Skin changes—sallow, brownish, pale, dry

Evidence of petechiae, bruising

Edema

Hypertension, signs of CHF

Intake and output—oliguria or anuria

TABLE 13-3 Summary of organ system involvement in patients with chronic renal failure

System	Manifestation	Cause
Integumentary		
Skin	Pallor	Anemia
	Gray/bronze pigmentation	Pigment retained
	Dry and scaly	Decreased size of sweat glands
		Decreased activity of oil glands
	Pruritus	Dry skin; phosphate deposits
Nails	Thin, brittle	Protein wasting
Hair	Dry	Decreased activity of oil glands
	Brittle	Protein wasting
Gastrointestinal		
Oral cavity	Halitosis (fetor uremicus)	Urea converted to ammonia by saline
	Bleeding of gums	Change in platelet activity
Stomach	Nausea, vomiting, anorexia	Serum uremic toxins
	Gastritis, ulceration	Serum uremic toxins
Lower bowel	Constipation	Aluminum hydroxide given as phosphate binders
Cardiovascular	Hypertension	Fluid overload
		Renin-angiotensin mechanism
	Congestive heart failure	Fluid overload, anemia
	Arteriosclerotic heart disease	Chronic hypertension
	Pericarditis	Calcification of soft tissues
		Uremic toxins in pericardial fluid
		Fibrin formation on epicardium
Pulmonary	Uremic "lung" or pneumonitis	Uremic toxins in pleural space and lung tissue
Neurologic	Fatigue, headache, sleep disturbance	Uremic toxins
	Muscle irritability	Electrolyte imbalances
	Seizures	Cerebral swelling resulting from fluid shifting
Hematologic	Anemia	Suppression of RBC production
		Decreased survival time of RBCs
		Loss of blood through bleeding
		Loss of blood during dialysis
	Bleeding	Mild thrombocytopenia
		Decreased activity of platelets
Metabolic	Carbohydrate intolerance	Decreased sensitivity to insulin in peripheral tissues
		Delayed production of insulin by pancreas
		Increased survival time of insulin
	Hyperlipidemia	Increased production of serum triglycerides
		Increased output of glycerides by liver as a result of elevated insulin levels
Endocrine	Hyperparathyroidism	Elevated serum phosphate results in decreased serum calcium which stimulates parathyroid
	Infertility	Mechanism unknown
	Sexual dysfunction	Mechanism unknown

From Long, B.C., and Phipps, W.J.: Essentials of medical-surgical nursing: a nursing process approach, St. Louis, 1985, The C.V. Mosby Co.

Dry hair and nails
Evidence of calcium deposits in skin
Ammonia odor to breath
Laboratory reports showing hyperkalemia and elevated BUN, creatinine and phosphate levels; metabolic acidosis, anemia

Nursing diagnoses
Diagnoses will depend on the degree of disease and the effectiveness of treatment control, but commonly include:

Activity intolerance related to generalized weakness
Alteration in comfort—bone pain, pruritus, or nausea

related to excess metabolic waste products and disordered metabolism

Actual or potential fluid volume excess related to the failure of renal regulatory mechanisms

Potential for ineffective individual or family coping related to life-style restrictions and dependence on dialysis for sustaining life

Knowledge deficit related to the treatment protocol necessary to sustain healthy functioning

Alteration in nutrition, potential for less than body requirements, related to multiple restrictions, anorexia, and nausea

Powerlessness related to the demands of the dialysis regimen

Disturbance in self-concept (body image, role performance) related to change in body and life-style associated with dependence on a machine

Expected outcomes

Patient's energy level will improve to the point where patient can complete normal daily activities without undue fatigue.

Patient will have less pruritus, anorexia, and nausea as condition stabilizes with dialysis. Patient's pain will not interfere with normal activities.

Patient will maintain an acceptable fluid and electrolyte balance on dialysis.

Patient and family will make adequate adjustments to the life-style changes caused by dialysis.

Patient will be knowledgeable about all aspects of treatment protocol: medications, diet, dialysis.

Patient will plan and consume a daily food intake that meets the body's nutritional needs and stays within prescribed restrictions.

Patient will maintain a sense of control over his or her life and participate in all care decisions.

Patient will adjust to body changes triggered by renal failure and maintain a positive self-concept.

Nursing interventions

Fluid and electrolytes

Maintain accurate intake and output records.

Weigh patient daily.

Restrict fluids as prescribed.

Plan with patient to distribute fluids effectively throughout the day.

Teach patient principles of sodium-restricted diet.

Encourage patient to read product labels carefully.

Monitor patient for edema; assess thirst.

Teach patient importance of restricting potassium in diet.

Explain which foods are high in potassium.

ALERT: Caution patient that most salt substitutes are high in potassium and should not be used.

Teach patient to avoid trauma and infection as tissue breakdown liberates potassium.

Administer aluminum hydroxide to bind excess phosphorus.

Administer vitamin D and calcium as prescribed to combat bone demineralization.

Azotemia and acidosis

Teach patient dietary protein restrictions as prescribed.

Ensure use of high-biologic value protein.

Restriction usually is not below 40 g daily.

Ensure adequate intake of carbohydrates and fats for energy.

Ensure adequate pulmonary function to assist in excretion of pCO_2.

Assess patient for changes in level of consciousness.

Ensure environmental safety.

TABLE 13-4 Indications and nursing interventions associated with vascular access for hemodialysis

Type	Indication for Use	Advantages	Nursing Interventions
External shunt	Long-term access Access within hours needed	Ease of access Can be used immediately	Do not place IVs or take blood pressure on affected arm. Assess for bleeding from insertion sites. Assess patency by observing continuous blood flow through shunt. Listen for bruit. Assess for infection; change dressing frequently, using institution's protocol. Keep clamps at bedside.
Arteriovenous fistula/graft	Permanent access needed	Easy access once graft has matured Least likely to develop infection	Assess for patency by palpating for thrill or auscultating bruit. Teach patient to avoid compression through tight clothing or positioning with arm bent. Teach patient to assess site for signs of infection. Do not place IVs or take blood pressure on affected arm.

Activity

Help patient plan and space activities to conserve energy.
  Plan for adequate rest.
  Assist patient with activities of daily living as needed.
  Assess patient for dyspnea and tachycardia, peripheral
    perfusion.
  Provide adequate warmth.

Comfort

Institute measures to control pruritus.
Teach patient importance of maintaining skin in-
  tegrity.
Attempt to relieve muscle cramps with use of heat and
  massage.
Provide frequent oral hygiene.
Make meals and environment as pleasant as possible.

Coping

Encourage patient to verbalize feelings about restrictions and treatment regimen.
Help patient maintain open communication with
  family.
Help patient explore financial and social resources in
  community.
Support all positive coping strategies employed by patient and family.
Support maintenance of family structure and desired
  roles.
Provide patient with opportunities to discuss issues
  involving sexuality and reproduction.
  Provide patient with accurate information.
Encourage patient to maintain hope and positive feelings about dialysis.

Dialysis

Assess for patency of vascular access (see Table 13-4
  and Figure 13-2).
Teach patient about peritoneal dialysis or hemodialysis
  if in use.

Evaluation

Patient has sufficient energy to participate in normal
  activities of daily living, hemoglobin and hematocrit
  levels are stable.
Anorexia, nausea, and pruritus are absent or controlled; skin is intact.
Patient's fluid and electrolyte balance is stabilized;
  there are no signs of peripheral edema; blood pressure is controlled.
Patient expresses positive attitude toward integrating
  successful dialysis regimen into life-style.
Patient can knowledgeably discuss treatment protocol
  and takes medications on schedule.
Patient plans and eats a diet that meets baseline nutritional needs and follows prescribed restrictions;
  positive nitrogen balance is maintained.
Patient acts as informed decision maker in all aspects
  of care planning and is consulted about proposed
  changes in treatment regimen.
Patient adjusts body image realistically but continues
  to refer to self in a positive way.

DIALYSIS

Dialysis involves the movement of fluid and particles
across a semipermeable membrane. It can help restore
normal fluid and electrolyte balance, control acid-base

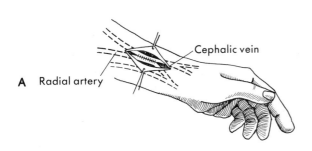

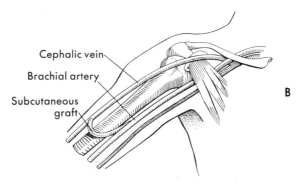

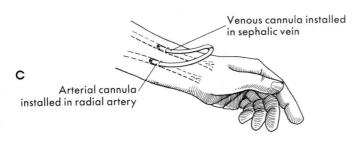

FIGURE 13-2 Frequently used means for gaining vascular
access for hemodialysis. **A,** Arteriovenous fistula. **B,** Arteriovenous graft. **C,** External arteriovenous shunt. (From Long,
B.C., and Phipps, W.J.: Essentials of medical-surgical nursing: a nursing process approach, St. Louis, 1985, The C.V.
Mosby Co.)

balance, and remove waste and toxic material from the body. It is used temporarily in acute failure and as a permanent substitute for the loss of renal function in patients with chronic end-stage disease. There are two main types: hemodialysis and peritoneal dialysis.

Hemodialysis

Shunts the patient's blood from the body through a dialyzer in which diffusion and ultrafiltration occur. He-

---

NURSING INTERVENTIONS FOR PATIENTS RECEIVING PERITONEAL DIALYSIS

PREDIALYSIS:

Take baseline weight and vital signs.
Have patient empty bladder before catheter insertion.
Provide meticulous skin and catheter prep per institution's protocol before connecting dialysis fluid line.

DURING DIALYSIS:

To initiate each cycle:
    Run prescribed amount of solution (usually 2 liters) into peritoneal cavity over about 10 minutes.
    Clamp tubing for prescribed time (usually 20 to 30 minutes).
    Drain cavity by gravity (usually takes 20 minutes).
Repeat procedure with fresh dialysate solution as many times as prescribed.
    Make sure solution is at body temperature.
    Maintain sterility during bottle changes.
Monitor patient continuously for:
    Changes in vital signs indicating hypotension or hypovolemia
    Pain
    Respiratory distress
    Signs of peritonitis
Maintain accurate intake and output records.
    Record amount of fluid instilled.
    Record amount of fluid drained.
    Note net gains or losses of fluid.
Discontinue dialysis following institution's protocol, keeping strict asepsis.

---

modialysis requires access to the patient's blood. The primary methods of vascular access include:

The external cannula or shunt, in which a Silastic cannula is implanted into an artery and adjacent vein in the forearm or elsewhere; the two ends are connected by a U shaped external connector. (See Figure 13-2.)

The internal arteriovenous fistula, in which a subcutaneous anastomosis is made between an artery and a vein. Fistulas may also be created using bovine or synthetic grafts.

The major nursing responsibilities for nondialysis nurses include:

Protecting the vascular access site (see Table 13-4)

Teaching the patient and family ways to manage the disease effectively

Assisting the patient to plan a work and activity schedule that is minimally disrupted by dialysis routine

Peritoneal Dialysis

The dialyzing fluid is instilled into the peritoneal cavity and the peritoneum becomes the dialyzing membrane. It may take up to 36 hours to complete the treatment. Dialysis may be done intermittently or on a continuous daily ambulatory basis with the insertion of a permanent peritoneal catheter. Nursing interventions are summarized in the box on this page.

RENAL TRANSPLANTATION

Kidney transplant offers the possibility of an improved quality of life without dialysis to patients with chronic renal failure. Problems of tissue rejection are serious; success rates 1 year after transplant stand at 50% when cadaver kidneys are used and 65% to 70% with sibling or parent donors. The associated nursing care is similar to that for other renal surgery with additional teaching and support concerning the surgery, treatment, and the uncertainty of outcomes. The box below describes types of rejection and their major symptoms.

KIDNEY TRANSPLANT REJECTION

TYPES:

Acute rejection—usually occurs 4 days to 4 months after transplant. May be successfully treated with immunosuppressive drugs.

Chronic rejection—usually occurs over months or years and is associated with gradual occlusion of renal blood vessels. There is no definitive treatment.

SIGNS AND SYMPTOMS

Decreasing urine output
Fever
Pain or tenderness over transplant site
Elevated serum creatinine and BUN levels
Edema, sudden weight gain
Hypertension
Developing hypertension
Proteinuria
Slowly rising creatinine and BUN levels
Malaise
Gradually deteriorating condition

BIBLIOGRAPHY

Cianci, J., *et al.*: Renal transplantation, Am. J. Nurs. 81:354-355, 1981.

Goldberger, E.: A primer of water electrolyte and acid-base syndromes, ed. 6, Philadelphia, 1980, Lea and Febiger.

Irwin, B.: Now—peritoneal dialysis for chronic patients too, RN 44:49-52, 98, 1981.

Leaf, A., and Cotran, R.: Renal pathophysiology, Cambridge, 1980, Oxford University Press.

Randolph, G.: Bringing them back out of renal shutdown, RN 44:34-39, 108-112, 1981.

Schrier, R.: Renal and electrolyte disorders, Boston, 1980, Little, Brown Co.

Sophie, L.R.: Meeting the immunologic challenge of transplant nursing, Heart and Lung 9:690-694, 1980.

Stark, J.: Acute renal failure, Nurs. 82 12:26-33, 1982.

Underwood, M.A.: Urinary tract infections, Crit. Care Q. 3:63-70, 1980.

NURSING CARE PLAN

ACUTE RENAL FAILURE

Nursing Diagnoses	Expected Patient Outcomes	Nursing Interventions
Alteration in patterns of urinary elimination related to falling urine production	Patient returns to a normal urinary elimination pattern without need for dialysis	1. Measure output carefully. Check urine pH. 2. Teach patient about dialysis procedures. 3. Assess vascular access sites during each shift. Protect from stress—no BP or blood drawing.
Alteration in fluid volume—excess or deficit related to failure of renal regulatory mechanism	Patient's fluid and electrolyte values are within normal limits Patient maintains a stable weight	1. Maintain IV at prescribed rate; restrict fluids as prescribed. 2. Keep accurate intake and output records. Weigh patient daily. 3. Monitor vital signs (including postural signs) frequently. 4. Assess neck veins, skin turgor, and mucous membrane; note peripheral edema. 5. Monitor for and report signs of hyperkalemia, hyponatremia or acidosis during oliguric phase. 6. Administer prescribed medications.
Potential impairment of skin integrity related to decreased mobility and tissue edema	Patient maintains an intact skin	1. Assess skin each shift. 2. Keep skin clean and dry. 3. Put pressure devices on bed—special attention to heels and sacrum. 4. Turn every two hours. 5. Avoid shearing force when moving patient.
Alteration in nutrition—less than body requirements; related to anorexia and multiple restrictions	Patient's diet conforms to needed restrictions and meets body needs for nutrients	1. Assess nutrient intake. 2. Give good mouth care prior to oral feedings. 3. Encourage eating of prescribed diet. 4. Restrict protein content as prescribed—ensure high biologic value.
Alteration in comfort related to nausea, thirst, or pain	Patient's thirst and nausea decrease	1. Use measures to decrease nausea (e.g., antiemetics, deep breathing). 2. Give mouth care. 3. Provide patient with a moist cloth to keep lips moist. Offer ice chips if allowed. 4. Plan with patient to distribute allowed fluid intake effectively throughout the day. 5. Bathe patient frequently, using bland soap and tepid water. 6. Give prescribed antipruritics as needed.
Alteration in thought processes related to the accumulation of waste products	Patient is fully oriented and able to problem solve effectively	1. Assess mental status for changes (confusion, somnolence). 2. Orient to person, place, and time as necessary. 3. Provide simple explanations and repeat instructions as necessary. 4. Ensure a safe environment. Keep siderails up and supervise ambulation. 5. Reassure patient that mental capacities will return with recovery. 6. Explain reasons for behavior to family and friends.
Activity intolerance related to fatigue of waste product accumulation	Patient gradually resumes independence in the activities of daily living	1. Promote maximal rest to lower metabolic load. 2. Assist with ADL as needed. 3. Employ active nursing measures to prevent complications of immobility. 4. Encourage ambulation as condition stabilizes. 5. Avoid exposing patient to persons with infections.

Knowledge deficit related to treatment and progression of disease process	Patient understands nature of disorder and therapeutic regimen	1. Teach patient:
		  a. Basis of symptoms and therapy.
		  b. Avoidance of preventable factors, if appropriate.
		  c. Prescribed medications and dietary regimens.
		  d. Signs of returning renal problems or infections.
		  e. Need for follow-up care.

CHAPTER 14

Disorders of the Reproductive System

Human sexuality is a complex biologic and psychologic phenomenon that is strongly influenced by society and culture. Disorders affecting sexuality and the reproductive system have a strong impact on an individual's self-concept and role performance. A wide variety of neurologic, cardiovascular, and metabolic disorders affect the patient's sexuality and require the nurse to be sensitive and alert to these problems. This chapter deals with specific major disorders in structure and function directly affecting the reproductive system.

FEMALE REPRODUCTIVE SYSTEM

The most common problems of the female reproductive system are problems of menstruation and menopause, contraception, and vaginal infection. With the exception of pelvic inflammatory disease, these disorders are usually treated on an outpatient basis. Nursing interventions involve careful teaching of patients to prevent recurrence where possible. Table 14-1 lists commonly encountered vaginal infections and their treatment. Sexually transmitted diseases are presented later in the chapter. Figure 14-1 shows the female internal organs of reproduction.

DISORDERS OF THE CERVIX AND UTERUS

The most common problems involving the cervix and uterus include structural problems, benign tumors, and cancer. Table 14-2 describes common structural problems and their treatment. Table 14-3 describes common benign tumors other than fibroid tumors, which are discussed below.

FIBROID TUMORS (MYOMAS)

Fibroid tumors are quite common. It is estimated that 20% to 25% of women over 30 years of age develop my-

omas. Their growth is stimulated by hormones so they tend to disappear at menopause.

Pathophysiology

The cause of myomas is unknown. They vary significantly in size and may affect the body of the uterus, cervix, or broad ligament. Larger tumors may cause uterine enlargement or impinge on the blood supply, but they rarely become malignant.

Medical Management

Treatment depends on the severity of symptoms and the age of the patient. Women nearing menopause who have completed their families are frequently treated by hysterectomy.

Nursing Management
Assessment
Subjective
   History of the condition
   Presenting symptoms and severity: menorrhagia or pain
   Feelings about hysterectomy
   Knowledge of procedure and its effects
   Constipation
   Menstrual history
Objective (Post-op)
   Vital signs
   Urinary output
   Vaginal bleeding
   Peripheral circulation

Nursing diagnoses
Diagnoses depend on the surgical approach used and the patient's response to surgery, but commonly include:
   Alteration in comfort—pain related to surgical incision and gaseous distention

TABLE 14-1 Common infections of the female reproductive system

Condition	Symptoms	Medical Management
Candidiasis	Vaginal itching and irritation Thick, white, cheesy discharge Frequent recurrence	Nystatin (Mycostatin) vaginal suppositories Miconazole (Monistat) vaginal cream
Trichomoniasis	Vulvar itching, burning, excoriation Yellowish to greenish discharge that is thick, foamy, and malodorous	Metronidazole (Flagyl) orally Floraquin vaginal tablets preceded by white vinegar douching
Simple vaginitis	Vulvar irritation Yellowish mucoid discharge	Appropriate antibiotic applied locally or taken systemically
Bartholinitis	Erythema around Bartholin's gland Swelling, edema, and pain	Appropriate antibiotics Surgical drainage or gland excision
Pelvic inflammatory disease (PID)	Ascending infection, which may affect ovaries, fallopian tubes, and other pelvic tissue. Symptoms include: Acute lower abdominal pain Fever and chills Purulent discharge Malaise, nausea, and vomiting	Appropriate antibiotics orally or IV Bed rest for acute cases Analgesics and local comfort measures as needed

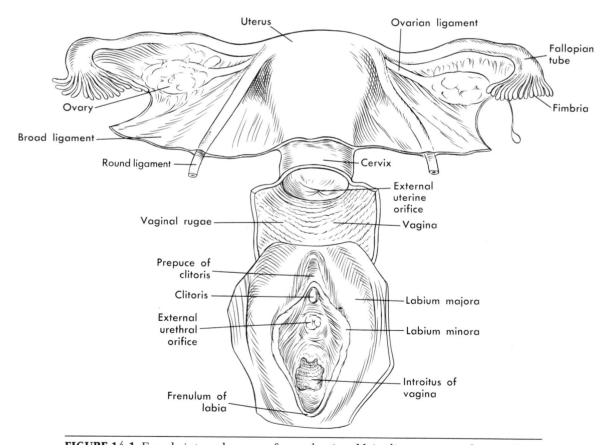

FIGURE 14-1 Female internal organs of reproduction. Major ligaments are shown. (From Long, B.C., and Phipps, W.J.: Essentials of medical-surgical nursing: a nursing process approach, St. Louis, 1985, The C.V. Mosby Co.)

TABLE 14-2 Structural problems of the female reproductive tract

Disorder	Signs and Symptoms	Medical Management
Uterine displacement or prolapse	Dysmenorrhea Chronic backache, pelvic pressure	Minor displacement may be treated with pelvic exercises Prolapse is treated by hysterectomy
Cystocele (weakening of anterior wall causes bladder to herniate into vagina)	Dragging pain in back and pelvis, worsened by prolonged standing or walking Stress incontinence	Surgical repair through tightening of the vaginal wall (anterior colporrhaphy)
Rectocele (weakening of the posterior wall causes rectum to herniate into vagina)	Dragging pain in back and pelvis, worsened by prolonged standing or walking Constipation and hemorrhoids	Surgical repair through tightening of the vaginal wall (posterior colporrhaphy)

TABLE 14-3 Benign tumors of the female reproductive tract

Disorder	Signs and Symptoms	Medical Management

Ovarian tumors and cysts (numerous varieties develop)	Early stages:
	  Asymptomatic or nonspecific
	Later stages:
	  Increasing abdominal size
	  Pelvic fullness or pressure
	  Menstrual irregularities
	  Pain if cyst twists
		Surgical removal, usually involving oopherectomy

Endometriosis (seeding of endometrial cells throughout the pelvis)	Pain and discomfort with menstruation Fullness in abdomen Menstrual irregularities Infertility	Oral contraceptives to produce endometrial atrophy In advanced cases with widespread adhesions, surgery may be necessary—hysterectomy, oopherectomy, or salpingectomy
Cervical polyps (proliferation of an area of cervical mucosa)	Small episodes of bleeding between menstrual cycles Contact bleeding with intercourse or examination	Removal of the polyp with biopsy forceps or sharp curette

Potential for ineffective individual coping related to the situational crisis of abrupt loss of childbearing potential

Potential alteration in peripheral tissue perfusion related to pelvic vessel congestion or thrombophlebitis

Expected outcomes

Patient will experience decreasing discomfort and resume normal activity.

Patient will make a positive adjustment to the loss of reproductive function and maintain a positive self-concept.

Patient will maintain adequate venous return and be free of phlebitis or thrombosis.

Nursing interventions

Preoperative

Teach patient about planned procedure.

Explain importance of early ambulation and leg exercises to prevent complications.

Perform douche or enema as ordered.

Postoperative

Maintain use of thigh-high TED stockings.

Encourage patient to ambulate and do leg exercises.
  Assess for Homans' sign.

Maintain patency of urinary catheter if used.
  Ensure adequacy of output after removal.
  Keep accurate intake and output records.
  Provide regular perineal care.
  Catheterize for residual if ordered.

Assess incision frequently if abdominal approach used.

Maintain perineal pad count.
  Assess for excess bleeding.

Auscultate abdomen for return of active peristalsis.
  Restrict food and fluid until patient passes flatus.
  Offer rectal tube for excess flatus if ordered.

Encourage patient to verbalize feelings and concerns.
  Offer support if depression occurs.

Teach patient before discharge.
  Patient should avoid driving for first weeks.
  Patient should avoid lifting or straining.

TABLE 14-4 Cancers of the female reproductive tract

Site	Incidence Rate (%)	Usual Age of Onset (yrs)	Signs and Symptoms	Medical Management
Cervix	4	30–50	Early stage: usually asymptomatic Later stages: foul vaginal drainage; spotting; pain	Conization of cervix for carcinoma in situ (considered 100% curable in early stages); hysterectomy, radiation for more advanced disease
Uterus	9	50–65	Early stage: postmenopausal bleeding Later stages: pain, uterine enlargement	Hysterectomy with salpingectomy and oophorectomy, supplemented by radiation and chemotherapy
Ovary	4	All ages	Early stage: asymptomatic Later stages: ascites, edema of legs, pain	Salpingectomy and oophorectomy, supplemented by chemotherapy and radiation Prognosis is generally poor

Patient can resume sexual intercourse after 4 to 6 weeks.

Vaginal sensation may be decreased initially.

Ensure that patient understands changes that will occur from onset of menopause.

Explain precaution for estrogen replacement if ordered.

Evaluation

Patient is free of discomfort and gradually resumes all preoperative activities.

Patient integrates body changes into self-concept and resumes preoperative familial and sexual roles.

Patient experiences no complications in the postoperative period.

CANCER OF THE REPRODUCTIVE TRACT

Cancer involving the reproductive tract may affect the cervix, uterus, or ovaries and is a significant cause of death. Table 14-4 outlines the symptoms and treatment of each major form of cancer. Nursing care for the hysterectomy patient was discussed in the preceding section. Patients who undergo salpingectomy and oophorectomy are treated like patients who have had other forms of abdominal surgery (see Chapter 2 for care of the patient receiving internal or external radiation or chemotherapy).

BREAST DISORDERS

Breast disorders, both benign and malignant, are significant health problems for women.

BENIGN DISORDERS

Fibrocystic disease causes thickened nodules, often bilateral, that become painful before or during menstruation and are believed to be related to cyclic hormonal imbalance. One distressing factor about fibrocystic disease is that it makes malignancies much more difficult to detect.

Fibroadenomas are tumors thought to result from hy-

RISK FACTORS ASSOCIATED WITH BREAST CANCER

Menarche before age 11
Menopause after age 50
Family history of breast cancer—especially mother or sister
Nulliparity or birth of first child after age 30
History of uterine cancer
Link with obesity, diabetes, and hypertension
Presence of benign breast disease

perestrinism (excess estrogen). The tumor is usually removed locally and carefully analyzed for malignant cells.

MALIGNANT DISORDERS

Breast cancers are the most common malignancies in women and the major cause of cancer deaths for women. The cause is not known although some risk factors have been identified and are listed in the box above. The incidence increases with age.

Pathophysiology

Breast cancer is not one disease but many, depending on the type of tissue involved, age of the patient at onset, and the degree of estrogen dependency of the tumor. Prognosis depends on the extent of disease present at the time of diagnosis. Classic symptoms that define breast cancers include:

Firm, nontender, nonmobile masses
Solitary, irregularly shaped mass
Adherence to muscle or skin causing dimpling effect
Involvement of upper outer quadrant or central nipple portion of breast

Medical Management

A variety of treatment plans are available, and controversy persists over the use of the various protocols. Surgery, radiation, and chemotherapy are the cornerstones of care. Surgical approaches may vary from lumpectomy, through partial or simple mastectomy, to modified radical mastectomy. Later breast reconstruction is an option being offered to increasing numbers of women.

Nursing Management

Assessment—subjective
Presence of risk factors
Breast self-examination routine
Symptoms and time period since discovery
Knowledge of treatment options
Patient's procurement of a second opinion
Knowledge of treatment protocol planned
Support systems and their adequacy and response
Usual coping patterns
Current state of anxiety
Feelings about surgery and future
Attitudes and knowledge of husband or partner

Assessment—objective
General health status
Presence of breast mass confirmed by mammography
   or biopsy

Nursing diagnoses
Diagnoses will depend on the extent of surgery and the woman's response, but commonly include:

Anxiety related to uncertainty of diagnosis or decisions
   about treatment protocol
Potential for ineffective individual or family coping related to body changes and perceived loss of attrac-
   tiveness
Alteration in self-concept (body image) related to mu-
   tilating aspects of the surgical procedure
Knowledge deficit related to postoperative rehabilitation and support groups
Alteration in comfort—pain related to surgical incision
   and alteration in chest wall musculature

Expected outcomes
Patient's anxiety will be reduced to a level where informed decision making and ongoing self-care are
   possible.
Patient and family will verbalize their feelings concerning the diagnosis and treatment, providing mutual support.
Patient will gradually integrate body changes into an
   altered but positive self-concept.
Patient will be knowledgeable concerning the exercises and self-care practices that will facilitate rehabilitation.
Patient will experience decreasing levels of discomfort
   and maintain full use of affected arm and shoulder.

POSTMASTECTOMY ARM EXERCISES*

EXERCISE: CLIMBING THE WALL
1. Stand facing wall with toes close to wall.
2. Bend elbows and place palms of hands against wall at
   shoulder level.
3. Move both hands parallel to each other up the wall as
   far as possible until incisional pull or pain occurs.
4. Move both hands down to starting position.
5. Goal is complete extension with elbow straight.
6. Activities that utilize the same action, reaching top
   shelves, hanging out clothes, washing windows, hanging curtains, setting hair.

EXERCISE: ARM SWINGING
1. Bend forward from waist, permitting both arms to relax
   and hang naturally.
2. Swing arms together left to right (motion comes from
   shoulder).
3. Swing arms in circles parallel to floor, clockwise and
   counterclockwise.
4. Stand up slowly.

EXERCISE: ROPE PULL
1. Attach a rope over a shower rod or hook.
2. Grasp each end of rope, alternately pulling on each
   end, raising affected arm to a point of incisional pull or
   pain.
3. Shorten rope over time until affected arm is raised almost directly overhead.

EXERCISE: ELBOW SPREAD
1. Clasp hands behind neck.
2. Raise elbows to chin level, holding head erect. Move
   slowly and rest when incisional pull or pain occur.
3. Gradually spread elbows apart. Rest when pull or pain
   occur.

*From American Cancer Society: Reach to recovery, New York, The Society.

Nursing interventions
Preoperative
Assist patient to verbalize feelings about meaning of
   impending surgery.
   Include husband and family as appropriate.
Encourage family to express fears and love to patient.
Support patient in whatever decisions she makes about
   treatment protocol.
Provide simple explanations of impending surgery and
   expected postoperative care.
   Explain use of Hemovac if planned.
   Teach exercises that will be used postoperatively.
Evaluate suitability of preoperative visit by Reach to
   Recovery volunteer.

Postoperative
Place patient in semi-Fowler's position, with arm el-
   evated on pillows.
Monitor Hemovac output.

BREAST SELF-EXAMINATION (BSE)

Perform BSE regularly each month.
   Premenopausal women: shortly after conclusion of the
      menstrual period
   Postmenopausal women: at a set time each month
      (such as the first day of the month)
Use a systematic approach (*one* of the three listed below)
   Palpate in concentric circles, beginning at outer rim of
      breast tissue and moving toward nipple.
   Divide breast into quadrants and examine area in each
      quadrant from outer perimeter toward nipple.
   Palpate inner half then outer half of breast.
Examine the entire breast tissue, including the tail and
   the nipple.
Carry out examination in both the horizontal and vertical
   body positions.
Use the flat parts of the fingers for palpation.

From Long, B.C., and Phipps, W.J.: Essentials of medical-surgical
nursing: a nursing process, St. Louis, 1985, The C.V. Mosby Co.

Check behind patient for bleeding.
Post signs warning against taking blood pressure,
   starting IVs, or drawing blood on affected side.
Initiate exercises to prevent stiffness and contracture
   of shoulder girdle.
   Immediate:
      Flex and extend fingers.
      Pronate and supinate forearm.
   Day 1 post-op:
      Squeeze rubber ball as tolerated.
      Brush teeth and hair.
Teach special mastectomy exercises as prescribed (see
   box on p. 193).
Provide adequate analgesia to promote ambulation and
   exercise.
Encourage regular coughing and deep breathing ex-
   ercises.
Continue to assist patient to explore and verbalize her
   feelings and grief.
Prepare patient for size and appearance of the incision
   and provide support when incision is viewed for first
   time.
Help family provide patient with appropriate love and
   support.
Arrange visit by Reach to Recovery volunteer.
Provide patient with detailed information concerning
   breast prostheses.
   Fitting is not possible for 4 to 6 weeks.
   A temporary prosthesis or lightly padded bra is worn
      until healing is complete.
Teach patient to avoid constrictive clothing and report
   persistent edema, redness, or infection of incision.
Teach patient importance of continuing monthly

breast examination on remaining breast (see box on
   p. 194).
Refer to Chapter 2 for appropriate interventions related
   to chemotherapy or radiation therapy.

Evaluation

Patient's anxiety is controlled; patient participates in
   decision making and acquires self-care skills.
Patient and family verbalize feelings with each other
   and provide mutual support.
Patient integrates mastectomy into self-concept,
   speaks positively of self, and resumes normal social
   and sexual activity.
Patient practices postmastectomy exercises and maintains full range of motion and strength on affected
   side.
Patient is free of discomfort and edema.

MALE REPRODUCTIVE SYSTEM

Disorders of the male reproductive system may affect any
structure, but by far the most common site is the prostate
gland. Prostatic enlargement affects 50% of men over 50
years of age and 75% of those over 70. Figure 14-2 shows
the male organs of reproduction.

BENIGN PROSTATIC HYPERTROPHY
Pathophysiology

Benign prostatic hypertrophy (BPH) appears to be related
to a hormone imbalance that occurs with aging. There
is overgrowth of smooth muscle and connective tissue
and an increase in glandular tissue. The enlargement
produces compression of the urethra and progressive urinary obstruction.

Medical Management

The initial treatment for BPH is frequently the relief of
urinary obstruction and retention by catheterization. The
actual problem is treated surgically. A variety of surgeries
are utilized, with transurethral resection (TUR) being the
most common. Table 14-5 describes procedures used for
prostate problems.

Nursing Management
   Assessment—subjective
   History of the disorder and symptoms
   Patient's knowledge of cause and proposed treatment
   Patient's feelings about proposed surgery
      Impact on sexuality and self-concept
   Patient's complaints of:
      Urinary frequency, nocturia
      Difficulty starting urinary stream
      Decrease in size or force of stream
      Symptoms of cystitis

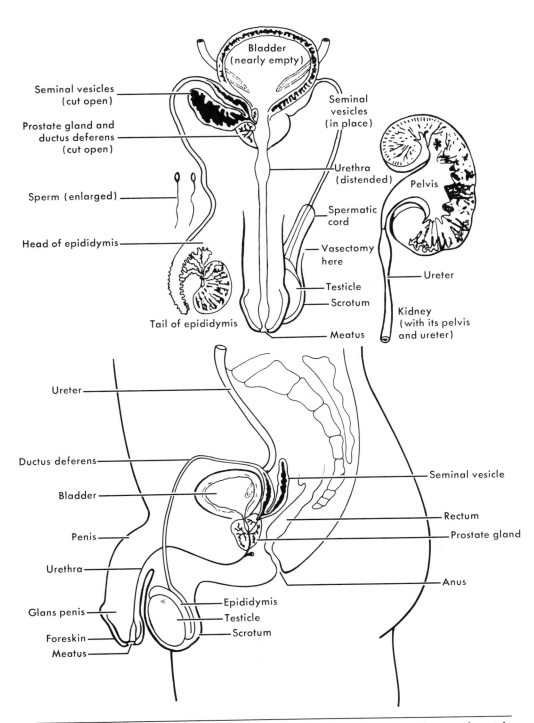

FIGURE 14-2 Male organs of reproduction. Note relatively large size of seminal vesicle as compared with testicle. (From Long, B.C., and Phipps, W.J.: Essentials of medical-surgical nursing: a nursing process approach, St. Louis, 1985, The C.V. Mosby Co.)

Assessment—objective

Hematuria

Acute urinary retention

Evidence of prostatic enlargement with digital examination or cystoscopy

Nursing diagnoses

Alteration in pattern of urinary elimination related to obstruction of urine outflow

Knowledge deficit related to the functions of the prostate gland and its role in sexual performance

TABLE 14-5 Comparison of types of prostatic surgery

	Transurethral Resection	Suprapubic Resection	Retropubic Resection	Perineal Resection	Radical Perineal Resection
Reason for surgery	Enlargement of medial lobe surrounding urethra	Extremely large mass of obstructing tissue	Large mass located high in pelvic area	Large mass located low in pelvic area	Cancer of prostate gland
Location of incision	No incision; removal by way of urethra	Low midline abdominal incision through bladder to prostate gland	Low midline incision into prostate gland (bladder not incised)	Incision between scrotum and rectum	Large perineal incision between scrotum and rectum
Drainage tubes	Three-way Foley catheter with 30 ml bag in urethra, constant irrigation for 24 hr	Cystotomy tube or drain through incision; Foley catheter with 30 ml bag in urethra	Foley catheter with 30 ml bag in urethra, constant irrigation for 24 hr	Foley catheter with 30 ml bag in urethra	Foley catheter with 30 ml bag in urethra; drain in incision
Bladder spasms	Yes	Yes	Few	Few	Few
Dressing	No dressing	Abdominal dressing; easily soaked with urinary drainage	Abdominal dressing; no urinary drainage	Perineal dressing; no urinary drainage	Perineal dressing; urinary drainage
Complications	Hemorrhage; water intoxication; incontinence	Hemorrhage; wound infection	Hemorrhage; wound infection	Hemorrhage; wound infection	Urinary incontinence; wound infection; impotence; sterility

From Phipps, W.J., Long, B.C., and Woods, N.F.: Medical-surgical nursing: concepts and clinical practice, ed. 2, St. Louis, 1983, The C.V. Mosby Co.

Potential for sexual dysfunction related to the perceived effects of prostatectomy on sexual potency

Expected outcomes
Patient will gradually return to a normal continent pattern of urinary elimination.
Patient will be knowledgeable about the role of the prostate gland and the impact of prostatectomy.
Patient will return to his preillness pattern of sexual activity and satisfaction.

Nursing interventions (for TUR procedure)
Preoperative
Ensure patency of urinary drainage.
Monitor intake and output.
Teach patient about procedure and expected care routines after surgery.
Encourage patient to express concerns about surgery and its impact on sexuality.
Reassure patient that procedures other than radical prostatectomy do not affect sexual potency.
Postoperative
Maintain patency of continuous bladder irrigation if utilized.
Solution should run rapidly enough to maintain urinary drainage of light pink-red color.

Monitor carefully for clot formation.
Maintain accurate intake and output records.
Maintain traction on catheter as prescribed.
Monitor vital signs frequently.
Teach patient that 30 ml catheter balloon triggers constant urge to void and bladder spasms.
Sensations decrease after 24 to 48 hours.
Administer analgesics and antispasmodics as prescribed.
Manually irrigate catheter if prescribed.
Encourage liberal fluid intake by mouth unless contraindicated.
Avoid use of rectal thermometer or tube, enemas.
Provide or teach patient scrupulous catheter care.
Monitor carefully for signs of infection.
Instruct patient not to attempt to void around catheter.
Assess for adequacy of voiding and bladder emptying when catheter is removed.
Teach patient perineal exercises to aid in full return of urinary control.
Dribbling is a common problem.
Teach patient about postdischarge care.
Patient should refrain from lifting, vigorous exercise, driving, and sexual activity for 3 to 6 weeks.
Patient should use stool softener to avoid straining.
Patient should keep fluid intake high.

TABLE 14-6 Inflammatory disorders of the male reproductive tract

Disorder	Signs and Symptoms	Medical Management
Urethritis	Urgency, frequency, and burning with urination Purulent urethral discharge	Appropriate antibiotics
Prostatitis	Perineal pain, fever, dysuria Urethral discharge	Appropriate antibiotics Rest, hydration, sitz baths, stool softeners
Epididymitis	Sudden scrotal pain and edema	Appropriate antibiotics Bed rest with scrotal elevation Analgesics
Orchitis	Same as for epididymitis Nausea and vomiting Pain radiating to inguinal canal	Same as for epididymitis

TABLE 14-7 Structural disorders of the testes and scrotum

Disorder	Description	Medical Management
Hydrocele	Benign, nontender collection of clear amber fluid within the outer covering of the testes; leads to scrotal swelling	Aspiration of the fluid
Spermatocele	Benign, nontender cystic mass attached to epididymis; contains milky fluid and sperm	Usually no treatment is needed—aspiration or excision
Varicocele	Dilation of spermatic vein, usually on the left side	Ligation of the vein
Torsion of spermatic cord	Kinking and twisting of spermatic cord and artery	Surgical fixation of testes to scrotal wall; excision of testes if gangrenous Spermatogenesis is usually destroyed although hormone production may continue

TABLE 14-8 Cancer of the testes and penis

Site	Incidence Rate (%)	Usual Age of Onset (yrs)	Signs and Symptoms	Medical Management
Testes	0.5	18–35	Painless enlarged testis Gynecomastia (breast development)	Surgery, orchiectomy, plus radiation and chemotherapy
Penis	1	50–70	Nodular growth on foreskin Fatigue, weight loss	Surgery—partial or total penectomy followed by plastic repair if feasible

Patient should contact physician if hematuria or signs of infection or cystitis occur.

Evaluation

Patient voids comfortably at regular intervals and does not experience dribbling.

Patient is knowledgeable about procedure, its effects on sexuality, and activity restrictions in postoperative period.

Patient returns to presurgical sexual functioning.

CANCER OF THE PROSTATE

Prostatic cancer is a common form of cancer in men over age 60. The symptoms initially are similar to those accompanying BPH. Radical prostatectomy procedures, outlined in Table 14-5, are utilized in treatment, and are accompanied frequently by radiation and chemotherapy. Urinary incontinence and sexual impotency are common complications of this surgery.

INFLAMMATORY DISORDERS

Urethritis, prostatitis, epididymitis, and orchitis are the most common infections affecting the male reproductive tract. The infecting organisms may reach the genital tract by direct spread up the urethra or be borne by blood or lymph. Table 14-6 describes these conditions.

STRUCTURAL DISORDERS

Structural disorders of the testes and scrotum are described in Table 14-7. Immediate medical attention is

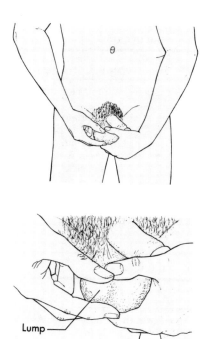

Lump

FIGURE 14-3 Self-examination of the testis. (From Phipps, W.J., Long, B.C., and Woods, N.F.: Medical-surgical nursing: concepts and clinical practice, ed. 2, St. Louis, 1983, The C.V. Mosby Co.)

TESTICULAR SELF-EXAMINATION (TSE)

Perform TSE after a bath or shower when scrotum is warm and most relaxed.

Grasp testis with both hands and palpate gently between thumb and fingers.

The testis should feel smooth, egg-shaped, and firm to touch.

The epididymis, found behind the testis, feels like a soft tube.

Any swelling that is not normal for the person should be examined by a physician.

From Long, B.C., and Phipps, W.J.: Essentials of medical-surgical nursing: a nursing approach, St. Louis, 1985, The C.V. Mosby Co.

TABLE 14-9 Sexually transmitted diseases

Organism	Diseases
Bacteria	Gonorrhea, chancroid, granuloma inguinale, *Gardnerella vaginalis*
Spirochete	Syphilis
Chlamydia	Nongonococcal urethritis, epididymitis, cervicitis, pelvic inflammatory disease, lymphogranuloma venereum
Virus	Herpes genitalis, hepatitis B, cytomegalovirus, AIDS, genital warts
Protozoa	Trichomoniasis
Yeast	Candidiasis
Parasites	Pediculosis pubis, scabies

TABLE 14-10 Syphilis, gonorrhea, and genital herpes

Disease	Incubation Period	Signs and Symptoms	Medical Management
Gonorrhea	Men: 3–30 days Women: 3 days to indefinite period	Men: purulent urethral discharge, dysuria, prostatitis, epididymitis Women: asymptomatic in early stages; cervicitis with purulent discharge, salpingitis (inflammation of fallopian tube), bartholinitis	Intramuscular penicillin G and probenicid by mouth; or ampicillin and probenicid
Syphilis	3 weeks (9 days to 3 months)	Positive serologic tests Stage I: chancre (hard sore or pimple that breaks and forms painless, draining erosion) Stage II: fever, headache, malaise accompanied by sores or generalized body rash Stage III: tumorlike masses, damage to heart and vessels, CNS involvement with paresis, loss of judgment and memory	Penicillin
Herpes genitalis	3–14 days	Vesicles that rupture and form ulcerations; pain; dysuria; flulike symptoms	Symptomatic, topical acyclovir

crucial because the degree of testicular damage may be influenced by the promptness of intervention.

TUMORS

Tumors of the male reproductive tract are almost always malignant. Except for tumors of the prostate gland, they occur quite rarely. Cancer of the testes and penis are described in Table 14-8. These disorders and their treatment may have devastating effects on the man's body image and sexual role. Testicular self-examination is considered an important health promotion technique to be taught to young adult males. The process is outlined in the box on p. 198 and shown in Figure 14-3.

SEXUALLY TRANSMITTED DISEASES

Sexually transmitted diseases encompass any disorder that is or can be transmitted from one person to another during sexual or intimate contact with the genitals, mouth, or rectum. Many of these disorders are significant health problems that are epidemic in the population. It is critical that accurate information about symptoms, treatment, transmission, and complications be communicated to the public. The highest incidence of these disorders is in the 15- to 29-year-old age group. Table 14-9 lists sexually transmitted diseases. Table 14-10 details the symptoms and treatment for syphilis, gonorrhea, and genital herpes.

NURSING CARE PLAN

FOLLOWING HYSTERECTOMY

Nursing Diagnoses	Expected Patient Outcomes	Nursing Interventions
Disturbance in self-concept: body image, self esteem related to loss of child bearing function	Patient verbalizes concerns about loss of uterus and maintains a positive view of herself	1. Give patient opportunities to express feelings and concerns about loss of uterus. 2. Be empathetic of patient's feelings that may include grief, guilt, shame, or remorse. 3. Encourage patient to continue activities associated with femininity, such as putting on makeup, arranging hair, wearing own apparel. 4. Help patient identify personal strengths. 5. Help partner understand rationale for behaviors expressed by patient and encourage him to demonstrate continued affection. 6. Correct any misconceptions about effect of surgery on sexual intercourse (normal relationships may be resumed after 4 to 6 weeks).
Alteration in comfort—abdominal pain related to surgical incision and gaseous distention	Patient experiences decreasing discomfort and successfully passes flatus	1. Use pain-relieving measures as needed during early postoperative period. 2. Encourage progressive ambulation to prevent abdominal distention. 3. If abdominal distention occurs, try a heating pad or rectal tube; give any prescribed enemas.
Potential alteration in patterns of urinary elimination related to pelvic edema and discomfort	Patient resumes a normal urinary elimination pattern	1. Monitor intake and output for at least 48 hours; assess for urinary retention, if appropriate. 2. Use measures to facilitate voiding if urinary retention occurs. 3. Provide catheter care if patient has an indwelling catheter.
Potential alteration in peripheral tissue perfusion related to venous congestion in the pelvis	Patient maintains an adequate venous return and is free of thrombosis or phlebitis	1. Monitor patient for leg or chest pain or for sudden dyspnea; assess for Homans' sign. 2. Encourage leg exercises and frequent turning in bed during early postoperative period. 3. Avoid using knee gatch or pillows under knees; encourage patient to keep knees flat while in bed. 4. Encourage patient to lie completely flat in bed for short periods every 2 hours during first 24 hours, then every 4 hours until ambulating well. 5. Encourage ambulation. Apply thigh-high TED stockings.
Knowledge deficit related to onset and management of menopause	Patient is knowledgeable about the effects of surgery and makes informed decisions about estrogen replacement	1. Teach patient: 　a. Physiologic effects of the hysterectomy. 　b. Psychologic reactions may continue for a few weeks. 　c. Possibility of slight vaginal discharge for 1 to 2 weeks. 　d. Avoid driving a car for 2 to 4 weeks (especially with standard shift drive). 　e. Avoid heavy activities and active sports for 4 to 6 weeks. 　f. Report to physician excessive or persistent vaginal drainage or signs of thrombophlebitis.

NURSING CARE PLAN

BENIGN PROSTATIC HYPERTROPHY FOLLOWING TUR PROSTATECTOMY

Nursing Diagnoses	Expected Patient Outcomes	Nursing Interventions

elimination related to obstruction of urine outflow or presence of Foley catheter	unobstructed and bleeding gradually decreases
	Patient returns to a normal continent pattern of urinary elimination
		1. Monitor urinary output and characteristics frequently.
		2. Monitor vital signs: report signs of shock or fever.
		3. Monitor appearance of urine for persistent bright red color rather than expected dark red beyond first few hours postoperatively.
		4. Maintain constant bladder irrigation as prescribed during first 24 hours at a rate sufficient to keep output pink to light red in color.
		5. Maintain patency of indwelling urinary catheter:
		  a. Irrigate manually as prescribed to keep catheter free of clots.
		  b. Maintain straight line closed drainage system.
		6. Encourage high fluid intake (2500 to 3000 ml/day) to promote increased urinary flow.
		7. After catheter is removed, monitor for signs of retention. Assess patient for dribbling. If dribbling occurs:
		  a. Tell patient this is a common occurrence but that continence will return.
		  b. Teach patient perineal exercises.

Alteration in comfort—bladder spasms related to placement of 30 cc catheter balloon	Patient experiences minimal discomfort from bladder spasms	1. Teach patient not to try to void around catheter. 2. Monitor patient at regular intervals for 48 hours to identify early signs of bladder spasms. Assess drainage system for patency if spasms occur. 3. Give prescribed medications (analgesics, antispasmodics). 4. Tell patient spasms will decrease in intensity and frequency within 24 to 48 hours. 5. Avoid use of rectal thermometers, rectal examinations, or enemas for at least 1 week.

Potential sexual dysfunction, related to perceived effects of prostatectomy on sexual functioning	Patient returns to his preillness pattern of sexual activity and satisfaction	1. Provide information as necessary:
		  a. TUR procedure does not affect sexual functioning
		  b. Occurrence of retrograde ejaculation (urine may have a milky appearance). Usually produces sterility.
		2. Give patient opportunities to discuss feelings about the effects of prostatectomy on sexual intercourse.
		3. Avoid sexual intercourse for 4 to 6 weeks after surgery.

Knowledge deficit related to activity restrictions for the post discharge period	Patient understands activity restrictions to be followed and need for medical followup	1. Teach patient:
		  a. Avoidance of heavy activities for 4 to 6 weeks.
		  b. Avoidance of straining at stool for 4 to 6 weeks; use stool softeners or laxatives as necessary; avoid Valsalva maneuver.
		  c. Patient should not drive a car or sit for prolonged periods for 4 to 6 weeks.
		  d. Ambulation is encouraged.
		  e. Fluid maintenance of at least 2500 ml/day to prevent complications.
		  f. Urine should remain clear; report onset of fresh bleeding to physician.
		  g. Instructions for medical follow-up.

Nursing Diagnoses

Activity intolerance
Activity intolerance: potential
Adjustment, impaired
Airway clearance, ineffective
Anxiety

Body temperature, altered: potential
Bowel elimination, altered: constipation
Bowel elimination, altered: diarrhea
Bowel elimination, altered: incontinence
Breathing pattern, ineffective

Cardiac output, altered: decreased
Comfort, altered: chronic pain
Comfort, altered: pain
Communication, impaired verbal
Coping, family: potential for growth
Coping, ineffective family: compromised
Coping, ineffective family: disabled
Coping, ineffective individual

Diversional activity, deficit

Family processes, altered
Fear
Fluid volume deficit: actual (1)
Fluid volume deficit: actual (2)
Fluid volume deficit: potential
Fluid volume excess

Gas exchange, impaired
Grieving, anticipatory
Grieving, dysfunctional
Growth and development, altered

Health maintenance, altered
Home maintenance management, impaired
Hopelessness
Hyperthermia
Hypothermia

Incontinence, functional
Incontinence, reflex
Incontinence, stress
Incontinence, total
Incontinence, urge
Infection, potential for
Injury, potential for
Injury, potential for: poisoning
Injury, potential for: suffocating
Injury, potential for: trauma

Knowledge deficit (specify)

Mobility, impaired physical

Noncompliance (specify)
Nutrition, altered: less than body requirements
Nutrition, altered: more than body requirements
Nutrition, altered: potential for more than body requirements

Parenting, altered: actual/potential
Post-trauma response
Powerlessness

Rape-trauma syndrome
Rape-trauma syndrome: compound reaction
Rape-trauma syndrome: silent reaction
Role performance, altered

Self-care deficit: bathing/hygiene
Self-care deficit: dressing/grooming
Self-care deficit: feeding
Self-care deficit: toileting
Self-concept, disturbance in: body-image
Self-concept, disturbance in: personal identity
Self-concept, disturbance in: self-esteem
Sensory-perceptual alterations: visual, auditory, kinesthetic, gustatory, tactile, olfactory
Sexual dysfunction
Sexuality, altered patterns
Skin integrity, impaired: actual
Skin integrity, impaired: potential
Sleep pattern disturbance
Social interaction, impaired
Social isolation
Spiritual distress (distress of the human spirit)
Swallowing, impaired

Thermoregulation, ineffective
Thought processes, altered
Tissue integrity, impaired
Tissue integrity, impaired: oral mucous membrane
Tissue perfusion, altered: renal, cerebral, cardiopulmonary, gastrointestinal, peripheral

Unilateral neglect
Urinary elimination, altered patterns
Urinary retention

Violence, potential for: self-directed or directed at others

From North American Nursing Diagnosis Association: Classification of nursing diagnoses: proceedings of the seventh conference, St. Louis, 1987, The C.V. Mosby Co.

Normal Laboratory Values

Blood, plasma or serum values

Reference range

Determination	Conventional	SI
Acetoacetate plus acetone	0.3–2.0 mg/100 ml	3–20 mg/l
Aldolase	1.3–8.2 mU/ml	12–75 nmol · s⁻¹/l
Alpha amino nitrogen	3.0–5.5 mg/100 ml	2.1–3.9 mmol/l
Ammonia	80–110 µg/100 ml	47–65 µmol/l
Ascorbic acid	0.4–1.5 mg/100 ml	23–85 µmol/l
Barbiturate	0	0 µmol/l
	Coma level: phenobarbital, approximately 10 mg/100 ml; most other drugs, 1–3 mg per 100 ml	
Bilirubin (van den Bergh's test)	One minute: 0.4 mg/100 ml	Up to 7 µmol/l
	Direct: 0.4 mg/100 ml	Up to 17 µmol/l
	Total: 1.0 mg/100 ml	
	Indirect is total minus direct	
Blood volume	8.5–9.0% of body weight in kg	80–85 ml/kg
Bromide	0	0 mmol/l
	Toxic level: 17 mEq/l	
Bromsulfalein (BSP)	Less than 5% retention 45 min after 5 mg/kg IV	<0.05 l
Calcium	8.5–10.5 mg/100 ml (slightly higher in children)	2.1–2.6 mmol/l
Carbon dioxide content	24–30 mEq/l	24–30 mmol/l
	20–26 mEq/l in infants (as HCO_3^-)	
Carbon monoxide	Symptoms with over 20% saturation	0 (1)
Carotenoids	0.8–4.0 µg/ml	1.5–7.4 µmol/l
Ceruloplasmin	27–37 mg/100 ml	1.8–2.5 µmol/l
Chloride	100–106 mEq/l	100–106 mmol/l
Cholinesterase (pseudocholinesterase)	0.5 pH U or more/h	0.5 or more arb. unit
	0.7 pH U or more/h for packed cells	
Copper	Total: 100–200 µg/100 ml	16–31 µmol/l
Creatine phosphokinase (CPK)	Female 5–35 mU/ml	0.08–0.58 µmol · s⁻¹/l
	Male 5–55 mU/ml	
Creatinine	0.6–1.5 mg/100 ml	60–130 µmol/l

Modified from Kaye, D.A., and Rose, L.F.: Fundamentals of internal medicine, St. Louis, 1983, The C.V. Mosby Co. Adopted by permission from the New England Journal of Medicine, Vol. 302, pages 37–48, 1980.
Abbreviations used: SI, Système International d'Unités (The SI for the Health Professions. World Health Organization, Office of Publications, Geneva, Switzerland, 1977); d, 24 hours; P. plasma; S, serum; B, blood; U, urine; l, liter; h, hour; and s, second.

Blood, plasma or serum values—cont'd

Reference range

Determination	Conventional	SI
Ethanol	0.3-0.4%, marked intoxication;	65–87 mmol/l
	0.4–0.5%, alcoholic stupor;	87–109 mmol/l
	0.5% or over, alcoholic coma	>109 mmol/l
Glucose	Fasting: 70–110 mg/100 ml	3.9–5.6 mmol/l
Iron	50–150 μg/100 ml (higher in males)	9.0–26.9 μmol/l
Iron-binding capacity	250–410 μg/100 ml	44.8–73.4 μmol/l
Lactic acid	0.6–1.8 mEq/l	0.6–1.8 mmol/l
Lactic dehydrogenase	60–120 U/ml	1.00–2.00 $\mu mol \cdot s^{-1}/l$
Lead	50 μg/100 ml or less	Up to 2.4 μmol/l
Lipase	2 U/ml or less	Up to 2 arb. unit
Lipids		
Cholesterol	120–220 mg/100 ml	3.10–5.69 mmol/l
Cholesterol esters	60–75% of cholesterol	
Phospholipids	9–16 mg/100 ml as lipid phosphorus	2.9–5.2 mmol/l
Total fatty acids	190–420 mg/100 ml	1.9–4.2 g/l
Total lipids	450–1000 mg/100 ml	4.5–10.0 g/l
Triglycerides	40–150 mg/100 ml	0.4–1.5 g/l
Lithium	Toxic level 2 mEq/l	2 mmol/l
Magnesium	1.5–2.0 mEq/l	0.8–1.3 mmol/l
5'Nucleotidase	0.3–3.2 Bodansky U	30–290 $nmol \cdot s^{-1}/l$
Osmolality	285–295 mOsm/kg water	285–295 mmol/kg
Oxygen saturation (arterial)	96–100%	0.96–1.00 l
P_{CO_2}	35–43 mm Hg	4.7–6.0 kPa
pH	7.35–7.45	Same
P_{O_2}	75–100 mm Hg (dependent on age) while breathing room air	10.0–13.3 kPa
	Above 500 mm Hg while on 100% O_2	
Phenylalanine	0–2 mg/100 ml	0–120 μmol/l
Phenytoin (Dilantin)	Therapeutic level, 5–20 μg/ml	19.8–79.5 μmol/l
Phosphorus (Inorganic)	3.0–4.5 mg/100 ml (infants in 1st year up to 6.0 (mg/100 ml)	1.0–1.5 mmol/l
Potassium	3.5–5.0 mEq/l	3.5–5.0 mmol/l
Primidone (Mysoline)	Therapeutic level 4–12 μg/ml	18–55 μmol/l
Protein: Total	6.0–8.4 g/100 ml	60–84 g/l
Albumin	3.5-5.0 g/100 ml	35-50 g/l
Globulin	2.3-3.5 g/100 ml	23-35 g/l
Electrophoresis	*% of total protein*	*Of total protein*
Albumin	52–68	0.52-0.68
Globulin:		
Alpha$_1$	4.2–7.2	0.042–0.072
Alpha$_2$	6.8–12	0.068–0.12
Beta	9.3–15	0.093–0.15
Gamma	13–23	0.13–0.23
Pyruvic acid	0–0.11 mEq/l	0–0.11 mmol/l
Quinidine	Therapeutic: 1.5–3 μg/ml	4.6–9.2 μmol/l
	Toxic: 5–6 μg/ml	15.4–18.5 μmol/l
Salicylate:	0	
Therapeutic	20–25 mg/100 ml; 25–30 mg/100 ml to age 10 yrs. 3 h post dose	1.4–1.8 mmol/l 1.8–2.2 mmol/l
Toxic	Over 30 mg/100 ml	Over 2.2 mmol/l
	Over 20 mg/100 ml after age 60	Over 1.5 mmol/l
Sodium	135–145 mEq/l	135–145 mmol/l
Sulfate	0.5–1.5 mg/100 ml	0.05–1.2 mmol/l
Sulfonamide	0 mg/100 ml	0 mmol/l
	Therapeutic: 5–15 mg/100 ml	
Transaminase (SGOT) (aspartate amino-transferase)	10–40 U/ml	0.08–0.32 $\mu mol \cdot s^{-1}/l$
Urea nitrogen (BUN)	8–25 mg/100 ml	2.9–8.9 mmol/l
Uric acid	3.0–7.0 mg/100 m	0.13–0.42 mmol/l
Vitamin A	0.15–0.6 μg/ml	0.5–2.1 μmol/l
Vitamin A tolerance test	Rise to twice fasting level in 3 to 5 h	

Urine values

Reference range

Determination	Conventional	SI
Acetone plus acetoacetate (quantitative)	0	0 mg/l
Alpha amino nitrogen	64–199 mg/d; not over 1.5% of total nitrogen	4.6–14.2 mmol/d
Amylase	24–76 U/ml	24–76 arb. unit
Calcium	150 mg/d or less	3.8 or less mmol/d
Catecholamines	Epinephrine: under 20 μg/d	<55 nmol/d
	Norepinephrine: under 100 μg/d	<590 nmol/d
Copper	0–100 μg/d	0–1.6 μmol/d
Coproporphyrin	50–250 μg/d	80–380 nmol/d
	Children under 80 lb 0–75 μg/d	0-115 nmol/d
Creatine	Under 100 mg/d or less than 6% of creatinine. In pregnancy: up to 12%. In children under 1 yr.: may equal creatinine. In older children: up to 30% of creatinine	<0.75 mmol/d
Cystine or cysteine	0	0
Follicle-stimulating hormone:		
Follicular phase	5-20 lU/d	Same
Mid/cycle	15–60 lU/d	
Luteal phase	5–15 lU/d	
Menopausal	50–100 lU/d	
Men	5–25 lU/d	
Hemoglobin and myoglobin	0	
5-Hydroxyindoleacetic acid	2-9 mg/d (women lower than men)	10–45 μmol/d
Lead	0.08 μg/ml or 120 μg or less/d	0.39 μmol/l or less
Phenolsulfonphthalein (PSP)	At least 25% excreted by 15 min; 40% by 30 min; 60% by 120 min	0.25 l
Phosphorus (inorganic)	Varies with intake, average 1 g/d	32 mmol/d
Porphobilinogen	0	0
Protein:		
Quantitative	<150 mg/24 hr	<0.15 g/d
Steroids:		

17-Ketosteroids (per day)

Age (yr)	Male (mg)	Female (mg)	Male (μmol/d)	Female (μmol/d)
10	1–4	1–4	3–14	3–14
20	6–21	4–16	21–73	14–56
30	8–26	4–14	28–90	14–49
50	5–18	3–9	17–62	10–31
70	2–10	1–7	7–35	3–24

Determination	Conventional	SI
17–Hydroxysteroids	3-8 mg/d (women lower than men)	8-22 μmol/d as hydrocortisone
Sugar:		
Quantitative glucose	0	0 mmol/l
Identification of reducing substances		
Fructose	0	0 mmol/l
Pentose	0	0 mmol/l
Titratable acidity	20–40 mEq/d	20–40 mmol/d
Urobilinogen	Up to 1.0 Ehrlich U	To 1.0 arb. unit
Uroporphyrin	0	0 nmol/d
Vanillylmandelic acid (VMA)	Up to 9 mg/24 hr	Up to 45 μmol/d

Special endocrine tests

Reference range

Determination	Conventional	SI
Steroid hormones		
Aldosterone	Excretion: 5–19 μg/24 h	14–53 nmol/d
Fasting, at rest, 210 mEq sodium diet	Supine: 48 ± 29 pg/ml	133 ± 80 pmol/l
	Upright: (2 h) 65 ± 23 pg/ml	180 ± 64 pmol/l
Fasting, at rest, 110 mEq sodium diet	Supine: 107 ± 435 pg/ml	279 ± 125 pmol/l
	Upright: (2 h) 239 ± 123 pg/ml	663 ± 341 pmol/l
Fasting, at rest, 10 mEq sodium diet	Supine: 175 ± 75 pg/ml	485 ± 208 pmol/l
	Upright: (2 h) 532 ± 228 pg/ml	1476 ± 632 pmol/l
Cortisol		
Fasting	8 AM: 5–25 μg/100 ml	0.14–0.69 μmol/l
At rest	8 PM: Below 10 μg/100 ml	0–0.28 μmol/l
20 U ACTH	4 h ACTH test: 30–45 μg/100 ml	0.83–1.24 μmol/l
Dexamethasone at midnight	Overnight suppression test: Below 5 μg/100 ml	<0.14 nmol/l
	Excretion: 20–70 μg/24 h	55–193 nmol/d
11-Deoxycortisol	Responsive: Over 7.5 μg/100 ml (after metrapone)	>0.22 μmol/l
Testosterone	Adult male: 300–1100 ng/100 ml	10.4–38.1 nmol/l
	Adolescent male: over 100 ng/100 ml	> 3.5 nmol/l
	Females: 25–90 ng/100 ml	0.87–3.12 nmol/l
Unbound testosterone	Adult male: 3.06–24.0 ng/100 ml	106–832 pmol/l
	Adult female: 0.09–1.28 ng/100 ml	3.1–44.4 pmol/l
Polypeptide hormones		
Adrenocorticotropin (ACTH)	15–70 pg/ml	3.3–15.4 pmol/l
Calcitonin	Undetectable in normals	0
	>100 pg/ml in medullary carcinoma	>29.3 pmol/l
Growth hormone		
Fasting, at rest	Below 5 ng/ml	<233 pmol/l
After exercise	Children: over 10 ng/ml	>465 pmol/l
	Male: Below 5 ng/ml	<233 pmol/l
	Female: Up to 30 ng/ml	0–1395 pmol/l
After glucose	Male: Below 5 ng/ml	<233 pmol/l
	Female: Below 10 ng/ml	0–465 pmol/l
Insulin		
Fasting	6–26 μU/ml	43–187 pmol/l
During hypoglycemia	Below 20 μU/ml	<144 pmol/l
After glucose	Up to 150 μU/ml	0–1078 pmol/l
Luteinizing hormone	Male: 6–18 mU/ml	6–18 u/l
Pre- or postovulatory	Female: 5–22 mU/ml	5–22 u/l
Midcycle peak	30–250 mU/ml	30-250 u/l
Parathyroid hormone	<10 μl equiv/ml	<10 ml equiv/ml
Prolactin	2–15 ng/ml	0.08–6.0 nmol/l
Renin activity		
Normal diet	Supine: 1.1 ± 0.8 ng/ml/h	0.9 ± 0.6 (nmol/l)h
	Upright: 1.9 ± 1.7 ng/ml/h	1.5 ± 1.3 (nmol/l)h
Low-sodium diet	Supine: 2.7 ± 1.8 ng/ml/h	2.1 ± 1.4 (nmol/l)h
	Upright: 6.6 ± 2.5 ng/ml/h	5.1 ± 1.9 (nmol/l)h
Low-sodium diet	Diuretics: 10.0 ± 3.7 ng/ml/h	7.7 ± 2.9 (nmol/l)h
Thyroid hormones		
Thryoid-stimulating-hormone (TSH)	0.5–3.5 μU/ml	0.5–3.5 mU/l
Thyroxine-binding globulin capacity	15–25 μg T_4/100 ml	193–322 nmol/l
Total tri-iodothyronine by radioimmunoassay (T_3)	70–190 ng/100 ml	1.08–2.92 nmol/l
Total thyroxine by RIA (T_4)	4–12 μg/100 ml	52–154 nmol/l
T_3 resin uptake	25–35%	0.25–0.35
Free thyroxine index (FT_4I)	1–4 ng/100 ml	12.8–51.2 pmol/l

Cerebrospinal fluid values

Reference range

Determination	Conventional	SI	Determination	Conventional	SI
Bilirubin	0	0 μmol/l	Glucose	50–75 mg/100 ml (30%–50% less than blood)	2.8–4.2 mmol/l
Chloride	120–130 mEq/l (20 mEq/l higher than serum)		Pressure (initial)	70–180 mm of water	70–80 arb. u.
Albumin	Mean: 29.5 mg/100 ml ± 112 SD: 11–48 mg/100 ml	0.295 g/l ± 112 SD: 0.11–0.48	Protein: Lumbar	15–45 mg/100 ml	0.15–0.45 g/l
IgG	Mean: 4.3 mg/100 ml ± 112 SD: 0–8.6 mg/100 ml	0.043 g/l ± 112 SD: 0–0.086	Cisternal	15–25 mg/100 ml	0.15–0.25 g/l
			Ventricular	5–15 mg/100 ml	0.05–0.15 g/l

Hematologic values

Reference range

Determination	Conventional	SI
Coagulation factors:		
Factor I (fibrinogen)	0.15–0.35 g/100 ml	4.0–10.0 μmol/l
Factor II (prothrombin)	60–140%	0.60–1.40
Factor V (accelerator globulin)	60–140%	0.60–1.40
Factor VII-X (proconvertin-Stuart)	70–130%	0.70–1.30
Factor X (Stuart factor)	70–130%	0.70–1.30
Factor VIII (antihemophilic globulin)	50–200%	0.50–2.0
Factor IX (plasma thromboplastic co-factor)	60–140%	0.60–1.40
Factor XI (plasma thromboplastic antecedent)	60–140%	0.60–1.40
Factor XII (Hageman factor)	60–140%	0.60–1.40
Coagulation screening tests:		
Bleeding time (Simplate)	3–9 min	180-540 s
Prothrombin time	Less than 2-s deviation from control	Less than 2-s deviation from control
Partial thromboplastin time (activated)	25–37 s	25–37 s
Whole-blood clot lysis	No clot lysis in 24 hr	O/d
Fibrinolytic studies:		
Euglobin lysis	No lysis in 2 h	0 (in 2 h)
Fibrinogen split products:	Negative reaction at greater than 1:4 dilution	0 (at > 1:4 dilution)
Thrombin time	Control ± 5 s	Control ± 5 s
"Complete" blood count:		
Hematocrit	Male: 45–52%	Male: 0.42–0.52
	Female: 37–48%	Female: 0.37–0.48
Hemoglobin	Male: 13–18 g/10 ml	Male: 8.1–11.2 mmole/l
	Female: 12–16 g/100 ml	Female: 7.4-9.9 mmol/l
Leukocyte count	4300–10,800/mm³	4.3–10.8×10^9/l
Erythrocyte count	4.2–5.9 million/mm³	4.2–5.9×10^{12}/l
Mean corpuscular volume (MCV)	80–94 μm³	80–94 fl
Mean corpuscular hemoglobin (MCH)	27–32 pg	1.7–2.0 fmol
Mean corpuscular hemoglobin concentration (MCHC)	32–36%	19–22.8 mmol/l
Erythrocyte sedimentation rate (Westergren method)	Male: 1–13 mm/h	Male: 1–13 mm/h
	Female: 1–20 mm/h	Female: 1–20 mm/h
Erythrocyte enzymes		
Glucose-6-phosphate dehydrogenase	5–15 U/gHb	5–15 U/g
Pyruvate kinase	13–17 U/gHb	13–17 U/g

Hematologic values—cont'd

Reference range

Determination	Conventional	SI
Ferritin (serum)		
Iron deficiency	0–20 ng/ml	0–20 μg/l
Iron excess	Greater than 400 ng/l	>400 μg/l
Folic acid		
Normal	Greater than 1.9 ng/ml	>4.3 mmol/l
Borderline	1.0–1.9 ng/ml	2.3–4.3 mmol/l
Haptoglobin	100–300 mg/100 ml	1.0–3.0 g/l
Hemoglobin studies:		
Electrophoresis for A_2 hemoglobin	1.5–3.5%	0.015–0.035
Hemoglobin F (fetal hemoglobin)	Less than 2%	<0.02
Hemoglobin, met- and sulf-	0	0
Serum hemoglobin	2–3 mg/100 ml	1.2–1.9 μmol/l
Thermolabile hemoglobin	0	0
L.E. (lupus erythematosus) preparation:		
Heparin as anticoagulant	0	0
Defibrinated blood	0	0
Leukocyte alkaline phosphatase:		
Quantitative method	15–40 mg of phosphorus liberated/h/10^{10} cells	15–40 mg/h
Qualitative method	Males: 33–188 U	33–188 U
	Females (off contraceptive pill); 30–160 U	30–160 U
Muramidase	Serum, 3–7 μg/ml	3–7 mg/l
	Urine, 0–2 μg/ml	0–2 mg/l
Osmotic fragility of erythrocytes	Increased if hemolysis occurs in over 0.5% NaCl; decreased if hemolysis is incomplete in 0.3% NaCl	
Peroxide hemolysis	Less than 10%	<0.10
Platelet count	150,000–350,000/mm³	150–350 × 10^9/l
Platelet function test:		
Clot retraction	50–100%/2 hr	0.50–1.00/2 h
Platelet aggregation	Full response to ADP, epinephrine and collagen	1.0
Platelet factor 3	33–57 s	33–57 s
Reticulocyte count	0.5–1.5% red cells	0.005–0.15
Vitamin B_{12}	90–280 pg/ml (borderline: 70–90)	66–207 pmol/l (borderline: 52–66)

Miscellaneous values

Reference range

Determination	Conventional	SI
Autoantibodies in serum		
Thyroid colloid and microsomal antigens	Absent	
Stomach parietal cells	Absent	
Smooth muscle	Absent	
Kidney mitochondria	Absent	
Rabbit renal collecting ducts	Absent	
Cytoplasm of ova, theca cells, testicular interstitial cells	Absent	
Skeletal muscle	Absent	
Adrenal gland	Absent	

Continued.

Miscellaneous values—cont'd

Reference range

Determination	Conventional	SI
Carcinoembryonic antigen (CEA) in blood	0–2.5 ng/ml, 97% healthy nonsmokers	0–2.5 µg/l, 97% healthy nonsmokers
Cryoprecipitable proteins in blood	0	0 arb. unit
Digitoxin in serum	17 ± 6 ng/ml	22 ± 7.8 nmol/l
Digoxin in serum		
0.25 mg/d	1.2 ± 0.4 ng/ml	1.54 ± 0.5 nmol/l
0.5 mg/d	1.5 ± 0.4 ng/ml	1.92 ± 0.5 nmol/l
Duodenal drainage:		
pH	5.5–7.5	5.5–7.5
Amylase	Over 1200 U/total sample	>1.2 arb. u
Trypsin	Values from 35 to 160% "normal"	0.35–1.60
Viscosity	3 min or less	180 s or less
Gastric analysis	Basal:	
	Females 2.0 ± 1.8 mEq/h	0.6 ± 0.5
	Males 3.0 ± 2.0 mEq/h	0.8 ± 0.6 µmol/s
	Maximal: (after histalog or gastrin)	
	Females 16 ± 5 mEq/h	4.4 ± 1.4 µmol/s
	Males 23 ± 5 mEq/h	6.4 ± 1.4 µmol/s
Gastrin-l in blood	0-200 pg/ml	0-95 pmol/l
Immunologic tests		
Alpha-feto-globulin	Abnormal if present	
Alpha 1-antitrypsin	200–400 mg/100 ml	2.0-4.0 g/l
Antinuclear antibodies	Positive if detected with serum diluted 1:10	
Anti-DNA antibodies	Less than 15 units/ml	
Complement, total hemolytic	150-250 U/ml	
C3	Range 55–120 mg/100 ml	0.55–1.2 g/l
C4	Range 20–50 mg/100 ml	0.2–0.5 g/l
Immunoglobulins in blood:		
IgG	1140 mg/100 ml Range 540–1663	11.4 g/l 5.5–16.6 g/l
IgA	214 mg/100 ml Range 66–344	2.14 g/l 0.66–3.44 g/l
IgM	168 mg/100 ml Range 39–290	1.68 g/l 0.39-2.9 g/l
Viscosity	1.4-1.8 expressed as relative viscosity of serum compared to water	
Iontophoresis	Children: 0–40 mEq sodium/liter	0–40 mmol/l
	Adults: 0–60 mEq sodium/l	0–60 mmol/l
Propranolol (includes bioactive 4-OH metabolite) in serum 4h after last dose	100–300 ng/ml	386–1158 nmol/l
Stool fat	Less than 5 g in 24 h or less than 4% of measured fat intake in 3–d period	<5 g/d
Stool nitrogen	Less than 2 g/d or 10% of urinary nitrogen	< 2 g/d
Synovial fluid:		
Glucose	Not less than 20 mg/100 ml lower than simultaneously drawn blood sugar	See blood glucose mmol/l
Mucin	Type 1 or 2	1–2 arb. u
	Grades as:	
	Type 1-tight clump	
	Type 2-soft clump	
	Type 3-soft clump that breaks up	
	Type 4-cloudy, no clump	
D-Xylose absorption	5–8 g/5 h in urine	33–53 mmol
	40 mg per 100 ml in blood 2 h after ingestion of 25 g of D-xylose	2.7 mmol/l

Abbreviations in Common Usage

ā	Before	CSF	Cerebrospinal fluid
aa	Of each	CT	Computed tomography
ac	Before meals	CVA	Cerebrovascular accident
ad lib	As desired	CVA	Costovertebral angle
A/G ratio	Albumin/globulin ratio	CVP	Central venous pressure
AK	Above knee	Cx	Cervix
aPTT	Activated partial thromboplastin time	Cysto	Cystoscopy
A/R pulse	Apical/radial pulse	D/C	Discontinue
ARDS	Adult respiratory distress syndrome	D & C	Dilation and curettage
ARV	Aortic valve replacement	Diff	Differential white blood cell count
ASCVD	Arteriosclerotic cardiovascular disease	DIP	Distal interphalangeal joint
ASHD	Arteriosclerotic heart disease	DJD	Degenerative joint disease
BaE	Barium enema	DM	Diabetes mellitus
BFT	Biofeedback therapy	DOA	Dead on arrival
b.i.d.	Twice daily	DOE	Dyspnea on exertion
BK	Below knee	DPT	Diphtheria, pertussis, tetanus toxoid
BMR	Basal metabolism rate	Dx	Diagnosis
BPH	Benign prostatic hypertrophy	ECG	Electrocardiogram
B.R.P.	Bathroom privileges	EEG	Electroencephalogram
BS	Bowel sounds	EENT	Eye, ear, nose, and throat
BSP	Bromsulphalein	EMG	Electromyogram
BUN	Blood urea nitrogen	ENT	Ear, nose and throat
Bx	Biopsy	ESR	Erythrocyte sedimentation rate
c̄	With	FB	Foreign body
CA	Cancer	FBS	Fasting blood sugar
CABG	Coronary artery bypass graft	FH	Family history
CAD	Coronary artery disease	FUO	Fever of unknown origin
CBC	Complete blood count	FWB	Full weight bearing
cc	Chief complaint	Fx	Fracture
CCK	Cholecystokinin	GI	Gastrointestinal
C.D.	Constant drainage	gtt	Drops
CDC	Centers for Disease Control	GTT	Glucose tolerance test
CHF	Congestive heart failure	GU	Genitourinary
CNS	Central nervous system	h	Hour
c/o	Complained of	HAV	Hepatitis A virus
COPD	Chronic obstructive pulmonary disease	HBV	Hepatitis B virus
CPK	Creatine phosphokinase	Hct	Hematocrit
CPR	Cardiopulmonary resuscitation	HCTZ	Hydrochlorothiazide
C & S	Culture and sensitivities	HCVD	Hypertensive cardiovascular disease

HDL	High density lipoproteins		NVD	Neck vein distention
Hgb	Hemoglobin		NWB	Nonweight bearing
HMO	Health maintenance organization		OD	Overdose
HNP	Herniated nucleus pulposus		O.D.	Right eye
HPI	History of present illness		OOB	Out of bed
HTN	Hypertension		O.R.	Operating room
h.s.	At bedtime		ORIF	Open reduction internal fixation
Hwb	Hot water bottle		O.S.	Left eye
hx	History		O.T.	Occupational therapy
IABP	Intraaortic balloon counterpulsation		O.U.	Both eyes
ICP	Intracranial pressure		p̄	After
ICS	Intercostal space		P & A	Percussion and auscultation
ICU	Intensive care unit		PAEDP	Pulmonary artery end-diastolic pressure
IDDM	Insulin-dependent diabetes mellitus		PAP	Papanicolaou smear
IHSS	Idiopathic hypertrophic subaortic stenosis		PAP	Pulmonary artery pressure
IM	Intramuscular		PBI	Protein bound iodine
IMB	Intermenstrual bleeding		p.c.	After meals
I & O	Intake and output		PCWP	Pulmonary capillary wedge pressure
IPPB	Intermittent positive pressure breathing		P.D.	Postural drainage
ITP	Idiopathic thrombocytopenic purpura		PEEP	Positive end expiratory pressure
IV	Intravenous		PERRLA	Pupils equal, round, reactive to light and accommodation
IVC	Intravenous cholangiogram			
IVP	Intravenous pyelogram		PFT	Pulmonary function test
LBP	Low back pain		Ph	Past history
LDH	Lactic dehydrogenase		PI	Present illness
LDL	Low density lipoproteins		PIP	Proximal interphalangeal joint
L.E. prep	Lupus erythematosus prep		Plt	Platelet
LLL	Left lower lobe		PMI	Point of maximal impulse
LLQ	Left lower quadrant		PMNs	Polymorphonuclear leukocytes
LMD	Local medical doctor		PMP	Past menstrual period
LMP	Last menstrual period		PND	Paroxysmal nocturnal dyspnea
LMP	Local medical physician		PNS	Peripheral nervous system
LOC	Level of consciousness		p.o.	By mouth
LP	Lumbar puncture		POD	Postoperative day
LVEDP	Left ventricular end-diastolic pressure		PPD	Postpartum day
L & W	Living and well		PPD	Purified protein derivative
lytes	Electrolytes		prn	According to necessity
ⓜ	Murmur		Pro time	Prothrombin time
MCH	Mean corpuscular hemoglobin		PSP	Phenosulphonphthalein
MCHC	Mean corpuscular hemoglobin concentration		PSRO	Professional standards review organization
MCP	Metacarpophalangeal joint		PT	Prothrombin time
MCV	Mean corpuscular volume		P.T.	Physical therapy
MGW	Magnesium, glycerin, and water enema		PTA	Prior to admission
MST	Mean survival time		PTT	Partial thromboplastin time
MTP	Metatarsalphalangeal joint		PVC	Premature ventricular contraction
MVR	Mitral valve replacement		PWB	Partial weight bearing
MWB	Minimal weight bearing		PZI	Protamine zinc insulin
NAD	No acute distress		qd	Every day
NIDDM	Noninsulin dependent diabetes mellitus		qh	Every hour
NMR	Nuclear magnetic resonance		qhs	At bedtime
NPH	Nonprotein Hagedorn (insulin)		qid	Four times a day
NPN	Nonprotein nitrogen		qns	Quantity not sufficient
N.P.O.	Nothing by mouth		qod	Every other day
			qoh	Every other hour

qpr	At earliest convenience	TBG	Thyroxine binding globulin
qs	As much as necessary (quantity sufficient)	TENS	Transcutaneous electrical nerve stimulator
RBC	Red blood cells	THA	Total hip arthroplasty
RLL	Right lower lobe	THR	Total hip replacement
RLQ	Right lower quadrant	TIA	Transient ischemic attacks
R/O	Rule out	t.i.d.	Three times a day
ROS	Review of symptoms	TKA	Total knee arthroplasty
RSR	Regular sinus rhythm	TKR	Total knee replacement
Rx	Treatment	TM	Tympanic membrane
s̄	Without	TP	Total protein
SBE	Subacute bacterial endocarditis	TPN	Total parenteral nutrition (hyperalimentation)
sc	Subcutaneous		
Sed rate	Sedimentation rate	TSP	Total serum protein
SGOT	Serum glutamic oxidase transaminase	TSS	Toxic shock syndrome
SGPT	Serum glutamic pyruvate transaminase	TURP	Transurethral resection of prostate
SLE	Systemic lupus erythematosus	Tx	Traction
SLR	Straight leg raising	ung	Ointment
SOB	Short of breath	URI	Upper respiratory infection
s.o.s.	Administer once if necessary	US	Ultrasound
S/P	Status post (occurred in past)	UTI	Urinary tract infection
SR	Systems review	UV	Ultraviolet
SSE	Soapsuds enema	VC	Vital capacity
stat	At once	VDRL	Venereal Disease Research Laboratory Test
STD	Sexually transmitted disease	VNA	Visiting nurse association
STS	Serologic test for syphilis	VS	Vital signs
T_3	Triiodothyronine	wa	While awake
T_4	Thyroxine	WBC	White blood count
tab	Tablet	WNL	Within normal limits
TBC	Tuberculosis		

Recommended Daily Dietary Allowances, Revised 1980

Mean heights and weights and recommended energy intake

Category	Age (years)	Weight		Height		Energy needs (with range)		
		kg	lb	cm	in	kcal		MJ
Infants	0.0-0.5	6	13	60	24	kg × 115	(95–145)	kg × .48
	0.5-1.0	9	20	71	28	kg × 105	(80–135)	kg × .44
Children	1–3	13	29	90	35	1,300	(900–1,800)	5.5
	4–6	20	44	112	44	1,700	(1,300–2,300)	7.1
	7–10	28	62	132	52	2,400	(1,650–3,300)	10.1
Males	11–14	45	99	157	62	2,700	(2,000–3,700)	11.3
	15–18	66	145	176	69	2,800	(2,100–3,900)	11.8
	19–22	70	154	177	70	2,900	(2,500–3,300)	12.2
	23–50	70	154	178	70	2,700	(2,300–3,100)	11.3
	51–75	70	154	178	70	2,400	(2,000–2,800)	10.1
	76 +	70	154	178	70	2,050	(1,650–2,450)	8.6
Females	11–14	46	101	157	62	2,200	(1,500–3,000)	9.2
	15–18	55	120	163	64	2,100	(1,200–3,000)	8.8
	19–22	55	120	163	64	2,100	(1,700–2,500)	8.8
	23–50	55	120	163	64	2,000	(1,600–2,400)	8.4
	51–75	55	120	163	64	1,800	(1,400–2,200)	7.6
	76 +	55	120	163	64	1,600	(1,200–2,000)	6.7
Pregnancy						+300		
Lactation						+500		

From Recommended Dietary Allowances, Revised 1980. Food and Nutrition Board National Academy of Sciences–National Research Council, Washington, D.C.

The data in this table have been assembled from the observed median heights and weights of children together with desirable weights for adults for the mean heights of men (70 in) and women (64 in) between the ages of 18 and 34 years as surveyed in the U.S. population (HEW/NCHS data).

The energy allowances for the young adults are for men and women doing light work. The allowances for the two older age groups represent mean energy needs over these age spans, allowing for a 2% decrease in basal (resting) metabolic rate per decade and a reduction in activity of 200 kcal per day for men and women between 51 and 75 years, 500 kcal for men over 75 years, and 400 kcal for women over 75. The customary range of daily energy output is shown for adults in parentheses and is based on a variation in energy needs of ± 400 kcal at any one age, emphasizing the wide range of energy intakes appropriate for any group of people.

Energy allowances for children through age 18 are based on median energy intakes of children these ages followed in longitudinal growth studies. The values in parentheses are 10th and 90th percentiles of energy intake, to indicate the range of energy consumption among children of these ages.

Daily dietary guide—the basic four food groups

Food group	Main nutrients	Daily amounts*
Milk		
Milk, cheese, Ice cream, or other products made with whole or skimmed milk	Calcium Protein Riboflavin	Children under 9: 2–3 cups Children 9–12: 3 or more cups Teen-agers: 4 or more cups Adults: 2 or more cups Pregnant women: 3 or more cups Nursing mothers: 4 or more cups (1 cup = 8 oz fluid milk or designated milk equivalent†)
Meats		
Beef, veal, lamb, pork, poultry, fish, eggs	Protein Iron Thiamin	2 or more servings Count as 1 serving 2–3 oz of lean, boneless, cooked meat, poultry, or fish 2 eggs
Alternates: dry beans, dry peas, nuts, peanut butter	Niacin Riboflavin	1 cup cooked dry beans or peas 4 tbsp peanut butter
Vegetables and fruits		4 or more servings Count as 1 serving ½ cup of vegetable or fruit or a portion such as 1 medium apple, banana, orange, potato, or ½ a medium grapefruit, melon Include
	Vitamin A	A dark-green or deep-yellow vegetable or fruit rich in vitamin A at least every other day
	Vitamin C (ascorbic acid)	A citrus fruit or other fruit or vegetable rich in vitamin C daily
	Smaller amounts of other vitamins and minerals	Other vegetables and fruits including potatoes
Bread and cereals		4 or more servings of whole grain, enriched or restored Count as 1 serving
	Thiamin	1 slice of bread
	Niacin	1 oz (1 cup) ready-to-eat cereal, flake or puff varieties
	Riboflavin	½–¾ cup cooked cereal
	Iron	½–¾ cup cooked pastas (macaroni, spaghetti, noodles)
	Protein	Crackers: 5 saltines, 2 squares graham crackers

*Use additional amounts of these foods or added butter, margarine, oils, sugars, etc., as desired or needed.
†Milk equivalents: 1 oz cheddar cheese, 3 servings cottage cheese, 1 cup fluid skimmed milk, 1 cup buttermilk, ½ cup dry skimmed milk powder, 1 cup ice milk, 1⅔ cups ice cream, ½ cup evaporated milk.

Recommended daily dietary allowances for growth

Category	Age (yr)	Weight kg	Weight lb	Height cm	Height in	Energy (kcal)	Protein (g)	Vit. A µg RE	Vit. A IU	Vit. D (µg*)	Vit. E (mgαTE)
Infants	Birth–0.5	6	13	60	24	kg × 115	kg × 2.2	420	1,400	10	3
	0.5–1	9	20	71	28	kg × 105	kg × 2.0	400	2,000	10	4
Children	1–3	13	29	90	35	1,300	23	400	2,000	10	5
	4–6	20	44	112	44	1,700	30	500	2,500	10	6
	7–10	28	62	132	52	2,400	34	700	3,300	10	7
Males	11–14	45	99	157	62	2,700	45	1,000	5,000	10	8
	15–18	66	145	176	69	2,800	56	1,000	5,000	10	10
Females	11–14	46	101	157	62	2,200	46	800	4,000	10	8
	15–18	55	120	163	64	2,100	46	800	4,000	10	8

*As cholecalciferol; 10 µg cholecalciferol equals 400 IU vitamin D.

Recommended daily dietary allowances of some selected nutrients for pregnancy and lactation

Nutrients	Nonpregnant girl 12–14 yr 47 kg (103 lb)	Nonpregnant girl 14–18 yr 55 kg (120 lb)	Nonpregnant woman 25 yr 58 kg (128 lb)	Pregnancy Added need	Pregnancy Girl 12–14 yr	Pregnancy Girl 14–18 yr	Pregnancy Woman 25 yr	Lactation (850 ml daily) Added need	Lactation Girl 12–14 yr	Lactation Girl 14–18 yr	Lactation Woman 25 yr
Calories	2,200	2,100	2,000	300	2,500	2,400	2,300	500	2,700	2,600	2,500
Protein (g)	46	46	44	30	76	76	74	20	66	68	64
Calcium (g)	1.2	1.2	0.8	0.4	1.6	1.6	1.2	0.4	1.6	1.6	1.2
Iron (mg)	18	18	18	‡	18+	18+	18+	‡	18+	18+	18+
Vitamin A (RE)*	800	800	800	200	1,000	1,000	1,000	400	1,200	1,200	1,200
Thiamin (mg)	1.1	1.1	1.0	0.4	1.5	1.5	1.4	0.5	1.6	1.6	1.5
Riboflavin (mg)	1.3	1.3	1.2	0.3	1.6	1.6	1.5	0.5	1.8	1.8	1.7
Niacin equivalent and tryptophan (mg)	15	14	13	2	17	16	15	5	20	19	18
Ascorbic acid (mg)	50	60	60	20	70	80	80	40	90	100	100
Vitamin D (µg)†	10	10	5	5	15	15	10	5	15	15	10

*Retinol equivalents.
†Cholecalciferol: 10 µg equals 400 IU vitamin D.
‡Required iron supplement 30–60 mg.

	Water-soluble vitamins						Minerals					
Vit. C (mg)	Folacin (μg)	Niacin (mg)	Riboflavin (mg)	Thiamin (mg)	Vit. B_6 (mg)	Vit. B_{12} (μg)	Calcium (mg)	Phosphorus (mg)	Iodine (μg)	Iron (mg)	Magnesium (mg)	Zinc (mg)
35	30	6	0.4	0.3	0.3	0.5	360	240	40	10	50	3
35	45	8	0.6	0.5	0.6	1.5	540	360	50	15	70	5
45	100	9	0.8	0.7	0.9	2.0	800	800	70	15	150	10
45	200	11	1.0	0.9	1.3	2.5	800	800	90	10	200	10
45	300	16	1.4	1.2	1.6	3.0	800	800	120	10	250	10
50	400	18	1.6	1.4	1.8	3.0	1,200	1,200	150	18	350	15
60	400	18	1.7	1.4	2.0	3.0	1,200	1,200	150	18	400	15
50	400	15	1.3	1.1	1.8	3.0	1,200	1,200	150	18	300	15
60	400	14	1.3	1.1	2.0	3.0	1,200	1,200	150	18	300	15

Signs of Malnutrition

Physical signs indicative or suggestive of malnutrition

Body area	Normal appearance	Signs associated with malnutrition
Hair	Shiny, firm, not easily plucked	Lack of natural shine; hair dull and dry, thin and sparse; hair fine, silky, and straight; color changes (flag sign); can be easily plucked
Face	Skin color uniform; smooth, pink, healthy appearance; not swollen	Skin color loss (depigmentation); skin dark over cheeks and under eyes (malar and supraorbital pigmentation); lumpiness or flakiness of skin of nose and mouth; swollen face; enlarged parotid glands; scaling of skin around nostrils (nasolabial seborrhea)
Eyes	Bright, clear, shiny; no sores at corners of eyelids; membranes a healthy pink and moist. No prominent blood vessels or mound of tissue or sclera	Eye membranes are pale (pale conjunctivae); redness of membranes (conjunctival injection), Bitot's spots; redness and fissuring of eyelid corners (angular palpebritis); dryness of eye membranes (conjunctival xerosis); cornea has dull appearance (corneal xerosis); cornea soft (keratomalacia); scar on cornea; ring of fine blood vessels around cornea (circumcorneal injection)
Lips	Smooth, not chapped or swollen	Redness and swelling of mouth or lips (cheilosis), especially at corners of mouth (angular fissures and scars)
Tongue	Deep red in appearance; not swollen or smooth	Swelling; scarlet and raw tongue; magenta (purplish color) tongue; smooth tongue; swollen sores; hyperemic and hypertrophic papillae; atrophic papillae
Teeth	No cavities; no pain; bright	May be missing or erupting abnormally; gray or black spots (fluorosis); cavities (caries)
Gums	Healthy; red; do not bleed; not swollen	"Spongy" and bleed easily; recession of gums
Glands	Face not swollen	Thyroid enlargement (front of neck); parotid enlargement (cheeks become swollen)
Skin	No signs of rashes, swellings, dark or light spots	Dryness of skin (xerosis); sandpaper feel of skin (follicular hyperkeratosis); flakiness of skin; skin swollen and dark; red swollen pigmentation of exposed areas (pellagrous dermatosis); excessive lightness or darkness of skin (dyspigmentation); black and blue marks from skin bleeding (petechiae); lack of fat under skin
Nails	Firm, pink	Nails are spoon shaped (koilonychia); brittle, ridged nails
Muscular and skeletal systems	Good muscle tone, some fat under skin; can walk or run without pain	Muscles have "wasted" appearance; baby's skull bones are thin and soft (craniotabes); round swelling of front and side of head (frontal and parietal bossing); swelling of ends of bones (epiphyseal enlargement); small bumps on both sides of chest wall (on ribs), beading of ribs; baby's soft spot on head does not harden at proper time (persistently open anterior fontanelle); knock-knees or bow-legs; bleeding into muscle (musculoskeletal hemorrhages); person cannot get up or walk properly

*From Christakis, G.: Am. J. Public Health 63(suppl):1–82, 1973.

Physical signs indicative or suggestive of malnutrition—cont'd

Body area	Normal appearance	Signs associated with malnutrition
Internal systems		
Cardio-vascular	Normal heart rate and rhythm; no murmurs or abnormal rhythms; normal blood pressure for age	Rapid heart rate (above 100, tachycardia); enlarged heart; abnormal rhythm; elevated blood pressure
Gastroin-testinal	No palpable organs or masses (in children, however, liver edge may be palpable)	Liver enlargement; enlargement of spleen (usually indicates other associated diseases)
Nervous	Psychologic stability; normal reflexes	Mental irritability and confusion; burning and tingling of hands and feet (paresthesia); loss of position and vibratory sense; weakness and tenderness of muscles (may result in inability to walk); decrease and loss of ankle and knee reflexes

INDEX

A